COLONIALISM IN AFRICA 1870–1960

GENERAL EDITORS

PETER DUIGNAN, *Director, African Program*
Hoover Institution, Stanford University
L. H. GANN, *Senior Staff Member, Hoover Institution*
Stanford University

VOLUME 1

HOOVER INSTITUTION PUBLICATIONS

WITHDRAWN

N 0010228 8

COLONIALISM IN AFRICA
1870–1960

VOLUME 1
THE HISTORY AND POLITICS OF
COLONIALISM 1870–1914

Edited by

L. H. GANN *and* PETER DUIGNAN

NEWMAN COLLEGE
BARTLEY GREEN
BIRMINGHAM, 32.

CLASS   960·2

ACCESSION   20325

AUTHOR   GAN

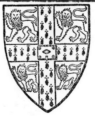

CAMBRIDGE

AT THE UNIVERSITY PRESS

1969

Published by the Syndics of the Cambridge University Press
Bentley House, 200 Euston Road, London N.W.1
American Branch: 32 East 57th Street, New York, N.Y. 10022
Cambridge University Press 1969

© Cambridge University Press 1969

Library of Congress Catalogue Card Number: 75–77289

Standard Book Number: 521 07373 1

Printed in Great Britain
at the University Printing House, Cambridge
(Brooke Crutchley, University Printer)

CONTENTS

CONTENTS

FIGURES

FOREWORD

Few questions have occupied modern intellectuals as much as the subject of imperialism. European colonialists in the past have been prone to make the most extraordinary claims concerning the accomplishments of white empire-builders. Men such as Cecil Rhodes were often depicted almost as demi-gods whose enterprise caused the deserts to bloom and transformed barbarism into civilization. Later on, critics of imperialism like Hobson and Lenin completely reversed these interpretations. Lenin viewed imperialism as the highest stage of capitalism; European imperialism, he maintained, marked a fateful step in modern history and was the source of innumerable evils for the whole of mankind. These and similar views exerted a profound influence on educated opinion of the time. Even today the evaluation of imperialism is a controversial topic not only among Marxist–Leninists, but among other historians in Africa, Asia, Europe and America as well.

The great debate is likely to continue for a long time. But as Hobson himself put the matter in his book *Imperialism: a study*, 'quibbles about imperialism are best resolved by reference to concrete facts'. The editors and contributors to this multi-volume study have followed Hobson's precepts and have assembled an impressive body of evidence. Some of them have summed up the existing state of knowledge in their particular subjects; others have reinterpreted conventional findings; still others have presented new material; all have helped to shed more light on this dramatic chapter in the interaction between Africa and the West. And all have placed future scholars in their debt.

W. GLENN CAMPBELL

Director
Hoover Institution
Stanford University

PREFACE

The history of Africa has in recent years begun to attract the attention of an ever-increasing number of professional historians. Research on even the limited subject of modern Europe's impact on Africa is far from exhausted. For many years investigations have mainly run along certain well-marked channels. Writers such as Rosa Luxemburg or G. W. F. Hallgarten devoted much effort to describing what they regarded as the economic and political mainspring of Western colonialism. In doing so, they investigated the financial aspect of imperialism in Europe without taking into account what actually happened in Africa. Others, such as Sir Reginald Coupland or H. R. Rudin, discussed imperialism in Africa as part of the 'expansion of Europe'; or the history of British, German or Arab imperialism in Africa, without, however, devoting much time to the indigenous African societies. A distinguished school of writers, many of them high officials, compiled works on the administration of the colonies. Scholars with special interests in southern Africa, among them W. M. Macmillan and C. W. de Kiewiet, broke new ground by investigating the relations between white, black and brown peoples in the southern part of the continent. Anthropologists such as Melville J. Herskovits and Max Gluckman concerned themselves with problems of change as well as of structure in African societies. A small number of Afro-Americans, such as W. E. B. Du Bois and other Negro scholars, dealt with the European occupation of Africa, as well as with other aspects of Negro history, from the black man's point of view.

The African historical scene is now changing. A new generation of scholars in Europe, Africa and North America is attempting to examine the subject from a fresh perspective and to write African history in a more Afrocentric fashion. In addition, scholars are now able to take advantage of a mass of new material that has become available in the archives of the former metropolitan powers and of the newly independent African states. Large numbers of specialized books and monographs are appearing. But the new research is hard to synthesize. Some investigators are not well acquainted with publications in languages other than their own. Many scholars devote their labours to one specific geographical region, and know little about work done with respect to other parts of Africa. Most research workers have not taken the time necessary to acquaint themselves with the findings of other disciplines that may have an indirect bearing on their own special fields. Our project concerns the imperial impact on sub-Saharan Africa only; yet the task is so complex as to require a team. We have planned four volumes, with a comprehensive bibliography to appear with Volume 2.

This study is intended to serve the specialist as well as the general reader. The volumes will try to summarize some of the best available knowledge relating to certain major fields concerned with the impact of European imperialism on Africa. They will also break new ground by presenting hitherto unpublished material based on original research. As is frequently the case in other disciplines, there is likely to be disagreement among the experts in many areas. The opinions expressed in these essays are therefore the writers' own, and do not necessarily correspond to those of the general editors nor of the Advisory Board. In selecting their collaborators, the editors have called upon leading scholars in various fields and have asked them in each case to write on the subject of most interest to themselves, provided the essay fitted within the general framework of the total project. Unavoidably, some gaps remain—partly because the contributors were rightly allowed a good deal of choice, partly for reasons of space, and partly because some scholars were prevented from contributing by other commitments.

In arranging this varied material, the general editors have had to steer a somewhat arbitrary course between a chronological and a topical arrangement. The first two volumes outline the history and politics of imperialism from the 'scramble for Africa' to decolonization. This first volume covers the period from about 1870 to the outbreak of World War I. The second volume will continue the story up to 1960. The production of these two volumes has been directly supervised by the general editors. An additional volume, edited by Professor Victor Turner of Cornell University and entitled *Profiles of change*, will treat of the impact of colonialism on African societies. The last volume in the series will deal with economic questions about colonialism.

Wherever possible, the editors have used the *Index-gazetteer of the world* of the London *Times* for the spelling of geographic names. They have consulted Joseph H. Greenberg, *The languages of Africa*; the International African Institute, *Handbook of African languages*; Malcolm Guthrie, *The classification of Bantu languages*; and George P. Murdock, *Africa: its peoples and their culture history* to establish uniformity in the employment of linguistic and ethnic terms. Where authors have expressed special preference for any particular version, the editors have tried to respect the writer's wishes. Editorial practices vary significantly from country to country and contributors often have a strong preference for their own standards. We have therefore allowed as much freedom as seemed consistent with standards set by the Cambridge University Press. As editors we have checked as many facts and bibliographical citations as possible, but we have left to each author the final responsibility for the accuracy of his own statements and citations.

The editors have conformed to the practice of Cambridge University Press in keeping footnotes to the minimum. Footnotes have been provided to give references for direct quotations used in the text, to cite the main authorities on disputed questions and to present evidence relied upon by contributors for novel or unusual conclusions that might appear strange unless thus supported. (We have tried to put a general interpretation on this latter provision by including references to archival sources which have as yet been little exploited, or which have not been previously available.)

The editors are much indebted for the valuable assistance they have received from the members of the Advisory Board for this series, including Professor P. T. Bauer of the London School of Economics, University of London; Professor Gordon A. Craig of Stanford University; and Professor J. D. Fage of The University of Birmingham, England. They are especially grateful to Professor Fage for permission to use Figures 4, 5, 6, 7, 14 and 15, adapted from his *Atlas of African History* (London, 1963). They similarly owe thanks to Professor Richard J. Hammond, formerly of Stanford University, who not only submitted an essay of his own but also translated all the French contributions into English.

The completion of this book owes much to the editing of Edna Halperin, to the organizational and administrative skills of Eve Hoffman and to the various bibliographic checking and typing chores performed by Karen Fung, Liselotte Hofmann and Benedicta Nwaozomudoh.

The editors appreciate the kind co-operation extended them by Dr W. Glenn Campbell, Director of the Hoover Institution. And they owe a great debt of gratitude to the Relm Foundation of Ann Arbor, Michigan, whose financial generosity has made this project possible.

PETER DUIGNAN, L. H. GANN *General Editors*

INTRODUCTION

The nineteenth century in Europe was an age of steam-power and of cultural and technological optimism. Railway builders covered Western Europe with a great network of iron tracks. In the United States, in Canada, in India and in Latin America, they inaugurated the age of great railways spanning a whole continent. Sub-Saharan Africa, on the other hand, long remained a backwater. Although railway development began on a small scale at the Cape of Good Hope during the years 1859 to 1864, it was not until 1867, with the discovery of the Griqualand West diamond deposits, that the first great impetus came. Later on, Europeans began to construct lines in some other parts of Africa—in Senegal, Kenya and the Gold Coast, for example. Goods could then be carried overland more cheaply and in greater bulk. For the first time in African history engineers were able to transport heavy machinery from the ports to the distant interior. Soldiers and their equipment were able to move at greater speed. Above all, railways did away with the need for human porterage. Without knowing it, railway builders struck a heavy blow at many traditional social relationships; and they played a major part also in mobilizing tribesmen for wage-labour.

The steam-engine similarly revolutionized transport by sea. Ships driven by steam-power increased in size, comfort and carrying capacity. Maritime traders no longer needed to confine their cargoes to goods of relatively small bulk and high value; instead they could move commodities such as coal, grain, peanuts and palm-kernels around half the world and still make a profit. The steamship thus vastly increased the volume of international trade. The Mediterranean once more assumed something of its former pre-eminence. Construction ventures such as the Suez Canal became commercially feasible. Vessels bound from Europe to the Cape of Good Hope could steam a straight course without making a long westerly detour in the South Atlantic. The steamship thus made Africa and Asia accessible to Europe in a way that would have seemed fantastic to merchants and shipowners of an earlier generation.

The development of the steam-engine was only part of a wider economic and scientific revolution that profoundly influenced relations between Africa and the West. The prophylactic use of quinine, for

I

instance, helped to remove the 'mosquito barrier' that had previously shut off the African interior. The rapid expansion of every branch of Western industry under the stimulus of power-driven machinery occasioned an ever-growing demand for tropical goods such as cotton, cocoa and edible oils. Above all, scientific and technological progress helped to produce an extraordinary feeling of cultural confidence among theoreticians and practical men alike. One might almost speak of 'steam-power optimism'. In this respect there was little difference between a socialist revolutionary like Marx and a bourgeois Christian reformer like Livingstone. Railways, Marx argued, would change the face of India:

You cannot maintain a net of railways over an immense country [he argued] without introducing all those industrial processes necessary to meet the immediate and current wants of railway locomotion, and out of which there must grow...the application of machinery to those branches of industry not immediately connected with the railways. The railway system will therefore become...the forerunner of modern industry...Modern industry, resulting from the railway system, will dissolve the hereditary divisions of labour... those decisive impediments to...progress.[1]

Livingstone's outlook was equally optimistic. Africa, he said, was ready for the Gospel. But commerce and Christianity must advance together. The slave-trade, the curse of Africa, would never be stopped by sermons or even by gunboats alone. In order to break the stranglehold of the slave-dealers over Central Africa, the Christian powers must introduce steam-powered transport by river and land. By doing so, they would develop the country, would enable Africans to produce crops for legitimate trade, would ensure social progress and would assist in the evangelization of Africa. Philanthropy and profits were bound to go hand in hand. This mood was commonly coupled with an all-pervading sense of Western cultural superiority and national self-confidence, not only on the part of militant imperialists but also of many socialists and even of anglicized or gallicized Africans at the time.

Doctrines of this kind provided a strong ideological justification for imperial expansion in Africa, while the industrial and scientific revolutions rendered tropical conquests more feasible than ever before. By the early 1870s the stage seemed set for the speedy partition of the continent. Yet few Europeans were paying much attention to African affairs. Portugal, the oldest European power in Africa, was a poor

[1] Quoted from Karl Marx in Rajani Palme Dutt, *India to-day* (Bombay, 1947), p. 81.

2

country. The Portuguese at this period controlled but a tiny portion of the territories now making up their empire. Much of their influence depended on the employment of African auxiliaries and on alliances with local African powers. The Portuguese were reluctant to emigrate to their colonies; they had practically no funds for overseas investments. Portuguese politicians dreaded colonial expenditure, and many regarded the future of their empire with the most profound pessimism.

The Germans were equally indifferent to colonial issues. By the middle of the nineteenth century, German merchants at Zanzibar, for instance, had already taken an important position in the island's trade. But there was no serious demand for German political protection. Many German writers were later to assert that the Reich had been created too late for Germany to secure her rightful place in Africa. But this interpretation had no basis in fact. Had there been a serious campaign for colonies, the North German Confederation (established in 1866) would have been perfectly capable of staking out territorial claims overseas; so would the united German empire after its inception in 1871. The Germans, however, were preoccupied with continental questions.

The French concern with tropical Africa was hardly greater than the German. As Brunschwig points out in his essay, the French were traditionally less interested in Africa than the British. They were never as fervent about the suppression of the African slave-trade as the Anglo-Saxons; abolition never became a popular issue with the French masses. The French navy, of course, had a traditional stake in West Africa. French sailors were always anxious to defend the honour of their flag against their British rivals. But French naval considerations were subordinated in the last instance to those of foreign policy in general. Constant budgetary deficits, a long history of guerrilla warfare in Algeria and the pitiful record of French intervention in Mexico had occasioned much distrust concerning colonial adventures. The French did, however, occupy a long-established position in the Senegal, where they tried to assimilate some Africans to French ways. The French traded extensively in peanuts; French-speaking mulatto merchants penetrated far into the interior and looked to France for protection against the exactions of local Muslim rulers. French soldiers and administrators like Faidherbe were only too anxious to provide the required assistance, and this combination of military and mercantile motives resulted in a local version of 'Senegalese imperialism'.

The British were no more inclined to a policy of large-scale expansion than the French. In Nigeria, for instance, as Flint puts it, the only people possessing a sense of the British 'imperial mission' were anglicized Africans. Educated or semi-educated black people—like their French-speaking counterparts in Senegal—looked to the imperial power to protect their trade inland. Literate Africans looked for promotion in the local public services, too. There were also a handful of highly cultured Africans, men like Reverend Samuel Johnson, Bishop Samuel Adjai Crowther and Surgeon-Major James Africanus Beale Horton, who attained some distinction in the realm of letters. Though they might criticize many aspects of white rule, nevertheless they welcomed European colonization for initiating a social revolution, for overthrowing slavery and expanding trade, for giving a chance to newly educated men irrespective of their ancestry, for destroying ancient superstitions and for depriving indigenous aristocracies of some ill-gained power.

By and large, the British did not consider alien colonization in itself inimical to British interests, provided always that foreigners would admit British merchants and investors on the same terms as other nationals. On the 'tribal frontiers', however, this policy often broke down. One alternative was to encourage white settlement. European colonization would create new markets. It would lead also to the creation of stable, self-governing British communities that would treat British merchants with fairness and that would themselves pay for maintaining law and order. The policy of granting local self-government to white colonists thus triumphed, for instance, at the Cape, which obtained representative institutions in 1853 and responsible government in 1872. A second alternative was to cajole backward rulers—be they Muslim or pagan, feudal lords or tribal potentates—into instituting reforms acceptable both to the British conscience and to British enterprise. A good deal of British history overseas during this period can be written in terms of such efforts, which extended all the way from Zanzibar to West Africa and to Turkey.

This policy did not necessarily preclude territorial expansion. 'Native' governments might prove hostile to British trade, or they might be unable to protect persons and property. British arms were used on the 'turbulent frontiers' of empire to protect existing commitments, to defend strategically placed naval stations or to establish what soldiers took to be more easily defensible boundary lines. The search

4

for secure frontiers was itself liable to provoke trouble. In South Africa, for instance, Boers and Britons competed for land with Bantu pastoralists; at the same time the colonists' cattle were often a temptation to warlike border tribes. In 1820 the British tried to cover the Eastern Cape by establishing English settlers on its exposed marches. The border, however, remained too thinly settled to afford real protection. Settlers and tribesmen could not be kept apart. Government officials then tried to gain added security by pushing forward the boundary. But each move further compressed the territory available to the indigenous tribes and nations and thereby often led to further conflict, with the result that the imperial power reluctantly kept adding to its commitments.

There were thus expansionist lobbies of all kinds. British settlers in South Africa commonly looked to the Queen's soldiers for protection against their African neighbours. Missionary writers like Livingstone called God's blessing on any power that would intervene in Africa to do away with the ravages of the slave-trade. Nevertheless there was as yet no influential British metropolitan lobby calling for vast colonial conquests. Even Disraeli's brand of imperialism was more concerned with considerations of international prestige and military defence than with large-scale expansion.

Some historians have therefore drawn a rigid distinction between the early and mid-Victorian period on the one hand and the 'new imperialism' of late Victorian and Edwardian days on the other. During the former period—they argue—free trade formed part of British imperial orthodoxy; no foreign power could challenge Britain's position as the workshop of the world. British capitalism had not yet entered into its monopolistic stage. British commercial policy was concerned with the export of commodities for trade, with removing restraints upon the international exchange of merchandise and with securing at best indirect influence over the backward parts of the world. The new imperialism, on the other hand, was supposedly characterized by financial monopolies, by massive export of capital and by vast territorial expansion.

There was no such historical caesura. Admittedly, no European state before 1871 deliberately aimed at vast imperial annexations. But the list of territories brought under European sway in the preceding half-century or so is an impressive one. Britain's Indian empire, for instance, continued to expand. The British acquired new naval stations such as Aden, Hong Kong and Singapore. In Africa, British soldiers fought as far afield as the Eastern Cape, Ethiopia and the Gold Coast. The French greatly extended their power in Senegal. Even the Portuguese tightened their grip on some outlying regions in Africa.

The export of capital during this period, on the other hand, did not necessarily lead to territorial expansion. Britain had already lent a good deal of money to foreigners before the inception of the new imperialism. Britain's most important debtors beyond the ocean were found not in the tropics but above all in the United States, in the self-governing British white colonies and in Latin America. Even in Africa there was no necessary link between capital exports and territorial annexations.

Nevertheless, from the 1870s onward, the pace of colonial expansion in Africa quickened. The reasons for this new outburst of imperial enterprise are complex, and can be only briefly touched upon here. We should, however, point to a few major issues. Brunschwig, for instance, places stress on the strident nationalism engendered in France by the catastrophe of 1871, and on the fear that France would sink to the level of a second-rate power unless she acquired more territory overseas. The great mineral discoveries in South Africa profoundly stirred public imagination in Great Britain and France alike. Many investors were firmly convinced that the great fortunes made at Kimberley would easily and quickly be equalled by similar gains in other parts of Africa. Contemporary literature on Africa produced an assortment of myths concerning the assumed El Dorados of the interior. The Suez Canal, opened in 1869, fired the dreams of a generation that had boundless faith in the wonders of technological progress. There were visionary projects for the creation of inland seas in Tunisia, for the construction of transcontinental railway lines with express trains running a hundred miles an hour from one end of Africa to the other! Schemes of this kind appealed not only to the imaginative but also to an army of dubious financial promoters who exploited none but their metropolitan shareholders.

Militant nationalism and visionary projectors' schemes blended with the outlook of real-estate speculators. Africa was thought to contain enormous potential wealth, and the value of its land and resources must surely rise. Patriots therefore ought to acquire a share for their country lest foreigners corner the lot! These assumptions often coincided with an aggressive variety of imperial philanthropy. Indeed, Western humanitarianism, whether of the missionary or of the secular kind, in many ways represented an overspill of domestic reform into the colonies—help the poor at home and the unbelievers in the African bush. Evangelism in all its forms commonly rested on the assumption that the Africans stood at the bottom of the evolutionary ladder and had to be lifted out of their sorry state. This view sometimes carried racist connotations—but not necessarily so.

The enterprise of geographers also contributed to the prevailing climate of opinion. During the second half of the nineteenth century Africa was still regarded as an open frontier, one of those few great regions where cartographers still left white spaces in place of rivers, lakes and mountains. There was the lure of the unknown. Scientific curiosity blended with romance, with the desire for self-advancement and for pioneering. De Brazza came to embody the very essence of the French explorer at his best. He was young; he was handsome; he was aristocratic, courageous and chivalrous. If De Brazza embodied the virtues of military gallantry, Livingstone represented the British non-conformist ideal. Livingstone was a self-made man, an ex-cotton spinner who had made good and came to be honoured by bishops and lords. When Livingstone died in the wilds of Africa, England buried a Protestant martyr of remarkable stature.

Several essays in this volume refer at some length to the scramble that followed upon the great journeys of discovery. In South Africa the British had originally been content with holding the Cape as a stepping-stone on the road to the Indies. They were on the whole averse to making further conquests but, as Krüger shows, events forced their hand. The British position was profoundly affected by the setting up of two independent Afrikaner republics beyond the Orange and the Vaal rivers and by the relations between white men and black. During the last quarter of the nineteenth century two additional motives came into play. The great diamond discoveries of 1867 and the gold finds of 1886 vastly enhanced the value of the interior. British imperial ambitions received a further stimulus from rivalry with other European powers, especially Germany.

Krüger shows how the British subsequently embarked on a forward policy and checkmated their competitors. By 1890 the doctrine of British hegemony in southern Africa was firmly established, and the Transvaal was cut off from further expansion inland.

The British had equally vital interests in Egypt, the other key area on the route to India. British intervention in Egypt was later to play a major part in causing Great Britain to acquire the Sudan and Uganda, both of which were regarded by many as strategic back doors to Egypt. (Indeed, these supposedly hard-headed military calculations often contained an element of the fantastic. Some European policy-makers imagined quite seriously, for instance, that the French, by gaining control over the upper reaches of the Nile and diverting its waters from their course, might render the British position in Egypt untenable. Such a mammoth project would, in fact, have exceeded the available resources of any European country.) British influence in East and East Central Africa owed a great deal also to the activities of missionaries, who were well established in parts of Uganda and in what is now Zambia, Malawi and Tanzania.

The British had a stake in West Africa, too. During the 1880s they greatly extended their possessions. British colonization received considerable support from educated Africans, from civil servants, traders and others, many of them Yoruba with Lagos connexions. But British empire-builders took little account of such African aspirations. As Flint shows, the British were initially concerned only to defend their commercial predominance against foreign encroachments; their motives were defensive; they acquired political control over the Nigerian coast and the banks of the Niger 'in a spirit of anti-imperialism and financial parsimony'. Nor were the British much interested in reforming African institutions. The British were, however, often affected by British traders on the spot. British merchants and the British Foreign Office were both determined to do away with local barriers to trade, to wipe out local African trade monopolies and to reduce or eliminate the middlemen's profits. The British also intervened in the hinterland for fear of French activities; they were able to make vast conquests with a relatively small military outlay partly because the Africans were disunited, partly because many communities actually welcomed the British advance. The Yoruba, for instance, with their people exhausted by internecine warfare and their rulers demoralized, were anxious for stable rule.

Anglo-French rivalry hung heavy over the period of the scramble. Having in effect been ousted from Egypt by the British, the French found some compensation in the western Mediterranean. Established in Algeria since 1830, they regarded Tunisia as a natural adjunct to their existing possessions, even though the British and Italians also had some interests there. In 1881 the French sent an army to Tunisia, with the result that Italian ambitions in the area were finally thwarted.

The most important French effort, however, was that in West Africa. Brunschwig's essay distinguishes three main drives. The French made extensive advances along the coast, where they competed to some extent with the British. They also expanded inland from Senegal. This was essentially the work of the French military who, in the late 1880s, turned the French Sudan into their game preserve. In the Congo, De Brazza's ventures were carried on for the most part in response to the colonial activities of King Leopold of Belgium. Support for De Brazza's endeavours came from various private French bodies and from French nationalist opinion, incensed at the French failure to intervene in Egypt and also at Leopold's maladroit attempts to impede the French in the Congo.

King Leopold's imperialism, on the other hand, was, in Stengers' words, 'the imperialism of a single man'. The creation of the Congo Free State was the king's brainchild; it owed nothing to Belgian governmental initiative. The State was politically independent of Belgium; it was run as an absolute monarchy. The king alone determined policy and in fact considered the State to be his private property. He was inspired by what J. A. Hobson, the British critic of imperialism, later stigmatized as 'kilometrisis' or 'milomania', the desire to own land for its own sake. Leopold imagined that all colonies were equally advantageous from the economic standpoint. He worked for self-aggrandizement; he wished to gain renown as a 'builder-king' and as the creator of Belgium's splendour. In the end his territorial acquisitions proved vastly disproportionate to the available resources, and his greed turned into a curse for his Congolese subjects.

Portuguese colonialism was equally prestige-conscious. Hammond has called it 'uneconomic imperialism'. Portuguese imperialism, however, had a much wider popular base than the Belgian variety. The Portuguese remembered the past glories of their crusaders, navigators and *conquistadores*. Once the scramble had begun, they stood in dread lest foreign powers should seize their possessions and Portugal should thereby lose her national independence. Portuguese colonialism was not in the main motivated by economic considerations. Her trade with the colonies was insignificant. Portuguese emigrants preferred to go to Brazil rather than to Angola, and the country had almost no capital available for investment abroad.

In 1890 the British inflicted on Portugal the humiliation of an ultimatum to enforce British claims in South East Africa. The ultimatum, however, led to a vigorous national reaction, and the Portuguese empire was saved—not by a system or a class but by a handful of determined individuals who gained support from a strong element of national quixotry. Because the great powers were unwilling to bring political turmoil to Portugal by wresting her colonies from her, the Portuguese empire in Africa managed to survive.

Up to this point we have discussed the scramble almost entirely in Eurocentric terms, once shared both by sturdy imperialists such as Sir Harry Johnston, a British administrator, and by militant critics such as Hobson and Lenin. The imperialists and their opponents argued furiously over whether the 'natives' benefited from the *Pax Britannica* or whether they were the victims of alien exploitation. But the indigenous people of Africa were always seen as the objects of outside manipulation, as helpless primitives who depended on a backward subsistence economy and whose institutions necessarily stood in the way of progress.

It is, however, mistaken to assume that all black Africans were wedded to a primitive patriarchical order that took no account of the cash nexus. Many communities of pre-colonial Africa engaged in trade, among them the Bisa, the Mbundu, the Ibo and countless others. All were capable of making rational economic decisions. African attitudes, however, were often obscured by unrealistic observations on the part of prejudiced observers. We owe our descriptions of pre-colonial Africa mostly to men to whom the precepts of Victorian morality seemed to be the only ones to be followed, who thought in terms of a Western mercantile ethos and a wage economy. Men of this stamp usually had little patience with African tribal systems and with what François Coillard, a French Protestant missionary, called 'kingly socialism'. Many, though by no means all, missionary writers mistakenly held that Africans lived in idleness, that their women did all the work and that African wives were nothing but the chattel of their slothful, drunken husbands.

In like manner many British imperialists argued that African rulers were unprogressive and that, in West Africa especially, British commerce could be vastly expanded by ousting the middlemen and by directly extending British rule into the interior. These convictions were often backed by what we call the 'tropical treasure house myth', a misconception that also came to be held by many critics of the imperial record. According to this interpretation, the verdant forests of Africa contained tremendous resources. Quick and easy profits were sure to reward the investor. Enormous fortunes would soon be made if only indigenous kingships were to make way for the *Pax Britannica*. These assumptions, of course, were often invalid. Many forms of African enterprise required an extensive 'infrastructure' that did not exist at the time. The African trade was generally risky; some businessmen made money, but others incurred heavy losses. At the time of the scramble the European trade in tropical Africa was still limited. As Newbury points out, the foreign commerce of West Africa increased rapidly from about 1850. Nevertheless, thirty years later Europe's trade with West Africa was still less than that with the Cape Colony. The extension of British rule inland, moreover, did not necessarily lead to an increase in the volume of traffic. Attempts to cut out black middlemen did not in all cases benefit the whites. The African middleman's role was indeed often grossly misunderstood. The Europeans commonly failed to appreciate the special knowledge possessed by black intermediaries or the value of the services rendered by black middlemen in collecting large quantities of different merchandise in small packets and distributing it over huge distances.

Many European theoreticians had similar misconceptions about African political institutions. All too often Africans were seen as an undifferentiated mass of savages, subject to the rule of bloodthirsty chiefs and superstitious witch-doctors. Cruelty and bloodshed there were indeed; nothing, in our view, is more mistaken than to romanticize the institutions of pre-conquest Africa. But as Miss Colson puts it, 'the assumed uniformity of savage life is but a foreign myth'. An African Aristotle intent on studying the political institutions to be found on the continent at the time of the scramble would have found as many varieties as did his Greek namesake. African polities included all kinds—from stateless societies held together by age-set or neighbourhood arrangements to city states and extensive kingdoms, the latter including both limited and absolute monarchies.

The most highly organized kingdoms were found in West Africa, where state-building had resulted from trade and permanent settlement. The production of sizeable agricultural surpluses, the evolution of relatively diversified economies, had helped to create a considerable degree of social stratification and complex political institutions. Strong rulers commonly attempted to expand the power of the state by gaining control over foreign trade and over local mineral deposits, by strengthening their armed forces and by improving their administrative machine. But even in the most highly centralized states the central government could perform only a limited number of tasks. Many functions that Westerners now associate with the state continued to be carried out by local authorities and kinship groups. Nevertheless, the century or so that preceded the partition was an age of rapid change. Foreign commerce grew in many parts of the continent. New commodities and new weapons came into use. New crops and new crafts were introduced, and the process of state-building gained considerable momentum in diverse regions, especially in West Africa but to some extent also in South Africa. Such indeed was the resultant diversity of political and economic institutions that Miss Colson refuses altogether to employ the term 'tribe', arguing that its use obscures rather than elucidates the complexities of African social organization.

Newbury's inquiry into the nature of West African trade before and during the scramble gives an additional dimension to Miss Colson's analysis. He emphasizes that specialized export products such as ivory, gold and slaves that were taken abroad by great caravans formed but a small proportion of the consumer goods offered for sale. The bulk of West Africa's internal commerce was in food. It developed from the interdependence of indigenous pastoralists, grain-growers, fishermen and root-croppers. It depended on an enormous number of small, unspectacular transactions. Methods of transport were slow. The amount of capital involved remained small. Goods had to be handled, so to speak, in 'penny packets'. Trade had to be carried on over large distances and costs were heavy.

Generally speaking, commerce contributed but a small proportion of the revenue accruing to indigenous African governments. There were exceptions, such as Dahomey and the Delta states, where the rulers acted also as merchants. By and large, however, the income received by African kings came from conquest and tribute rather than from commerce. Much of West Africa's wealth was spent in conspicuous consumption, on lavish hospitality, on gifts to kinsmen and followers. Great men on the whole 'invested' their riches in political power. Wealth was channelled into complicated systems of gift exchanges rather than into purely economic enterprises. Though the indigenous societies of West Africa conducted a good deal of trade, they did not produce a new class of merchant princes.

Nevertheless, the impact of foreign trade in palm-oil, ground-nuts, kola-nuts and similar commodities was great. Commerce, from the Senegal down to the Niger, came to rest on a series of interlocking markets that linked food-gatherers and food-importers with purveyors of Western goods. The new 'trader's frontier', properly speaking, lay along the vague limits between European and African jurisdiction over markets. Many African rulers tried to control commerce. Barriers to trade, which were political rather than geographical or fiscal in character, were harshly resented by many businessmen. According to Newbury, the frontier came to embody a search for authority, not a search for trade. At the same time the expansion of West Africa's export economy gave employment to a new class of anglicized or gallicized Africans. These new men participated in many aspects of commerce. Various educated Africans thus began to accumulate some capital of their own and, in turn, to play an active part in shaping the pattern of African development and imperial penetration.

Both Hargreaves and Ranger apply this Afrocentric interpretation to other aspects of the scramble. The partition was affected in some ways by African responses to new economic opportunities, for instance by the way in which the Wolof of Senegal took up peanut growing. It was influenced also by the 'African partition of Africa' during the nineteenth century, including such major state-building ventures as the great Muslim jihads. The imperial rulers possessed not only Mausers and Maxim guns but the vast resources of a great industrial civilization. However, as Ranger points out, they could employ only a tiny proportion of their strength on the colonization of Africa. Besides, they laboured under a mass of internal restraints. The colonizers had to cope with financial stringency, with diplomatic complications abroad and opposition at home. Missionary and humanitarian lobbies often censured the white men on the spot. So sometimes did white merchants who were dependent on the goodwill of African customers.

African military power was by no means always negligible. In East and Central Africa, for instance, the fighting potential of the stronger African societies had in fact increased during the nineteenth century. Hence Africans were not necessarily helpless in their relations with the white man. The British in Uganda, for instance, depended on an alliance with the Ganda aristocracy. In Kenya the British had an implicit understanding with the Masai; in what is now Zambia they co-operated closely with the Lozi (Barotse). Some powerful African groups managed to set up their own 'subimperialismus' within the colonial framework. Ranger points out that many African communities thus experienced British colonial rule more through their Ganda or Lozi overlords than through the British themselves.

Both Ranger and Hargreaves stress the positive role of African resistance to the whites during and after the partition. Both emphasize that resistance and collaboration were not mutually incompatible; the resisters and the collaborators were not fundamentally distinct. Samory, for instance, both negotiated with the French and fought against them. Neither was resistance to European rule necessarily coupled with reluctance to modernize. Resistance was not always a gallant anachronism, nor did it necessarily prove disastrous to the African societies involved in it. Under certain circumstances, protracted warfare might indeed improve the Africans' subsequent bargaining power under white rule. African resistance movements might also occasion major internal changes and lead the insurgents to search for new principles of political solidarity as well as for new techniques of warfare. In the long run, resistance movements may even have influenced post-colonial politics.

It is equally dangerous to dogmatize concerning African accommodation to colonial rule. Accommodation might follow along with 'Christian revolutions' of the kind attempted by the indigenous rulers of Barotseland, Bechuanaland and Uganda. But accommodation did not necessarily entail modernization. Some societies, such as the Masai, thus peacefully adjusted themselves to British rule while refusing to alter their way of life. Accommodation, on the other hand, was equally capable of turning into armed resistance. Menilek of Shoa, for example, as shown in Marcus's essay, first collaborated with the Italians and later smashed them on the battlefield.

Clearly, indigenous as well as European actors played their part in the scramble. Nothing would be more unjustifiable than to look upon pre-colonial Africa as a *tabula rasa*. In our opinion, however, the range of decisions open to most indigenous peoples was nevertheless limited. Even the most highly organized states of sub-Saharan Africa laboured under severe limitations. All of them depended on fairly simple forms of agriculture, supplemented to a greater or lesser degree by trade. Urban life was restricted to a few areas. Many of the larger centres of population were 'agro-towns' which drew their sustenance mainly from farming, fishing and tribute. Even the most highly developed cities, including those of the Sudanic belt, had not advanced beyond the handicraft stage of production. Literacy was confined to a limited number of regions and, within these regions, to small minority groups, including white settlers in southern Africa, europeanized Africans in West Africa, and the Islamic intelligentsia of the Sudanic belt and the east coast, as well as their opposite numbers in Christian Ethiopia. On the eve of the partition even a backward European state such as Portugal was immeasurably superior in science and technology, in its educational institutions, literary traditions and industrial arts to the most advanced states in Africa, whether white, brown or black. Politically speaking, no African state managed to acquire full legitimacy in Western eyes—not even Zanzibar or the Transvaal, both of which attempted to gain recognition in the wider system of world diplomacy.

In the military sphere the indigenous states of Africa generally laboured under comparable difficulties. The means of production available to tribal communities sufficed for the manufacture of shields, lances and knobkerries. Advanced Muslim craftsmen in the Sudanic cities could fashion swords and bullets. But no African state could produce a bomb, much less a battleship. The British might suffer occasional disasters, such as the battle of Isandhlwana where in 1879 the Zulu wiped out a small British force. But such defeats could usually be reversed. However weak a colonizing state might be on the spot at any given time, its potential power was generally much superior to that of its opponents in sub-Saharan Africa. Even kingdoms completely dedicated to war, such as the 'Black Sparts' formed by the Zulu and kindred peoples in South and East Central Africa, all succumbed to the arms of British and Portuguese soldiers in the 1890s.

The colonizers made only two major military miscalculations in sub-Saharan Africa, both of which had far-reaching consequences. Both involved warlike minority groups that were capable of using European arms on a large scale and of taking advantage of the local terrain. The first Europeans to suffer a crushing defeat were the Italians, who tried to turn Ethiopia into a dependency. They met their match in Menilek II, one of Ethiopia's greatest rulers. Menilek was able to assert the crown's authority over his country's 'over-mighty subjects', the great feudal lords; he successfully played off the British, French, Italians and Mahdists against one another, and he finally bested the Italians in battle. The Ethiopians thus succeeded in maintaining their independence and in obtaining diplomatic recognition from Europe. What is more, they took an active part of their own in the scramble, competing effectively with the French, Italians and British along Ethiopia's borders.

As for the British, they underestimated the Afrikaners as badly as the Italians had underestimated the Amhara. Behind Anglo-Boer quarrels over the Uitlanders' franchise in the Transvaal, Kruger's dynamite monopoly and the dispute over the Transvaal's constitutional position, there was always the greater question of whether Boers or Britons should be the dominant white minority in South Africa. War broke out in the end, and the Boer War came to mark a watershed in military history. It began as a British imperial venture of the limited liability kind, financed on a shoestring and fought against an enemy whom many British professional soldiers hardly considered to be on a par with warlike Indian mountaineers. It ended as the greatest military effort on land hitherto put forth by Great Britain. The British at long last gained a decisive victory in the field, but they failed to win the peace. A few years after the conclusion of the Peace of Vereeniging (1902), the British—unwilling to maintain a large occupation army in South Africa—restored self-government to the two Boer republics.

The Boer War had not, therefore, prevented the ultimate devolution of imperial power to the locally dominant white groups. The war had played an important part also in shaping anti-colonial opinion at home. For a short period the British masses were intoxicated by the assumed splendour of empire; but the war-fever did not last. On the contrary, the war produced a bitter reaction. J. A. Hobson, whose critique of imperialism was later taken over and elaborated by Lenin, was deeply influenced by events in South Africa, a country he had visited as a journalist.

At the turn of the present century, however, in many parts of Africa the colonizers had yet to make their rule effective. Cartographers might colour the map in Prussian blue or British red. But over vast stretches of the interior the white man's writ did not actually run, and European power was enforced only in the first decade of the twentieth century— sometimes even later. Apart from a few territories such as the Cape or Sierra Leone, the bulk of Africa experienced white rule for only a brief period, for no more than two generations or so. In establishing their rule, the various colonial powers all had their national style. In theory, at any rate, the French stood for administrative centralization; their approach was inclined to be military and bureaucratic. The British had a more pragmatic outlook; they favoured administrative decentralization and gave much latitude to the man on the spot. The Germans, although they had a strong military and bureaucratic tradition, often tried to imitate the British. For instance, they attempted to copy the British device of governing cheaply through chartered companies; but German endeavours in this respect were no more successful than those of the British in Rhodesia and East Africa.

Nevertheless, the colonizers' approach depended more on local circumstances than on their nationality. In an age of tiny administrative cadres and inadequate communications, the *broussard*, be he a British district commissioner or a French *commandant du cercle*, wielded immense powers for good or evil. Some went to pieces, falling victim to the morphine habit or sexual debauchery. The great majority, however, displayed a surprising degree of toughness and common sense. And the best of them developed comparable doctrines of government. The rulers should 'govern to serve'; they should act as trustees for their subjects; they should develop Africa in the interests both of the Africans and of the world at large. Whether these doctrines are to be considered as rationalizations of class interests or as an autonomous ideology, they did influence the tone of colonial administration in many different ways; and they embodied what might be called an outlook of cautious, conservative reform.

The colonial era produced bitter controversy over the real or assumed record of rival powers. Some nationalities were considered better colonizers than others. But in truth the performance of each European nationality varied a great deal according to time and place. As Cornevin shows, for instance, there were many German imperialisms. In large parts of South West Africa the Germans practised a ruthless policy of white settlement. Togo, on the other hand, became a *Musterkolonie* that depended on indigenous peasant agriculture rather than on foreign planters. In Kamerun the Germans began to form the nucleus of a semi-germanized African élite. In East Africa, on the other hand, the Germans encouraged the spread of Swahili and placed much power into the hands of Muslim auxiliaries.

It is hard to make general statements with regard to even a single territory under the sway of any one colonial power. There was not one, but several 'German East Africas'. There were also two Kameruns. German policy in northern Kamerun had much in common with British policy in northern Nigeria. As Cornevin points out, the Germans admired Islam; they considered the Fulani horsemen a superior race.

Hence the Germans employed a system of indirect rule in the north. Christian schools and missions did not penetrate to the north; there was no European economic development, and the country remained administratively separated from the southern forest belt.

In Nigeria there was a similar division between imperial policy in the north and south respectively. In the south the British co-operated to some extent with educated Christian Africans. In the north their rule was based on an alliance with the Muslim emirs. The northern policy finally prevailed over Nigeria as a whole, and Lord Lugard's indirect rule doctrines became an accepted part of British imperial orthodoxy. But even indirect rule was not all of a piece. The term itself, as explained by Flint, covered several different policies that differed greatly from one another even within a single territory.

Just as there were many political imperialisms, so there were many imperialisms in the economic field. One of the harshest forms of exploitation was what the Germans call *Raubwirtschaft*, entailing the direct appropriation of goods or the destruction of irreplaceable wealth. Looting, especially cattle-rustling, characterized several predatory indigenous economies such as those of the Matabele and the Ngoni. Nor were the Europeans above such practices. The British South Africa Company's régime in early Southern Rhodesia and in North-Eastern Rhodesia confiscated herds from the defeated Matabele and Ngoni. By and large, however, the whites did not loot. For one thing, proceedings such as those of the chartered company aroused the wrath of humanitarians and radicals at home. For another, African economies with their backward modes of production rarely provided the goods that the whites most desired.

In order to make profits, the Europeans were forced to wage war on predatory African societies such as the Zulu or the Ngoni who raided their neighbours for captives. Backward agricultural export economies depended on slaves. But slave-catching, slave-trading and slavery had long since become abhorrent to the great European powers by the time of the scramble. European, and to some extent American, sea power largely eliminated the sea-borne traffic. The European colonial economies gradually came to depend on free wage-labour; European entrepreneurs regarded slavery both as an affront to human dignity and as a challenge to their own economic system. The British, French, Belgians and Germans all combined to stamp out slave-trading within their respective dominions, doing away thereby with what a senior

British police officer called 'the iniquitous abduction of valuable labour'.[1]

Still another form of early enterprise depended on the unplanned destruction of natural wealth. At the time of the scramble, Arab, African and European hunters all took their part in chasing elephants in order to supply the luxury industries of Europe, India and North America with a highly prized raw material. These hunters destroyed a great many animals, for only a few of the more powerful and far-sighted chiefs, such as Khama, paramount of the Bamangwato, and Lobengula, head of the Matabele, took any steps to safeguard the game. But like the fur-traders and trappers of the early Canadian frontier, the ivory-hunters could operate quite well within the framework of tribal polities; frontiersmen such as Carl Wiese among the Ngoni thus achieved high positions as advisers to indigenous chiefs.

Ivory-hunters at worst 'shot out' big game. The search for wild rubber was apt to have more serious consequences. Hunting elephants was a highly skilled job; but any one could collect wild rubber, and unskilled workmen could therefore be conscripted in large numbers. The industrial revolution in Europe produced a steadily increasing demand for rubber, and for a time merchants looked to Africa to supply their needs. The worst type of exploitation occurred in the Congo Free State (ironically enough the only African colony having its origin in an attempt at international colonization under humanitarian auspices). The Congo Free State monopolized both the country's ivory and wild rubber. It relied on private enterprise only for the development of mines and railways, that is to say, for those undertakings calling for heavy investment and high risk. Standing in desperate need of additional revenue to meet its growing administrative expenditure, the Congo Free State put the harshest possible pressure on local Africans to gather rubber. Exploitation was not universal, being necessarily confined to regions where rubber-trees flourished. It was further limited by the weakness of the Free State's administrative machinery, which had to rely on a handful of men to control huge areas. But where coercion was employed, the Free State's monopolistic system led to bloody terror. The Congo, as Stengers points out, was unique among European colonies in Africa in that its revenues were used directly to subsidize the mother country. Leopold employed Congolese money for

[1] Quoted by L. H. Gann in 'The end of the slave trade in British Central Africa: 1889–1912', *Rhodes-Livingstone Journal*, 1954, no. 16, p. 41.

conspicuous expenditure on public buildings at home, thereby offending against the unwritten convention that disapproved the colonial powers' diverting colonial state revenue into the metropolitan exchequer.

In the end, humanitarian, missionary and diplomatic pressure from outside as well as a good deal of publicity concerning Congolese abuses forced the king to abandon his estate. In 1908 the Congo was annexed to Belgium. Congolese and metropolitan finances were separated; the domanial régime and forced labour were suppressed; the Congo became a colony of the classical variety. The Congolese reforms had the unintended effect, moreover, of facilitating the Congo's subsequent mineral and industrial development. Before annexation, impassioned reformers such as E. D. Morel and others of his stamp had had no conception of the Congo's enormous mining wealth. And without the changes forced upon the Congo by such men, the rational exploitation of the Congo's minerals would hardly have been possible. *Raubwirtschaft* had interfered with the free flow of labour. Congolese monopolies had impeded economic enterprise, and had thereby run counter to the king's aspirations in the long run. The annexation of the Congo and the consequent social and administrative reforms were followed by economic development on an impressive scale.

Although the Congo stands out as the worst instance of colonial exploitation in tropical Africa under the aegis of the new imperialism, abuses were to be found in many other colonies. In the Portuguese colonies, in early Rhodesia and elsewhere, obligatory labour services were imposed on Africans. And as Mme Coquery shows, forced labour was employed on a large scale in French Equatorial Africa. Nor were concessionary monopolies confined to the Congo. The British South Africa Company in Southern Rhodesia and the French in Equatorial Africa similarly operated at first on the assumption that outside capital could be secured only by the granting of large territorial concessions on easy terms. This approach, however, did not work. The grantees usually failed to invest sufficient funds or to do much serious development work; many concessionary companies indeed suffered heavy losses.

The coercive and monopolistic approach soon met with bitter criticism in the metropolitan capitals and sometimes encountered hostility also from white people on the spot. In Germany both the Catholic Centre and the Social Democratic parties denounced colonial malpractices; in London the Aborigines Protection Society, missionary bodies and similar groups were able to mobilize considerable support.

Many mine-owners and some farmers in Rhodesia, for instance, preferred freedom of employment for a variety of economic reasons. Coercion was widely unpopular within colonial administrations too. Few district commissioners liked the unpleasant work of forcing villagers to work for white men, nor did the senior officials in colonial ministries at home. The combination of economic self-interest, humanitarian pressure, political campaigning and official trusteeship doctrines thus helped to bring about major changes.

The first decade of the twentieth century might thus be called in many ways an age of capitalist self-criticism and reform in the African colonies. In Southern Rhodesia extensive administrative and social improvements were made under the administration of Sir William Milton, who ran the country from 1898 to 1914. The appointment to the German Colonial Office in 1906 of Bernhard Dernburg, a liberal-minded banker and a believer in efficiency, was symptomatic of a desire to right abuses. In French Equatorial Africa, as Mme Coquery explains, extensive changes for the better were made after 1910. The French Equatorial colonies were federated; administration improved; encouragement was given to the cultivation of peasant-grown export crops; steps were taken to end concessionary abuses. The Congo entered upon a reforming period in 1910. Even Portugal, the most backward of all the colonial powers, the country most addicted to forced labour policies, tried to improve the lot of its indigenous subjects when the country became a republic in 1910. The impact of these various reforms was distinctly uneven. Many abuses persisted; many colonies continued to experience much popular discontent. Nevertheless there were improvements; and during the First World War neither the British, the Germans nor the French had to cope with any large-scale African rising at a time when all their military strength was fully committed against white rivals.

As regards overall economic progress during the period under review, it is difficult to generalize. Our series devotes an entire volume to economic questions of colonialism, but we may here point to a few salient features. Economic development was very uneven. Some regions were hardly affected by the new currents, while a few of the more favoured areas increased their output rapidly. Development was confined largely to the production of raw materials. The most dramatic expansion took place in the mineral industries of southern Africa and the Congo, on peasant holdings in West Africa and, to a much smaller extent, on white-run farms and plantations established in parts of Rhodesia and of East and South Africa. But development was not confined to these sectors alone. The colonizers, for instance, created new port facilities. The bulk of Africa's existing railway-network came into being before 1914. In addition, the colonizers founded a great number of new cities during the half century or so preceding the First World War, including Dakar, Salisbury and Johannesburg. They introduced also a host of new urban management techniques, including provision for such facilities as sewerage, insect control and clean water. The colonizers indeed were Africa's town-builders *par excellence*.

It is difficult to assess the Europeans' imperial record as a whole. Contemporary discussion on the subject indeed bears some resemblance to the interminable debates concerning the war-guilt question after the First World War. We can hardly deal here with all the charges regarding the economic and psychological exploitation of Africans made by critics of the European record. As editors we have made no attempt to impose our views on our contributors. But at least we should like to make our own bias clear. We do not share the widely-held assumption that equates colonialism with exploitation. Neither do we believe that profits necessarily imply exploitation. In our view, economic exploitation occurs only when the exploited have to pay more for their purchases than the price at which other sellers would be willing to supply the required merchandise. Exploitation likewise takes place when people have to supply goods or services for less than they would be able to receive on the open market. Exploitation, in our opinion, must imply the contrived denial by coercive means of alternatives that would otherwise have been available and preferred. We thus consider the enforced growing of crops, or forced labour of the Congo Free State, of the early Rhodesian and Kenyan variety or of the French and Portuguese kind to be forms of exploitation. But we do not believe that, say, a bush trader exploits his customers simply by charging high prices in his store. The prices charged have to be seen in terms of the trader's own costs, the risks he shoulders, his own labour time and the demand that exists for his merchandise.

We thus take a more favourable view of white (and of course also non-white) entrepreneurship than some of our contributors. We should also be more inclined than some of them to stress the immigrants' technical and technological contributions. (Elsewhere, for instance, we have referred to the way in which white farmers increased the value of their properties by improving the land and by introducing new agricultural methods.) We also argue that European immigration to Africa, while occasioning all manner of new social problems, represented at the same time a much-needed transfer of modern skills. We accordingly interpret European imperialism in Africa as an engine of cultural transfusion as well as of political domination. We thus regard the European era as most decisive for the future of Africa.

We likewise look favourably on many of the Europeans' political achievements. By 1914 the colonial rulers had established peace, rule of law and inexpensive but honest government for much larger units than had existed in Africa previously. In our own view, for instance, the pacification and administrative unification of a huge territory such as Nigeria—a country never previously united under the same flag—was in itself a major achievement.

Imperialism, according to our interpretation, acted as a means of cultural transformation. Among other things, the whites brought to Africa modern forms of education, medical facilities and a host of economic techniques. In this connexion Reverend C. P. Groves rightly stresses the special role of the missions. In modern Africa, as in mediaeval Europe, the churches pioneered most of the social services. They contributed greatly to the spread of literacy; they also played an important part in linguistic and other kinds of research. Many have argued with much justice that, whatever the missionaries' subjective intentions may have been, objectively they helped to serve European bourgeois interests. The missionaries' opposition to traditional forms of serfdom, their hostility to sumptuary legislation and other restraints on consumption existing in some of the more highly stratified indigenous societies, their creed proclaiming aristocrats and bondsmen alike in the sight of God, their economic and moral individualism, their hostility to indigenous witchcraft beliefs and magical practices of course all brought revolutionary economic as well as religious consequences. Putting the matter in its simplest form, a literate African who had been trained as a printer, a clerk or a carpenter at a mission school was certainly more useful to his white employer than an illiterate heathen. But the advantages for the white men did not necessarily entail disadvantages for the black. The mission pupil also benefited from the diversification of skills, and the missions are therefore entitled to moral as well as economic credit for their enterprise, however limited their efforts may have been and however uneven their impact.

Missionary influence, however, went further. Ecclesiastical lobbies combined with secular pressure groups in denouncing imperial abuses and proposing reforms. Seen as a whole, the European rulers in Africa—for all their malpractices—were forced to set themselves standards of a kind unknown to ruling races from a different cultural background, such as the Zanzibari or Matabele. Humanitarian pressure groups often managed to reduce or eliminate evils, especially when the reformers were able to benefit from dissensions within the imperial ranks.

But whatever their political complexion, even the most advanced humanitarians during this period did not think in terms of creating independent black states. Trusteeship was not a formula for nation-building. On the contrary, the abuses that flourished in Liberia and Haiti were commonly taken as proofs for the assertion that 'the black man...is incapable of the art of government...and that [whatever] the negro may become after centuries of civilized education...he is not fit to govern now'.[1] The Europeans thus developed a doctrine of imperial rule which, in the Livingstonian missionary tradition, justified white governance by linking pacification, economic development, technological innovation and moral uplift as part of a coherent philosophy. At the Brussels Conference of 1890 the powers thus promised to fight the slave-trade, to build roads, railways and telegraphs, to prevent the unrestricted traffic in fire-arms and to 'diminish inland wars between the tribes...to initiate them into agricultural works and in the industrial arts so as to increase their welfare; to raise them to civilization and to bring about the extinction of barbarous customs such as cannibalism and human sacrifice'.[2]

These doctrines expressed the best of imperial aspirations at the time. They also became standards by which the imperial performance and imperial failures could be judged. They made little appeal to black rural radicals of the Messianic kind. But they did influence the attitudes of the emergent élite. The black intellectuals and politicians assembled at the Pan-Africanist Congress held at Paris in 1919 thus put forward demands which in many respects differed little from the views of the more enlightened colonial rulers. Ultimately the humanitarian and reformist programme of the African intelligentsia merged with popular varieties of rural radicalism and with nationalist and socialist strands. These

[1] Sir Spenser St John, *Hayti or the Black Republic*, 2nd ed. (New York, 1889).
[2] *General Act of the Brussels Conference, 1889–1890, with annexed declaration*, Great Britain, *Parliamentary Papers*, C. 6048 (London, 1890).

new forms of political thought will be treated by contributors to subsequent volumes in this series.

The present volume is concerned only with the period of the scramble and its aftermath to 1914. Some of the material presented here is new; other essays are syntheses of what is known. Inevitably gaps remain. For instance, many metropolitan and colonial archives have as yet hardly been touched, and there is still wide scope for researchers using primary sources. In addition, much work remains to be done by synthesizers willing to reappraise the more orthodox interpretations.

As regards specific topics, the present study does not attempt to cover the internal organization of various European colonial offices. It provides only scanty detail concerning local administrations or great empire-builders like Rhodes. We have not dealt with the outlook and social background of the various administrative officers. More might have been said concerning the role of individual governors in situations where the man on the spot wielded tremendous power. The history of administrative and technical services offers much scope for further study. So do African military, political and economic reactions to European rule.

Historians will in addition have to ask new questions. For instance, how should we assess what Coillard called 'kingly socialism'? Was Coillard right in arguing that a system of tributary kingship that 'managed' the exchange of goods between different provinces for political and prestige reasons was incompatible with economic progress? Others may wish to inquire into the role of economically active alien minorities such as the Indians and Arabs in East Africa, the Levantines in West Africa and the Europeans in East and East Central Africa. The black middlemen of West Africa, the lusitanized, gallicized, anglicized or americanized black people of West Africa also played a major part in the development of the region. There is need both for detailed investigation and for more general comparative study concerning their role. How far can one speak of a black bourgeoisie? What was the connexion between kinship and capitalism? Are the conventional critics of capitalism right in claiming that capitalism was bound to shatter traditional family links? Or did kinship links in fact facilitate the emergence of wealthy entrepreneurs, as they may have done in the history of the house of Rothschild?

The military history of Africa likewise remains to be reinterpreted. The existence of colonial empires, for example, to some extent affected world strategy. Certain areas of Africa became reservoirs of military manpower and thereby played a part in world history. African development in general might be reinterpreted on the lines earlier sketched out by Sir Keith Hancock, in terms of moving 'frontiers', including those of the trader, the miner and the farmer, all of which impinged both upon one another and upon more traditional economies. The role of cities in African development remains to be written. Further investigation is required on the origins and growth of African nationalist movements and proto-nationalist movements. Indeed few fields offer the modern historian more opportunities than the African continent. The present volume and those to follow in this series are therefore part of a wider effort to evaluate the colonial period of African history.

L. H. GANN
PETER DUIGNAN

CHAPTER I

AFRICAN SOCIETY AT THE TIME
OF THE SCRAMBLE

by ELIZABETH COLSON

Nineteenth-century Africa supported a greater variety of political and social institutions than Europe. In a few regions simple bands with rudimentary economic institutions made a meagre living from a difficult land. Elsewhere, highly developed states supported a richly varied life. The majority of African peoples lived in societies which lay somewhere along the continuum between the two extremes.

These societies, whatever their complexity, were not static fossils surviving from an earlier era. Political units were being radically revised throughout the nineteenth century; for the impact of foreign trade, the spread of new crafts and new materials, the adoption of new food crops, the acquisition of new armaments, all helped to alter the balance of power among the old polities. In some areas the new influences favoured the rise of new and more powerful political alignments; in others they brought old régimes crashing into ruins. The emergence of more powerful states was perhaps the usual denouement in West Africa, where the impact of foreign trade and the development of communications had gone farthest and where long centuries of state-building had familiarized people with the role of remote authority. East, Central and South Africa were more vulnerable. Raids and invasions had devastated wide areas formerly occupied by small political communities dependent for their government on a minimal elaboration of office. Yet even here new states had been built in the early part of the century, and a few were building at the time of the scramble.

Few of the newly expanded polities had had time to become rooted in tradition before they were engulfed by European colonialism. Nor had the new régimes such as the Fulani empires been able to stamp a uniformity of culture upon their subjects. Differences in language, ideology, legal rules, and social institutions characterized the kingdoms and principalities and demonstrated the difficulties of communication between capital and hinterland, between one small region and another. Where no centralized government existed and each small community regulated its own affairs, heterogeneity was even more apparent.

Political Africa in 1870

PROBLEMS OF TERMINOLOGY. European visitors of the 1870s—like subsequent colonial officials—were likely to misinterpret African institutions and to find in them a generalized uniformity. The romantic emphasis upon savagery and exotic custom, and the opposite failing of interpreting local institutions in the light of European precedent, helped to mislead the observers.

The common classification of African political units as 'tribes' downgraded the extent of political development in many regions and implied that African polities were of a lower order than those of Europe. The term 'chief' for a ruler or ranking official produced much the same effect.

In common parlance, 'tribalism' usually refers to a continued allegiance to units smaller than the new states created during the colonial period. 'Tribe' is used for both political and non-political groupings, even though these may have none of the characteristics usually connoted by the term, which variously conveys the sense of a people under its own government, with a homogeneous culture, speaking a common language, occupying its own territory, and having a common history, but too few in numbers to provide the base for a complicated governmental structure. A 'tribe' is too small to be a 'nation'. It shares with 'nation' the implications of common language, common culture and common descent. Many so-called African tribes are not distinguished by these traits. This was as true in 1870 as it is today.

Much of south-eastern Nigeria has long been occupied by the Ibo people, who today number something like five and a half million. In 1870 the Ibo lived in small autonomous village communities that warred on one another. They recognized no common political leaders, though adherence to a few popular shrines provided a means of exerting widespread influence, as did the existence of a number of voluntary associations with chapters throughout south-eastern Nigeria. The Ibo communities may have felt some common identification as against communities of non-Ibo speakers, but this was probably minimal since they had no common name for themselves nor any tradition of a former unity. The various Ibo dialects were usually but not always mutually intelligible. Some Ibo communities preserved traditions of descent from non-Ibo speaking immigrants. The various communities shared a common culture only in the loosest meaning of the term. They differed radically from one another even with regard to fundamental institutions such as family organization, inheritance, land rights, village political organization, religious beliefs and rituals. The Ibo became a self-conscious unity only after they had been identified as such by foreigners who perceived common features of language and custom despite the many manifest differences. Foreigners gave the Ibo their name, and, by treating them as though they were a single people, encouraged them to become one. By 1870 an Ibo nationality or an Ibo ethnic group may have emerged, but the Ibo had not yet organized themselves into an Ibo political group.

The mobilization of other so-called tribes of the twentieth century occurred in much the same fashion. Tribal organizations were created during the colonial period when the desire for orderly administration led administrators to amalgamate formerly independent communities into larger units under officially appointed leaders. Wherever possible, European officials drew political boundaries to coincide with language or cultural boundaries, since they assumed this would provide a natural cohesion and stability to the administrative unit. The importance given to 'language' and 'nationality' as political factors in nineteenth- and twentieth-century Europe no doubt encouraged such endeavours.

The creation of the Tonga 'tribe' in southern Zambia is only one illustration of what was happening throughout Africa. In the 1870s, Tonga-speakers lived in many small independent neighbourhoods that treasured slight differences in dialect and custom. They recognized no common name and had no feeling that they belonged to a common polity. Foreigners who settled among them were easily absorbed into local society. Each small community knew that its members were of heterogeneous origin, but since their relationships were not governed by a dogma of common descent this did not matter. The name 'Tonga' was first applied to them by other Africans. Colonial administrators in the twentieth century bestowed upon them 'tribal organization'.

Some present-day 'tribes' do represent pre-colonial political units. In that case almost invariably they are composed of people who claim diverse origins, retain distinctive customs, and perhaps speak distinctive languages. The Barotse 'tribe' in western Zambia belongs in this category. It descends from a kingdom of some magnitude which existed for centuries on the upper Zambezi river. At times it held sway over areas today divided among Angola, Zambia, South West Africa and Botswana. In 1839 Barotseland was conquered by the Kololo, a band of raiders who had fled from the turmoil then prevalent in southern Africa. Before 1839 and again after the Kololo were expelled in 1864, an aristocracy known as Lozi or Luyi ruled the region. Their subjects were of diverse origin. Some claimed to be long-established residents of the Zambezi plain, like the Lozi themselves. Others were captives or the descendants of captives, though these usually merged with the free population within a generation or two. Refugee groups, sometimes of considerable size, had sought safety under Lozi rule. When strong enough in numbers, they retained their languages and customs, but gave allegiance to the Lozi king. The Lozi intermarried with most of the subject peoples. Both aristocrats and royalty were of mixed ancestry, though they spoke the Lozi language of the court and maintained the courtly customs regarded as typical of the Lozi. Barotse-land was a miniature melting pot with many peoples incompletely assimilated to any common model, though it had a political unity and a common language used for public affairs.

If the word 'tribe' means common culture, common tongue, and a sense of ethnic unity based on a belief in common descent, the Barotse do not fit the definition. No more do the people of many another pre-colonial state where an aristocratic nucleus claiming perhaps a common origin ruled over a heterogeneous population with a different history. In such cases the people saw no reason to adopt the language and customs of the court to the total extinction of their own ways and languages, which continued to be used at home or in local affairs. Heterogeneity characterized all the larger states and many of the principalities in existence in the nineteenth century; for political stability drew followers, and boundaries shifted with fluctuations in power.[1]

[1] See Ian Cunnison, *The Luapula peoples of Northern Rhodesia* (Manchester University Press, 1959), pp. 30–61, for the heterogeneity within the Lunda kingdom of Kazembe, which straddled the Congo–Zambia border; M. G. Smith, *Government in Zazzau, 1800–1950* (London, Oxford University Press, 1960), p. 2, for the complexity of a Hausa kingdom; Elliott P. Skinner, *The Mossi of the Upper Volta: the political development of a Sudanese people* (Stanford University Press, 1964), pp. 7–12, for the same pheno-menon in the Mossi states of Mali; and Aidan Southall, *Alur society: a study in processes and types of dominations* (Cambridge, 1956), pp. 14–25, for the ethnic diversity found within very small Alur principalities on the Uganda–Congo border.

The word 'tribe' carries an implication of homogeneity which is at odds with African history. Large- and small-scale migrations had created mixed populations in every region. Those who claimed a common ancestry might be widely scattered, accepting more or less willingly the dictates of different political authorities. To call such dispersed groups 'tribes' is surely a misnomer, though there are those prepared to use the term even for the Fulani. Over the centuries, Fulani-speaking groups have spread across the savannah from Guinea and Senegal in the west to Bornu and Bagirmi in the east, and had continued their migration south into the northern Cameroons. In some places they lived as small independent bands of herders; in others they had become settled villagers. Some became subjects of whatever political régimes they encountered. Others imposed themselves as lords of established states. Still others created new Fulani kingdoms.

In fact, political and ethnic boundaries rarely coincided in pre-colonial Africa. Human ambitions were too pressing to allow people to remain static over long periods. States expanded when they were sufficiently powerful to do so. Communities competed with one another to attract settlers and thereby gain supporters. Whether newly attached persons were treated as serfs, as second-class or full citizens depended both on the incentives that attracted them and on the amount of force that could be marshalled to prevent their escape. Men moved to find better land or more favourable opportunities in their crafts, to engage more profitably in trade, to escape difficulties at home, to build a political following in a region without powerful rivals. According to their purposes they looked for stable communities and powerful patrons, or for power vacuums. They sought proximity to trade routes, or distance from unruly bands who preyed upon the routes. These considerations rather than the desire to be associated with others of the same stock might determine where the uprooted settled.

Classifying the various political and ethnic groupings which made up the mid-nineteenth-century African scene under the term 'tribe' obscures their differences and minimizes the complexity of many of the states of the period. The term would still be appropriate for designating the many small principalities or communes of equals whose ideology stressed unity based on common ancestry, no matter what the known facts may have been. Yet because of the general confusion about its implications, it is probably best abandoned. I shall describe the

31

nineteenth-century political units in terms which make some token acknowledgement to their bases of organization.[1] Ethnic groupings based on common culture or common language will be referred to by name. Thus I shall write of Yoruba when I refer to the people who shared a common language, and of the Yoruba states and cities when I refer to Yoruba polities.

BANDS, STATES, STATELETS OR PRINCIPALITIES. In 1870 only a few desolate regions in the deserts of southern Africa or remote pockets of the Rift Valley in East Africa were populated by people living permanently in bands. These were small autonomous political groups composed sometimes of no more than a score of people. The band provided for the organization of common action by a population large enough to maintain the daily round of subsistence activities. The political policy of such a band revolved around questions of how to exploit the various local resources and of how to plan an itinerary through the common territory.

Occasionally a band fought with neighbouring bands in an attempt to preserve its own resources or to encroach on resources claimed by others. Bands might also form alliances helped by the fact that intermarriage was usually necessary given the limited size of any one band. Hence all bands within a region were likely to be linked by ties of kinship. Such ties permitted men and women to move rather freely from one band to another. The band organization was stable; membership was not. More formal long-term political links between bands were not envisaged and were probably impossible, given the harshness of the environment. The only formal political office that existed was band headmanship; and since the band had minimal purposes, the office had minimal authority. There is no evidence that any such localized band began a career of conquest or attempted the development of a larger polity. But in the mid-nineteenth century, localized bands were

[1] Political terminology applicable to pre-colonial Africa has been argued at length in many places. For an insight into the problems of terminology and the varieties and complexities of political organization, see Meyer Fortes and E. E. Evans-Pritchard, eds., *African political systems* (London, Oxford University Press, 1940), the pioneer attempt to produce a classification or typology; John Middleton and David Tait, eds., *Tribes without rulers: studies in African segmentary systems* (London, 1958), a collection of essays dealing only with so-called segmentary societies; I. Schapera, *Government and politics in tribal societies* (London, 1956), a general discussion of kinds of political order in southern Africa; Lucy Mair, *Primitive government* (Baltimore, 1962), a discussion of the varieties of political organization found in East Africa.

found only in areas where difficulties of terrain and scanty rainfall made small dispersed populations almost a necessity.

Rather comparable band organization was frequently adopted by rovers of one kind or another. Groups of traders joined together for distant commercial ventures, and refugees who had been uprooted by slave raids or invading armies formed bands who roved the countryside. Bands of refugees formed under the leadership of any man who was prepared to take action in an emergency. Then in turn they preyed upon one another or upon the small settled communities which had until then escaped devastation. Bands of traders were tempted to usurp power as they moved through regions where no indigenous political force could subject them to control or offer them protection. These bands in some respects resembled the *condottiere* bands of the European middle ages or the armies of war-lords in early twentieth-century China.

Marauding bands consisted of the personal following of a leader rather than of men united by residence within a common locality or by hereditary loyalties. They were prepared to hire themselves to any employer or to ally themselves with any other group so long as such a course seemed to their advantage. Members were linked by ties of comradeship and allegiance to a common leader, who maintained his hold so long as he led them profitably and settled their inevitable disputes. Bands were frankly opportunistic in purpose and in method. Several might be joined in any particular raid or might form an uneasy alliance to dominate a countryside. But alliances tended to be brief. They soon broke up into the constituent followings, though sometimes with an exchange of members.

The roving bands were mixed in membership, since they recruited as they raided or perhaps traded. They named themselves for their leader or sometimes sought legitimacy by using the name of the old community from which the leader and perhaps some of his following had originally sprung. They might retain one or more old emblems or customs as symbolic assurances that they had an identity with greater dignity than that possessed by a mere pirate gang.

Most of the roving bands known to us from the mid-nineteenth century were short-lived. Nevertheless, a few able leaders succeeded in becoming rulers of territorial states before the Europeans seized the continent and outlawed local marauders. Some men imposed themselves and their lieutenants as the new lords of established régimes. Others organized a number of bands into a new political unit which then dominated the settled populace. They did so by tactics which allowed them to lift themselves above their coevals and to demand a loyalty overriding that due to the leaders of now subordinate groupings. They thus created a nucleus of centralized power based on a court and an incipient hierarchy of officers who could bind formerly independent bands and settled communities to a common purpose.

In East Africa, caravans led by coastal Arab or Swahili traders, or by headmen of communities lying behind the coast, began to carve out inland principalities or to seize power over small states in the interior. In the absence of powerful indigenous political rulers, caravans became bands of raiders and then took control of favoured localities. By mid-nineteenth century, Yao bands from eastern Tanzania controlled much of northern Moçambique and eastern Malawi. At much the same period, Swahili and Arab traders established themselves as rulers in Ugogo and around the shores of Lake Nyasa. They were following a precedent already established by Arab traders in central and western Tanzania. The same pattern was later to reappear in the Arab state founded in the eastern Congo by Hamed ben Mohammed ben Juma, also known as Tippu Tib.

Trading bands imposed themselves on a number of the old political units of the Congo. Chokwe bands from Angola, who appeared sometimes as traders and sometimes as raiders, overran Lunda country early in the century. Between 1852 and 1887 they began to infiltrate into the Kasai. The Nyamwezi trader Msidi, from Tanzania, seized an old kingdom or principality in the Katanga copper region about 1856. Eventually he fell before the rival adventurers employed by the Congo Free State, who killed him and took his kingdom.

Refugee Ndebele and Ngoni bands from southern Africa terrorized Rhodesia, Zambia, Malawi, Tanzania and Moçambique during this same period. They created new states in preference to seizing power within old political units. As they raided, they incorporated droves of captives. Their leaders then faced the problem of control occasioned by the rapidly snowballing size of each band. Ngoni leaders experimented with a variety of methods of delegating authority and organizing their greatly expanded followings. A number were successful. They created the small Ngoni kingdoms that dominated the border zone of Zambia, Malawi and Moçambique from mid-century. Farther north, Ngoni bands that raided Tanzania failed to solve the problems of internal organization posed by expansion. As they increased in size or met misfortune, the band broke up into smaller units that continued their career as bandits.[1]

Occasionally an established ruler enlisted bands of raiders to expand his own territory. Mirambo, ruler of two small Nyamwezi principalities in the 1860s, hired Ngoni and Masai mercenaries to help him subject much of Nyamwezi–Sukuma country, and thus became the dominant power in central Tanzania. Mirambo could appeal to a tradition of ancient unity in giving legitimacy to the Nyamwezi state he sought to create, but this alone did not win acceptance of his rule. The availability of raiding bands provided him with the personal army he needed.

The trading band that turned raider before usurping political power was a common phenomenon in the Africa of this period; so was the refugee band which succeeded in finding a new political role. But both the bands and the new states they created retained an air of improvisation. Few band leaders were able to hand power to a legitimate successor. Even where a band leader had become the ruler of a state, succession remained a problem. Leadership was a personal role rather than an established office. The death or decline of a leader might well lead to the break-up of his following. Here was a major distinction between the roving bands and the band-dominated states and the old kingdoms that still controlled wide areas of Africa.

The largest kingdoms with the most complex organization were in West Africa, where ancient states had developed in conjunction with the centuries-old trade that linked sub-Saharan Africa with the Mediterranean and the centres of Islamic culture. It was in the savannah belt that West African states attained their maximum size and stability; only here could horses and camels be used to speed the movement of armies and to permit large-scale trade between the various regions. By the early nineteenth century, most of the old states of the western savannah had fallen under the sway of various Fulani overlords. The alliance of Fulani states of Niger, Nigeria and the northern Cameroons under the aegis of the ruler of Sokoto provided the largest area of unified political action found in sub-Saharan Africa during this period.

[1] J. A. Barnes, *Politics in a changing society: a political history of the Fort Jameson Ngoni* (London, Oxford University Press, 1954), pp. 6–63, describes the history of Zwangendaba's band, which developed into the Ngoni kingdom of Mpeseni on the Zambezi-Malawi border. See also M. Read, *The Ngoni of Nyasaland* (London, Oxford University Press, 1956), pp. 3–15, 29–100, for descriptions of other Ngoni kingdoms of Malawi; and J. D. Omer-Cooper, *The Zulu aftermath: a nine-teenth-century revolution in Bantu Africa* (Evanston, Northwestern University Press, 1966).

In the forests south of the savannah, tsetse fly prevented the introduction of livestock. Goods had to travel on the backs or heads of porters or by river boat. Here states were smaller in extent, though some were of ancient origin. The Yoruba had been forced back upon the forests of western Nigeria, beyond the range of Fulani cavalry, in the early part of the century. Here they had created a large number of small independent city states. The Yoruba looked back to the sacred city of Ife as the centre from which they had sprung. They acknowledged the more recent hegemony of the city of Oyo, whose ruler still held the right to confirm the kings of a number of other cities. Still the cities fought one another for territory, or more particularly to gain control of the trade routes to the coast. They also battled against the rival kingdoms that flanked them on either side. On the east lay Benin, an ancient city of the forest region. On the west was the upstart Dahomey, a product partly of the trade wars of the seventeenth and eighteenth centuries, which had fought its way to the sea only recently. Beyond Dahomey lay the Ashanti Confederacy, dominated by the state of Kumasi, which was gradually consolidating its control.

Along the coastal belt, numerous small commercial towns, each with its dependent territory, maintained their independent policy, much as did city states in ancient Greece and mediaeval Italy. These towns had grown up in conjunction with the development of overseas trade. They were dominated by oligarchies of merchants who served as middlemen between European traders and the hinterland. At the time of the scramble, some of the small coastal towns on the Oil Rivers of Nigeria or along the coasts of Dahomey, Ghana and Senegal were already a century and more old, with established institutions and a patina of tradition.

Few ancient states of any size were still extant in other regions of Africa by the 1870s. There is, however, evidence that states of some stability had existed in many regions at an earlier period, probably along commercial routes or near workable mineral deposits. The history of Africa is probably dominated by the rise and fall of such kingdoms. In Ethiopia and in the Great Lakes region of East Africa, the European explorers found powerful rulers with impressive courts who ruled large territories. Elsewhere they found only shadows of former splendour. In Rhodesia, Karanga and Rozwi, which had derived their prosperity from the gold-trade with the east coast, had long since begun to decay. They finally disintegrated in mid-century under the onslaught of Ngoni raiders.

On the west coast and along the Congo river, the kingdom of Kongo was a hazy memory. The Luba and Lunda kingdoms of Kasai and Katanga were on the decline or already broken by Yeke and Chokwe marauders; their offshoots in Angola and Zambia were in difficulties. In Central Africa, the Lozi, Bemba and Kuba states remained to reflect the institutions and greatness of earlier African monarchies; neither in territory nor in population did they compare with the large West African régimes.

Far northward, the still expanding Azande and Mangbetu kingdoms spent their strength in endemic warfare while still encroaching on the small settled communities of the north-eastern forest. In the far south, European settlers had begun to curtail the freedom of the warrior kingdoms founded earlier in the century when Chaka had devastated a sub-continent to build the Zulu kingdom and other rulers of tiny principalities had gathered survivors of his wars into a number of small kingdoms. These last were already diminished in power, and by 1870 the Zulu kingdom was past its zenith, though its régime was still intact and it still ruled perhaps half a million subjects.

PROBLEMS OF POLITICAL ORDER IN STATE RÉGIMES. African states varied enormously in territory, population, and organization. What they shared was centralization of power under a ruler who controlled outlying districts or provinces through a hierarchy of officials responsible to himself. All the states had common problems related to the fact of centralization: (1) the risk involved in the delegation of power to distant officials who might obtain local support for rebellion or secession; (2) the possibility that a strong ruler might develop into a tyrant unless subject to checks which might leave him without the authority necessary to control disaffection; (3) the difficulty of collecting sufficient revenue to support the court and provide rewards to loyal adherents; (4) the necessity of providing for continuity of government through the regulation of succession. These problems were compounded by the difficulties of communication, which made control from the centre difficult, and by the general poverty of resources. Different states found different solutions, which in turn affected other aspects of government. African states and kingdoms conformed to no single form, despite a recent attempt to define such a type.[1]

[1] See Roland Oliver and J. D. Fage, *A short history of Africa* (Harmondsworth, Middlesex and Baltimore, 1962), pp. 44–52. For general treatment of African state

West African states showed a variety of political patterns, as the following instances illustrate. The Fulani kingdoms in Niger and Nigeria, which ruled the most extensive territories, also had the most complex organizations. They derived their political institutions in part from earlier Hausa régimes they had replaced and in part from Islamic sources. Their Islamic rulers based their claims to legitimacy upon the orthodoxy of their religion as well as upon the right of conquest. They favoured the council of Muslim scholars and saw themselves restricted by Islamic law. They employed scribes for the keeping of records and judges trained in Islamic law. At the same time, military considerations tended to determine overall policy, since the Fulani rulers drew the large revenue needed for the support of an elaborate state structure from the sale of captured slaves or from the use of slave labour on large estates assigned to the various state offices.

The Yoruba, too, may have borrowed political institutions from the old Hausa states, but in the nineteenth century some Yoruba cities were experimenting with new institutions. The majority were ruled by kings, but in the nineteenth century several came to be governed by councils of more or less equal officials. In those cities ruled by kings, a royal lineage had the right to supply successive monarchs. The king's power was severely limited by a council of officials representing major craft guilds, various trade associations, and the great lineages held to have been joined with the royal lineage in the foundation of the city. Offices of government were distributed among the great lineages, which had the right to provide the successive incumbents. The king had only a limited voice in the selection of either major or minor officials and little power to dismiss members of his council. When united the council could depose the king, but could only replace him with another member of the royal lineage. In some cities the royal lineage was split into several branches, which alternated in supplying the ruler.

An elaborate etiquette prevented easy association between Yoruba kings and their subjects. The king symbolized the state and its continuity. He was held responsible for its welfare; but he had little to do with day-to-day administration. Most of his officials were not dependent on his favour since they were supported either by fees attached to

organization, see Peter Lloyd, 'The political structure of African kingdoms', in Conference on New Approaches in Social Anthropology, Jesus College, Cambridge, 1963, *Political systems and the distribution of power* (New York, 1965), pp. 63–112; Audrey I. Richards, ed., *East African chiefs* (London, Oxford University Press, 1960), pp. 344–58.

their offices or by the resources of their own lineages. It was they, rather than the king, who recruited and controlled the armies.

Some Yoruba cities were dominated by secret societies whose senior officials also held high government office. Such societies claimed the right to legislate for their members and sometimes for the rest of the populace. Junior members formed a police force for the enforcement of society orders. Disputes between members might be heard by society officials rather than in the secular courts. Some offences, no matter by whom committed, were offences against a particular society and were punished by that group rather than by the state. In all Yoruba cities the power of the state was affected by the authority exercised over their own members by large lineages, craft guilds, and trade associations. Perhaps in Yoruba eyes a man was first a member of such a grouping and only secondarily a citizen of the state. The complex distribution of power and authority among a series of institutions and offices meant that no single one held any great monopoly of force.

This system contrasted sharply with that of the Fulani kingdoms to the north and of Dahomey to the west. In Dahomey the kingship increased in power through the several centuries during which Dahomey was fighting its way into a dominant position on the trade routes to the west of Yoruba country. In nineteenth-century Dahomey, as in most Yoruba states, the government was exercised by the king-in-council. But in Dahomey it was the monarch rather than the council who held the reins of government. Lineages had lost their claim to provide the holders of state offices, and retained only the right to administer their own internal affairs. Even then they were subject to the controls of public law and the interests of the state. The king controlled appointments to office throughout his domain and could promote, dismiss or transfer officials. He controlled also a well-developed network of spies to keep watch over officials both in the capital and in the provinces. The standing army and the militia were officered by men appointed by the ruler and dependent upon him for advancement. To support his elaborate court, staff of civil officials and army (which included the famous corps of women soldiers known as the Amazons), the king systematically taxed his subjects. His revenues were supplemented by fines and confiscations, by the spoils of war and by trading profits which fell to him by virtue of his role as chief merchant of the kingdom. Dahomean kings prevented the growth of secret societies which might provide a cover for political disaffection.

They also subjected the priests of established religious cults to the royal power. If the Yoruba states are reminiscent of the oligarchies of ancient Greece, Dahomey more nearly resembled an absolute monarchy. Within Dahomey, each person was first of all a citizen of the state and only secondarily a member of some other group.

West of Dahomey, the Ashanti towns were allied in a confederacy organized on still other principles. The towns were independent in most respects but recognized the leadership of the Asantehene, ruler of Kumasi town. As among the Yoruba, each town was ruled by a council upon which sat representatives of the great lineages. The council was therefore composed of the senior men of the important lineages. One lineage held the right to provide the town king, whose appointment was subject to confirmation by the council. Council members then swore an oath of allegiance to the new king. Each town also had a Young Men's Association composed of men who held no office. The Young Men swore no oath to the king. They could therefore demand his deposition and otherwise influence the decisions of the council. Kumasi and its ruler took ritual precedence over other towns and rulers: these swore an oath of allegiance to Kumasi which required them to accept Kumasi guidance in some policy matters, to cede to Kumasi the exclusive use of the death penalty, to provide troops for both offensive and defensive wars and to help finance the Kumasi government through the regular payment of tribute. During the nineteenth century, Kumasi used this tribute to finance a standing army, which it then used to establish greater control over the other towns. Even so, the Ashanti Confederacy remained a decentralized state. A high degree of local autonomy was vested in the various local councils, whose officials were not subject to appointment or dismissal by Kumasi. They were directly responsible to the people whom they ruled and represented. Kumasi could reach the people of other towns only through the official channel of their councils.

Other West African states had still other types of political institutions. All were associated with trade and permanent settlement and with populations dense by African standards. In the savannah country animal husbandry could be combined with agriculture, and farmers could till the same fields over long periods. Hence people remained attached to the fields of their fathers. Stability was also encouraged by the development of economic tree crops, already especially important in the forest zone. Here the cocoa tree had not yet arrived to tie people to the land, but the kola-nut and the palm-oil trade were already important. They served to stabilize settlement near stands of long-lived trees. Cash crops for export, a highly developed trading system, a relatively dense population and the development of towns and cities that could support a varied group of specialized crafts provided the stable base for the complex social and political institutions so characteristic of the region.

In this setting, titles and offices proliferated; rank and status flourished. The rulers of such states were no longer personal leaders, in close touch with their followers, existing on the same standard of living as their subjects, but remote beings, screened from common life by palace walls and by numerous servants and officials.

A few fertile areas apart, the soils elsewhere in sub-Saharan Africa favoured shifting cultivation with frequent changes of residence and a dispersal of population. Exceptions were found in the interlacustrine region bordering on Lake Victoria with its rich volcanic soils and banana plantations, and in the flood plain of the upper Zambezi, where soil fertility was renewed by the annual flood. Both regions were occupied by states of some stability and elaboration, those of the Ganda and the Lozi, respectively.

Elsewhere kingdoms and principalities might arise whenever an able adventurer, royal or commoner, was able to attach people to his interests; but such states tended to be short-lived. Especially in places where ecological conditions prevented large numbers of people from dwelling permanently in any one area, difficulties of communication encouraged local interests and loyalties. These in turn led to the break-up of kingdoms whenever a ruler was weak or when other circumstances led to the lessening of the central power. Such states seldom built up more than an embryonic administrative structure, perhaps because the lack of revenue made it impossible to reward officials. Trade tended to be sporadic and less profitable than in West Africa, though everywhere rulers tried to control trade as a source of revenue and to enhance their own authority. The scanty tribute in labour and in kind reaching the court reflected the general poverty of the country. Rulers could not support an elaborate court on the West African style; the wealth they did obtain was likely to be rapidly expended to provide hospitality and gifts to supporters. Kings were known by their liberality rather than by the splendour of their capitals.

Given a system of shifting cultivation and the general availability of land, rulers could rarely reward officials and followers by gifts of landed estates. In most of the continent, land was free, easily taken up and as easily abandoned. Landed estates attached to office, found in some of the West African states, seem to have been created only in the Ganda and Lozi kingdoms where special conditions encouraged generations of men to cultivate the same land. Where livestock flourished, supporters could be rewarded with gifts or loans of herds; in effect, estates in cattle supported the state officials. For the most part, officials received their reward by recognition as territorial rulers with the right to receive allegiance and tribute from a body of followers. This discouraged the development of specialized functions.[1]

In the south kings customarily recognized local hereditary rulers as territorial officers through whom they administered their dependencies outside the capital. At the same time, they sought to identify the local lords with the interests of the royal house through political marriages. Central African monarchs more commonly appointed royal princes or princesses as territorial rulers. But territorial magnates of whatever kind were liable to assert their power against the distant king. Indeed, royal princes who saw no legitimate chance of succession to the throne were only too ready to declare themselves independent on the death of the ruler who had appointed them.

At best it was difficult for the central government to extract more than a token allegiance from those who lived at a distance from the court. Boundaries between political units were fluid; some regions, in fact, gave nominal allegiance to two distant courts.

On the other hand, the court was not tied to a permanent capital city as was usually the case in West Africa, where the investment in labour and materials made shifting the site of authority a serious matter. Permanent towns existed only on the East African coast, though ancient towns had existed in Ethiopia and probably in Rhodesia. Even royal villages moved periodically as soil became exhausted or buildings deteriorated or as bad fortune indicated that the old site had lost its virtue.[2] A ruler might also disperse his wives and children through a

---

[1] Elizabeth Colson, 'The role of bureaucratic norms in African political structures', in American Ethnological Society, *Systems of political control and bureaucracy in human societies: proceedings of the 1958 annual spring meeting of the American Ethnology Society*, Verne F. Ray, ed. (Seattle, 1958), pp. 42–9.

[2] See Peter Gutkind, 'Note on the Kibuga of Buganda', *Uganda Journal*, 1960, 24, 29–32, for the movable capital of the Ganda; Max Gluckman, *Politics, law and ritual in tribal society* (Oxford, 1965), for the same phenomenon among the Lozi.

number of royal villages among which he and his personal retinue moved. This brought him into at least intermittent contact with different parts of the kingdom and may have slowed its disintegration. The court provided a training centre in manners and government for youths sent in from outlying areas. While at court they were hostages for the good behaviour of their own people. Once more at home and they became emissaries of the court who spread its values.

Continuity in these states, as in the more highly developed kingdoms of West Africa, was achieved by vesting the kingship in royal lineages sometimes held to be of divine descent. On the death or deposition of a king, his successor was chosen from among the eligible princes. Occasionally the matter was referred to what the people held to be the will of the gods. Nyoro and Nkole princes in two of the interlacustrine states were expected to enlist a following and to fight for the throne. The victor was installed as king while his rival brothers were killed to prevent further threat to his reign. In other kingdoms a succession council chose the most suitable of the candidates, guided by various criteria. Eligible Lozi princes had to be sons of a king born after his accession. Swazi princes were eligible only if they were the eldest sons of a wife chosen for the king by the state council. It was common practice not to designate a specific heir during the life of a ruler lest the crown prince usurp power or form the centre of a rival party.

Where a succession council was recognized, it usually included one or more senior women of the royal lineage, perhaps a widow of the dead king, various priest officials, and the more important secular officers of the state. The chief minister of the dead king was almost always a member. He was a commoner appointed by the king and could not himself be a candidate for kingship. He served as regent during the interregnum and presided over the installation of the new king. Having ensured the continuity of rule, he was then expected to retire, perhaps to become a priest at the shrine associated with his dead master. Whatever the system of selection, succession to the throne was not automatic but depended upon popular support in some form. Unpopular princes could be and were bypassed.[1]

Every ruler, therefore, was selected from among many princes; but the rituals of installation set him apart both from his subjects and from

[1] See Audrey I. Richards, 'Social mechanisms of the transfer of political rights in some African tribes', Royal Anthropological Institute, *Journal*, 1960, **90**, 175–90, for a general discussion of the problem.

other members of the royal line, making him as well as his office unique. In a few states, the new monarch acquired the divine essence of kingship by partaking of a portion of the body of his predecessor. Such a ruler could be deposed only by death from natural causes, or from assassination or execution; for only upon his death could the divine essence be handed on to legitimate a successor. In most kingdoms, royal power was defined in different terms which allowed the people to depose and exile an unpopular ruler. A new king merely took powerful medicines which gave him the strength to withstand the envy and magic of malevolent subjects, rivals within the royal lineage, or foreign potentates. Most kings by definition were the great magicians in their domains, having been given the secrets of the most potent medicines on their installation. In addition, they were regarded as the chosen representatives of the royal ancestors and thus their intermediaries with living men. A king's medicines and his favour with unseen powers were to be used for the benefit of the people, but it was expected that a bad king or one angered by ingratitude or neglect might turn his power against them. Checks upon a king's authority usually prevented his full exercise of the power implied by the rituals of installation. A monarch almost always had difficulty exerting control over outlying provinces. He could exercise full control only in his own immediate vicinity. Nevertheless, even here a variety of circumstances held tyranny in check. Very few rulers had the means to support a loyal standing army of any size which could be used against dissenters. Armaments were simple. The weapons of the people were as good as those wielded by the king's men, though imports of guns and gunpowder were already beginning to strengthen the king's hold over his subjects. Rebellions and secession were frequent enough so that every ruler had to consider them as a possibility if he became unpopular.

Breakaway movements were common even in West Africa and the few other favoured regions where men made material improvements upon the land. Elsewhere they formed part of the history of every state. The general level of technology encouraged frequent moves. Given provocation, subjects could migrate beyond the borders as well as within the boundaries of a kingdom. Malcontents either joined some pre-existing polity, or they rallied behind a leader of their own, a junior member of the royal line or a commoner who established a new dynasty by founding a new state.

In the central portion of any long-established state, arbitrary power was checked by the existence of one or more great offices whose incumbents shared power with the king, often through a separate hierarchy of minor officials. In a few places the division of power was so marked that observers spoke of a dual kingship. Frequently the person sharing rule was a royal woman, either sister or mother of the king, who was installed with him and continued to reign so long as he held power. The royal woman might or might not be a member of the advisory council, which customarily discussed important political decisions and also served as a judicial body to hear appeals to the king. The council was usually composed of secular officials, priests, heads of great lineages resident at the capital, and any other notables of the kingdom. At its head stood a commoner who served the king as chief adviser. Where the administration was highly developed, he became the prime minister in charge of government. Any ruler rash enough to act against the views of his council was likely to find himself at odds with his subjects and faced with imminent revolt. The smaller states of southern Africa usually had a further advisory body composed of all responsible men, who were expected to assemble at least once a year to show their allegiance to the ruler and to give him their counsel.

Rituals that underlined the king's unique position and his right to exercise authority also provided checks on despotism. Subjects usually held their king responsible for the prosperity of the realm. The king was expected to protect it against invasion and to ensure his subjects sufficient land for crops and pastures. He was also expected to prevent drought, plague, insect infestations and similar disasters. If catastrophe struck, it was the king who was held accountable. His subjects accused him of having angered the divinities by failure in his royal duties or of himself invoking the divinities or his own magical powers to show his anger. In either case, they called upon him to restore good health to the country by carrying out the sacred ceremonies appropriate to the situation. The elaborate ceremonies required the co-operation of the ritual experts of the kingdom. In most of the states, these same men carried out periodic rituals to ensure the well-being of the country. They were priests. They were also official representatives of powerful factions, lineages or territorial groups, who shared among themselves the secrets of rule. Each priest knew a different portion of the total ritual and might hold a particular piece of regalia required for its performance. He could only be replaced by another member of the body he represented to whom he had taught the secrets of his office.

When the priests stood together, they could hold the king in check; for if they refused to carry out their duties, they prevented him from giving ritual security to the nation. Since the king could neither replace them with his own appointees nor act without their help, he had to give way.

Pre-colonial Africa did know despots, such as Chaka the Zulu and Mwanga the Ganda. Kings could be cruel and arbitrary. But the greatest tyranny seems to have occurred either in newly formed states where the usual controls had not been introduced or in those few places where able rulers had subverted the old controls. Chaka was a military genius bent on creating an empire. In Buganda a series of forceful kings had managed to free themselves from most of the ritual controls that elsewhere characterized African monarchies. They secularized their own office. They also attacked the hereditary basis of other offices and obtained control over most appointments. But even they failed to secure absolute power.

In many regions, kingship was interpreted as of divine origin, though only rarely was the actual ruler regarded as divine. Effective exercise of kingship, however, rested upon the consent of the governed, which usually meant the general population. Permanent class distinctions were little developed outside the highly organized states of West Africa and in a few interlacustrine states. The economic base was too meagre, wealth too quickly dispersed, lineage organization with its emphasis upon the reciprocal obligations of kinship too pervasive, for political opposition to form on class lines in most areas. Opposition, if it existed at all, had a territorial or personal basis. Slavery, which existed almost everywhere, was mitigated by personal contacts between slave and master; and within a generation or two slaves were likely to become absorbed into the free population. Usually their descendants formed branches of the lineage of the old master. Slaves, or their descendants, thus acquired institutionalized kinship ties with others in the community at the same time that they acquired citizenship. The kingship, which symbolized government and nation, in effect represented the whole population, though it did not represent all aspects of life. Many functions assumed by modern governments either did not exist or were left to local communities, kinship groups, or individuals. The primary duty of the state was the maintenance of an overriding framework of order, but even this might be handled in different fashions.

The more centralized and elaborate systems of government had a

hierarchy of judicial courts attached to the different levels of administration. Some matters were reserved to the highest court at the capital.
More commonly local communities or kinship groups held the right
to adjudicate; the king and his officials intervened only when requested.
Much of the regulation of daily life was left to local or kinship groups,
which might have their own particular codes of conduct. Few African
states emphasized legislation. It was assumed that people could and
should live by the well-known rules of their ancestors. Change was
more likely to be introduced by administrative order, or by some
process of local consensus. Many important recurrent activities were
regulated by the ruler, who yearly performed the rituals that initiated
planting, harvesting, the movement of herds, game drives or the
opening of the fishing season. Detailed regulation of such pursuits, as
well as the regulation of an individual's access to local resources,
commonly fell to local groupings rather than to the state. If land was
regarded as a form of property, it was almost always a local or a
kinship group that held rights to a particular area. The king was lord of
the country, not owner of its surface. As lord, he almost invariably had
the right to call upon his people for tribute in kind and in labour. He
used the labour to cultivate the royal fields, to build the royal capital
and the headquarters of territorial officials, for porterage and for war.
In large, loosely structured states that lacked a highly developed
administrative hierarchy, a king usually could not maintain a monopoly
on warfare. Subordinate officials in distant regions felt free to attack the
surrounding people without permission from the ruler, and sometimes
in direct opposition to his policy.

Throughout the nineteenth century, as no doubt had happened
before, strong rulers apparently tried to increase their control over
their subjects and their subjects' possessions. This may well be related
to the attempts they made to regulate long-distance trade. As people
became more dependent upon imported goods, control of such trade
became a major policy objective. Rulers sought control also over local
products that could be exported. Ivory, gold and valuable skins were
common royal monopolies. As these goods became depleted in any
area, rulers tried to control other commodities produced by their
subjects or by their neighbours. West African states often claimed a
share in local mineral resources and sometimes seized the producing
areas. During the mid-nineteenth century the rulers of Katanga strove
to assert their right to the local copper mines, though previously anyone

who wished had been free to work the deposits. Despite the attempt at monopoly, free access continued to be the rule until Europeans seized the region.[1] The need for exports led other nineteenth-century rulers to engage in slave wars, while yet others became dealers in their own people.

NON-CENTRALIZED POLITICAL SYSTEMS. However greatly African states differed from one another, they shared in common the concept of office and a regard for centralized authority. In this respect they differed still more profoundly from the many communities that maintained a minimal political order based on other principles. Some organized themselves through the existence of associations that drew their membership from a larger population than the local community. Others used segmentary lineage systems to the same purpose. Finally there were large areas that depended upon an amorphous network of personal relationships for the ordering of public life. These communities had in common their refusal to concentrate authority in the hands of individuals holding political office; to this extent they may be said to have lacked governments though they possessed political structure.

Most East African communities, between the Swahili-speaking coast and the interlacustrine kingdoms, were organized into polities ruled through age-set associations. Both agriculturalists, such as the Kikuyu and the Arusha, and pastoral peoples, such as the Masai and the Suk, used age-sets to provide a minimal organization capable of providing for the adjudication of disputes between local districts, the performance of large-scale rituals, and the waging of wars. Some effective polities encompassed only a portion of a linguistic or cultural grouping; others included sections of several different ethnic groups. Pastoral Masai and agricultural Arusha in Tanzania, for example, shared a common system of age-sets and thereby organized themselves for some purposes into a common polity.

Such polities were based on territorial districts, or local communities, cross-cut by age-set associations, each of which was composed of men of about the same age who had been initiated during the same period. Each age-set had its name, insignia, songs and dances. Men were

[1] Lars Sundström, *The trade of Guinea* (Studia Ethnographica Upsaliensia, no. 24, Uppsala, 1965), pp. 127–8 (salt trade), 188–9 (iron), 217–22 (copper). Sundström comments (p. 218), 'Where there was little commercial gain involved in the exploitation, custom definitely forbade the chief to show any but the most cursory interest in the mines'.

expected to offer assistance and hospitality to their age-mates and were constrained to submit to their arbitration. Men spent much of their time with age-mates as in a common club. Refusal to join in the activities or to accept common decisions could result in ostracism, beatings, or the confiscation of property.

Those members residing in a district formed a local chapter, as it were, of the association. It was this chapter which in fact regulated most day-to-day activities. A chapter had its officers, usually chosen by the members at the time of initiation. They continued to lead their fellows as they matured and assumed new responsibilities. They organized age-set activities, heard disputes, represented their set in negotiations with other age-sets in the district. A man belonged primarily to his local chapter, but wherever he went he was free to join the local activities of his set and could expect to receive its protection. The system provided also a means of regulating formal behaviour between all males of the countryside. Every man owed respect to those of senior sets. Each had the right to expect respect and service from members of junior sets. At the bottom of the social hierarchy were the uninitiated boys.

East African societies with developed age-sets also recognized a series of ranks through which the age-sets were promoted as corporate groups: initiates, warriors, elders. The ranks may be regarded as collective offices: each had its particular role in public life which was performed by the members of the incumbent age-set. Elders had ritual power and the right to adjudicate in difficult matters. They formed the local council, which decided general policy. They negotiated with the elders of other districts and settled such vital matters as the timing of the transfer of ranks from one age-set to another. Warriors served as the executive arm of the elders. Younger warriors raided cattle and provided the most easily mobilized fighting force against foreign raiders. At fifteen- to twenty-year intervals, a series of great ceremonies transferred the ranks in turn to the junior sets which had been demanding new responsibilities. All members of a set moved forward together and thereby acquired the right to new privileges. The most senior set retired from the rank or office of senior elders and abandoned direct concern with public life, making way for the promotion of the other sets in turn. The promotion of the most junior set left room for the creation of a new set through the opening of a new initiation period. All youths who had begun to mature since the last initiation period were formed into a new set and began their slow progression as a corporate group through public life.

In these societies, no man could call himself a ruler; none had hereditary claim to rank or office. Age-set officers played a predominant role in the regulation of public life, but they did this as representatives of their set and under the surveillance of the set. Some men acquired personal followings because of wealth or ability, but they created no office. They simply had qualities which led their fellows to respect them beyond others who were regarded as belonging to the same rank. The emphasis was upon equality among age-mates, and upon the importance of good fellowship and mutual counsel.

Strong leadership did have one legitimate channel, but this existed outside the age-set system. On occasion, men who claimed personal inspiration from the divinities announced themselves as prophets. As divine representatives, they had the right to give orders. The Masai had hereditary prophets who spoke under inspiration. Early European visitors misinterpreted them as political rulers. Other East African communities relied upon the divinities to inspire men anew when it was necessary for a prophet to arise.[1]

Political communities organized by age-sets faced the European explorers only in eastern Africa. Elsewhere, if age-sets existed at all, they lacked political functions or were subordinated to other forms of control. In West Africa, secret societies dominated some of the small states, and also provided a degree of political order in a number of regions whose people recognized no central power. Here widespread secret associations used their local chapters to regulate the life of formally independent communities. They could co-ordinate activities to facilitate trade, settle disputes, and ensure a great many other results usually associated with specialized political institutions. The Poro Society organized activities through much of Sierra Leone and Liberia; Egbo facilitated trade and political alliances in the Niger Delta.

Such associations maintained minimal government in many regions. Less effective co-ordination existed where segmentary lineage systems provided the basis of organization, for these lacked permanent offices which could maintain continuity of action. Lineages are small corporate

[1] See Mair, *Primitive government*, pp. 78–106, for a general description of age-set systems. She calls them systems of diffused government. P. H. Gulliver, *Social control in an African society: a study of the Arusha, agricultural Masai of northern Tanganyika* (Boston University Press, 1963), is a fine study of social control at work in a contemporary society of this type (the Arusha).

groups composed of kinsmen who trace their relationship to one another through descent from a common ancestor, through either a line of men or a line of women. In Africa lineages commonly occur as a form of organization that may provide the nucleus for a small local community, control property in land or stock or title to office, or undertake a great many other services. In the absence of a strong centralized régime which could safeguard life and property, lineages often took responsibility for protecting their members and exacted retribution if members' rights were infringed upon by outsiders. A man was identified with other members of his lineage. The offence of one was the offence of all, and any member could be punished for the crimes of another.

Loose political organizations for offence and defence could be constructed on a lineage model. In much of the southern Sudan, northern Uganda, northern Kenya and Somalia, and again in central Nigeria, early European visitors found themselves dealing with political systems which have been termed 'segmentary lineages'. Large-scale political organization existed only in the form of short-term alliances between local groups which expressed their mutual relationships in terms of an ideology of kinship. They described themselves as bands of kinsmen joined together through a genealogy. The whole polity was seen as united through its common descent from some common founding ancestor, perhaps six to seven generations removed from the oldest living members of the society. At the same time, it was divided into smaller units which traced descent from various sons and grandsons of the founder. Each small local community, the only political unit continuously in existence, bore the name of some assumed ancestor who fitted into the general genealogy. Commonly the local community relied upon itself, quarrelled and settled its own affairs. In a dispute with outsiders, internal differences were forgotten. The community became one for purposes of defence or offence and sought allies among others with whom it claimed common descent. The momentary grouping that thus came into existence took the name of its putative common ancestor, and for the moment stressed its common identity. Once the emergency was over, the united front broke up into small communities prepared to quarrel among themselves and apt to emphasize differences in interests and in descent. Group identification was situational. A foreign power in contact with such a polity might well see it as a large united population with a single purpose and perhaps even with a single ruler. It might be all of these things when temporarily mobilized against an outsider. But there were no permanent leaders except on the local level, and even here power was usually personal rather than derived from any office. The man who one day spoke for a hundred thousand people might the next represent no more than a hundred, and receive from them no greater deference than any other man of his age and wealth.

Segmentary lineage systems thus provided a framework for warfare and raid, and for retaliation. But they had even less formal government or public policy than the systems organized through associations. Their political boundaries were transient, their political communities ephemeral. But both types of systems resembled states in having the rudiments for territorial organization. At any one time people probably knew who did and who did not belong to their body politic. This was not true in areas where political organization beyond the local community was completely amorphous. Here, personal networks existed, along which influence could operate, but there were no political units above the small local community. Societies with amorphous polities were widely scattered through Africa. The Tonga of Zambia, the LoDagaba of northern Ghana belonged to their number. The residents of each small local community, perhaps numbering five hundred persons, recognized that their interests overlapped with those of people in neighbouring communities to whom they were individually connected by kinship, clientship or bond friendship. Each ceremony, dispute or particular occasion was likely to mobilize a different group of participants drawn from the surrounding countryside. Ritual leaders usually had a sphere of influence rather than a fixed congregation.

Amorphous polities, like segmentary lineage polities, stressed the extremes of egalitarianism, a disregard for authority and an acceptance of only highly specific leadership. Rich men could use their resources to create influence, but great distinctions of wealth were absent. No organizational framework provided for the mobilization of manpower. Amorphous polities were therefore easily subdued by invaders. Once conquered, they were hard to rule. They bowed to force and did not easily legitimate it as authority. The Zambia Tonga at least made explicit their attitude towards claims to rule when they said, 'Anyone may call himself a ruler (*mwami*), but that does not mean that we will follow him'. Armed strangers moved easily through territory occupied by such people. But since no one could guarantee safe passage, white explorers were likely to regard the inhabitants as treacherous. Associational and segmentary lineage polities, on the other hand, were able to co-ordinate and mobilize large forces. They were known for their belligerent willingness to meet force with force. Warfare was a sport and a principal interest of young men. Travellers, who were fair game, usually tried to avoid such communities. In either victory or defeat, the large associational and segmentary polities tended to fall apart into their smallest constituent territories; but it was the segmentary systems which carried this to the extreme. Nevertheless, either form of social order had incipient structures through which organized large communities could be brought into existence when the need arose. Given the right circumstances, such systems had the minimal equipment for a shift in the direction of centralized government. The amorphous systems had not.

At least some of the people who had amorphous systems seem to represent the oldest settled populations of their regions. Their social systems may represent an early but tough and resilient form of organization which had been able to survive through all vicissitudes. Another explanation is equally possible. Their territories had usually been devastated during the nineteenth century by stronger neighbours or by invaders. It may be that the loosely structured network of relationships constituted an adaptation to the days of violence.

The non-political order

Whatever their form of political order, most African societies maintained continuity through certain basic institutions. These continued to function despite the fate of larger political units. Almost everywhere people belonged to corporate lineages based on either patrilineal or matrilineal descent. Kingdoms might rise and fall, but lineages or other kin groups continued to care for their members in illness and distress. They provided protection against enemies and a measure of internal discipline. Where overall political organization was weak, lineages might assume important political functions. Where central government waxed strong, lineages might continue as corporations controlling property rights in land, stock, or political and religious office.

In a few areas where the ruler had established his right to dispose of the available land and had assigned estates in reward for service, lineages might have disappeared or become attenuated. The Lozi of Zambia had landed estates and no lineages. The Ganda of Uganda put little stress on lineage membership, emphasizing rather the development of client relationships with political superiors from whom they received land and other favours. In most regions, if land could be divided into permanent holdings, it was usually held by lineages or local communities who based their claim on the right of first settlement or on a transfer from previous holders. The land-holding group, whether lineage or local community, allocated particular fields to its members, or loaned them to desirable strangers. It claimed the right to resume vacant land or land whose occupant refused to carry out his duties to the group. Transfer of land, except to other members of the community, was restricted by the rights of the group. Transfers had to be validated by the elders, or perhaps by all adult members. The only person who could freely dispose of his rights to the soil was the man who pioneered a new area of unoccupied waste. On his death, his rights passed to his heirs, who then formed a new land-holding corporation, usually also at the same time a new branch of the older lineage.

European adventurers and the later colonial governments sought to recognize the ruler of a region as the owner of its land and other resources. They then treated with him to obtain particular pieces of land they wished to exploit. In the early years, probably few subjects would have questioned a ruler's right to dispose of waste land. It was another matter if he attempted to sell land used by his subjects. The question became increasingly controversial in the years to come. Pre-colonial rulers, territorial officials and local communities often expected or demanded presents from strangers who sought to settle in their area or to use its resources. Such gifts were seen as an acknowledgement of sovereignty, a plea for protection, an expression of goodwill. It was not the purchase price or rent for land. In fact, most newcomers in the 1870s were given access to land as a matter of course simply as a result of their acceptance by a community. When a large group arrived in a kingdom, the ruler usually indicated an area with vacant land open to settlement where the newcomers would not impinge upon the rights of others. Where all land was in use, the ruler or senior official had to ask a previously settled community to share its resources with the newcomers. Single refugees or travellers joined an existing community which either allocated land to them or pointed out unclaimed land. Land rights were more rigidly defined in a few regions, especially in the densely settled areas of West Africa. Where population pressure, cash crops, or other factors encouraged a demand for land, people had begun to rent, mortgage and even sell land; but developments were channelled into characteristic patterns by the continued claims of lineages and other land-holding corporations.

Besides the lineage, many African societies gave importance to another grouping based on descent. This was the clan. Clan traditions frequently traced the institution to the beginnings of human history. Each clan had a name, sometimes derived from a natural species. Usually clans were exogamous and marriage with a fellow clansman was forbidden. Since clan members were dispersed over the countryside and sometimes across political and ethnic boundaries, corporate clan gatherings or other activities were rare. Nineteenth-century clans usually lacked clearly demarcated functions other than exogamy, though fellow clansmen often recognized they had the obligation to assist one another. This led early observers to argue that the clans were rapidly decaying vestiges of some earlier order. The continued existence of clan systems, with the same vague functions, during the following century suggests another interpretation as more appropriate. The very vagueness of its functions may have permitted the clan to become a symbol of important values. A clan system stood to the people as a recurrent reminder of the basic verities of their heritage and of their membership in some larger community. It symbolized the importance of descent, the obligations of kinship, the interdependence of kinship groups which had to rely upon one another for marriage partners. In a sense the clan could represent the common concerns of all men. The clan names, easily remembered, the clan slogans, dramatic to recite, served to place people in a wider social context and to remind them of their manifold responsibilities to one another.

Local communities, kinship groups, age associations, sometimes secret societies, helped to regulate social life and converted simple existence into something much richer. Additional associations based on occupational specialization and shared professional interests added still further diversity. In West Africa, craft guilds and trade associations were well organized and very much in evidence. They played a part in political and religious life, in production and exchange, in education and family life. In the towns and cities they might occupy their own quarters and choose officials through whom they governed themselves and dealt with the town authorities and the people at large. Endogamous castes of specialists had appeared in a few localities.[1]

[1] In some cases the origins of these castes may be traced back several centuries. [Eds.]

West Africa possessed also a system of regular markets controlled by market officials, where both local and imported goods were available. Most people frequented the market-place, either selling or buying and often both. Such markets, which made it possible for a man to buy his daily requirements from strangers, spread the idea of impersonal economic transactions. It is this emphasis upon trade and the market-place, and so upon the existence of specialized economic institutions, which most distinctively characterizes West Africa. It differentiates the region from other areas where people did not regularly meet for the exchange of goods. In such areas associations of hunters, or blacksmiths, or smelters were common enough. Traders organized in caravans for long-distant journeys and foreign trade. But these occupational groupings were of secondary importance. Local produce was exchanged through occasional acts of barter, or through the system of reciprocal obligations that tied together those of equal status, or through the political hierarchy which provided for the redistribution of tribute and other goods. Local economic exchanges were thus regulated by institutions which had other purposes and by an ethic which emphasized the maintenance of the long-term relationship between participants rather than immediate gain.

Economic activity was therefore strongly conditioned by religious beliefs which reflected the complex interweaving of multiple social relationships and pervaded most aspects of life. In general, African religions stressed the values placed on kinship, the significance of membership in local territorial communities, the legitimacy of any existing hierarchy of authority. They also recognized the moral significance of the primary economic activities upon which the society rested. In this they had no quarrel with Islam, nor with Christianity. The first had long since become the established religion over much of the savannah belt and in the coastal towns of eastern Africa. In the nineteenth century it was rapidly advancing, carried by Muslim traders and by the armies of Muslim rulers. Christianity lagged far behind, with few adherents beyond the coastal areas.

Both Islam and Christianity were opposed to other aspects of African religions. Most of these religions recognized the continued existence and importance of the spirits of the dead. The dead were supposed to participate in the community just as much as did the living. A person's influence as a spirit was held to be related to the role played during his lifetime. Those who had held political or ritual office supposedly still intervened in the communities or congregations subject to that office, as well as among their own kin. Those who had held no office were invoked only in the ancestral cults of their kin. The long series of funeral rites which dramatized the separation of the deceased person from the living also served to readmit him in his new status as a spirit. From then on he had the obligation of protecting and advancing the interests of those to whom he was attached. He could also be expected to punish those who neglected his memory or sinned against the rules of morality, particularly by ignoring the rights of his living representative.

Where agriculture was the basis of subsistence, or perhaps everywhere, men recognized their reliance upon the earth, to which they attributed mystical powers. The pervasive universal power of earth was invoked by living communities at local shrines which represented men's attachment to particular sites. Regular annual rituals celebrated the agricultural cycle. Occasional rituals dealt with emergencies. Shrine custodians represented the first settlers, who had converted an uninhabited waste into a community of living men. These custodians, usually drawn from lineages held to be descended from the earliest pioneers, were the well-known earth priests found throughout West Africa and in other areas where people stressed long-term occupation of the land. Conquerors or creators of new states customarily respected their priestly office, since this derived from the ancient dead.

In those states which had not fallen to Muslim rulers, the principle that gave ritual authority to the earth priests and also governed inheritance led to a proliferation of royal shrines dedicated to the spirits of dead rulers. The dead were identified with what they had created in life and were expected to exert control over the current use of that which they had brought into being: a state, office, property, descendants. A new régime quickly received spiritual legitimation with the death of its first ruler. Spirits of dead kings and princes supposedly still ruled over the realms they had created or governed, just as the first settlers continued their control over the earth they had brought into human use. Sometimes a hierarchy of shrines paralleled the political and territorial hierarchy. Shrines of kings were ritual centres for the kingdom; shrines of district rulers served the district; shrines of local headmen were effective within the village area. Officiants at the shrines were either the present incumbents of the founding office or hereditary priests descended from officials who had served the dead ruler. The dead also

figured in cults that stressed the importance of lineages and of kinship
in general, rather than the political order. Each lineage usually had its
ancestral cult; often it had a shrine or shrines for all its members.
Where lineages were most strongly organized for corporate action, the
right of appeal to the ancestors was usually monopolized by lineage
elders, who could use it to entrench their control over junior members.
Elders thus exerted strong ritual sanctions against rebels; so did the
ruler who controlled access to the royal dead. In any crisis of authority
the spirits were expected to support elders and rulers unless these were
blatantly at fault.

Principles of collective responsibility that applied in the relations
among the living were considered to hold good also for dealings
between the living and the dead. Men who roused the anger of the
spirits supposedly also involved their associates. An offender against the
earth and its spirit guardians could be blamed for general drought or
for the lightning bolt that struck some other member of the community.
Provocation to the royal spirits brought retaliation against king or
kingdom as well as against the original criminal. One who swore
falsely or who broke a ritual oath could cause the death of other
members of his lineage. To the spirits, the particular communities with
which they dealt were unities. This principle lay behind the common
dislike for experiment or for blatant disregard of existing custom.
Either course might be interpreted as sacrilege. This was the most
commonly recognized public offence because it might occasion general
disaster. Crimes against persons could be left to the discretion and adjudication of the victim's kin group.

African religions varied in the emphasis they gave to spirits who had
never been living men. East African religions were likely to give
greater attention to such spirits than to ancestors, possibly because
age-set systems so often overshadowed the importance of lineages and
kinship. Men joined in the worship of divinities or spirits who had not
originated within the kinship structure—ancient heroes, or perhaps a
single creator deity who ruled all men equally. Elders still controlled
access to the divinities, but they did this as representatives of the most
senior age-set, not because they belonged to the senior generation of a
lineage.

West Africa possessed both the most intricate social institutions and
the most complex religions of the sub-continent. In addition to cults
of the earth, of lineages and of the royal dead, West African religions

recognized gods who represented different aspects of nature or different human attributes. Men might associate themselves with the cult of some particular deity, attend its shrine and support its priesthood, in addition to participating in kinship and local rituals. Cult membership was open to any who wished to join, while priesthood was frequently a full-time profession requiring the novice to spend some years learning the complex rituals and myths associated with the divinity. Elsewhere only the Ganda had a similarly elaborated religion; and they too had a complex state and a developing economic system based on trade. The rest of Africa held to simpler doctrines. A creator god was known but little worshipped. Personified spirits other than the dead were few in number. Pantheons and professional priesthoods did not exist. However, almost everywhere, men believed in a universe full of impersonal power which they could learn to control to their own advantage. Here lay the realm of magic and medicine. Here also lay the common explanation for differences in fortune. Magic powers were sought for many purposes: to bring economic prosperity or political advancement, to afford protection against enemies, or to increase vital forces. They were invoked also for malicious use against enemies.

Probably no magic was regarded as completely innocuous. Men who claimed to have acquired magic only to bring personal advantage were still accused of injuring others. Some of the more powerful medicines, in fact, supposedly became effective only when vitalized by the spirit of a kinsman sacrificed for this purpose. Men who succeeded while their kinsmen or neighbours suffered were likely to be regarded as sorcerers or witches who sacrificed others for their own gain. Men who won political office or other favour in competition against their rivals were assumed to have used magical means. So long as their rule was fortunate, this was of no concern to their followers, who expected rulers and leaders to have strong medicine to protect their people from sorcerers and witches. Let a series of disasters strike, and the following was likely to vanish as its members put a safe distance between themselves and the now supposedly destructive magic of the ruler. Loss of power was also attributed to the loss of magic. Political and residential instability were common in Africa before 1870. Instability was encouraged by the short life of arable fields under existing cultivation methods, by the difficulties of creating permanent improvements, by the problems of maintaining effective communication. Recurrent natural disasters, wars, slave raids, frequent illnesses, and high mortality also played their part in speeding the splintering of communities; for they took place among people who attributed misfortune to human failures or human malice. The distribution of surpluses was encouraged by the insistence that the good man must share his advantages with his followers and fellows or be suspect of sorcery. At the same time, this insistence on sharing tended to discourage the development of marked inequalities among those joined by enduring social ties.

Beliefs in magic, sorcery and witchcraft existed also in West Africa, but their impact was different. Here men remained in long-term association on the land, tried to accumulate property, engaged in conspicuous consumption, and knew at least incipient class differences. Perhaps a different view of fate had also developed. Multiplicity of offices encouraged people to use initiative in seeking personal advantages through cultivating a series of patrons. The large number of gods and spirits encouraged worshippers to look among them too for possible patrons. The ambitious worshipper could enhance his chances by acquiring different patron spirits just as he could enhance his chances by pleasing various human patrons. He was no longer dependent upon the small world of kinsmen and ancestral spirits, of neighbours and the spirits of the earth. The number of possible explanations for variations in fortune increased, and men had less reason to blame their close associates for their failures. They may also have felt less hostility towards the institutions that channelled their lives, and thus have had less incentive to solve their immediate difficulties by flight or rebellion.

Whatever the explanation, most West Africans were already involved in complex stable societies before the scramble started. Other regions found it more difficult to pit their simpler institutions against the onslaught of the European invasion.

BIBLIOGRAPHY

Abraham, D. P. 'Ethno-history of the empire of Mutapa: problems and methods', in *The historian in tropical Africa: studies presented and discussed at the Fourth International African Seminar at The University of Dakar, Senegal, 1961*, Jan Vansina, R. Mauny and L. V. Thomas, eds. London, Oxford University Press, 1964.

Alagoa, Ebiegberi Joe. *The small brave city-state: a history of Nembe-Brass in the Niger Delta*. Madison, University of Wisconsin Press, and Ibadan University Press, 1964.

Arnot, Frederick. *Garenganze: or seven years' pioneer mission work in Central Africa*. London, 1889.

Barnes, J. A. *Politics in a changing society: a political history of the Fort Jameson Ngoni*. London, Oxford University Press, 1954.

Bascom, William R. 'The sociological role of the Yoruba cult-group', American Anthropological Association, *Memoirs*, no. 63, 1944 (issued also as **46**, no. 1, pt. 2, of *American Anthropologist*).

Beattie, J. 'Bunyoro: an African feudality?' *Journal of African History*, 1964, **5**, no. 1.

Bennett, Norman. *Studies in East African history*. Boston University Press, 1963.

Biobaku, S. O. *The Egba and their neighbours, 1842–1872*. Oxford, Clarendon Press, 1957.

Bohannan, Laura. 'Political aspects of Tiv social organisation', in *Tribes without rulers*, J. Middleton and D. Tait, eds. London, 1958.

Bohannan, Paul. 'The migration and expansion of the Tiv', *Africa*, 1954, **24**, no. 1.

Bohannan, Paul, and George Dalton, eds. *Markets in Africa*. Evanston, Northwestern University Press, 1962.

Bradbury, R. E. *The Benin kingdom and the Edo-speaking peoples of south-western Nigeria*. London, International African Institute, 1957.

Busia, K. *The position of the chief in the modern political system of Ashanti: a study of the influence of contemporary social changes on Ashanti political institutions*. London, Oxford University Press, 1951.

Codere, Helen. 'Power in Ruanda', *Anthropologica*, n.s., 1962, **4**, no. 1.

Colson, Elizabeth. *The Plateau Tonga of Northern Rhodesia: social and religious studies*. Manchester University Press, 1962.

  'The role of bureaucratic norms in African political structures', in American Ethnological Society, *Systems of political control and bureaucracy in human societies: proceedings of the 1958 annual spring meeting of the American Ethnological Society*, Verne F. Ray, ed. Seattle, 1958.

Cunnison, Ian. *The Luapula peoples of Northern Rhodesia*. Manchester University Press, 1959.

Delafosse, Maurice. *Negroes of Africa*, trans. from the French by F. Fligelman. Washington, D.C., 1931.

Dike, Kenneth O. *Trade and politics in the Niger Delta, 1830–1885: an introduction to the economic and political history of Nigeria*. Oxford, Clarendon Press, 1956.

Evans-Pritchard, E. E. *The Nuer: a description of the modes of livelihood and political institutions of a Nilotic people*. Oxford, Clarendon Press, 1940.

  'The organization of a Zande kingdom', *Cahiers d'Etudes Africaines*, 1960, **1**, no. 4.

Fage, John D. *An introduction to the history of West Africa.* Cambridge University Press, 1962.

Forde, Daryll. *African worlds: studies in the cosmological ideas and social values of African peoples.* London, Oxford University Press, 1954.

The Yoruba-speaking peoples of southwest Nigeria. London, International African Institute, 1951.

Fortes, Meyer. *The dynamics of clanship among the Tallensi: being the first part of an analysis of the social structure of a trans-Volta tribe.* London, Oxford University Press, 1945.

Fortes, Meyer, and E. E. Evans-Pritchard, eds. *African political systems.* London, Oxford University Press, 1940.

Gluckman, Max. *The ideas in Barotse jurisprudence.* New Haven, Yale University Press, 1965.

'The Lozi of Barotseland in northwestern Rhodesia', in *Seven tribes of British Central Africa*, Elizabeth Colson and Max Gluckman, eds. London, Oxford University Press, 1951.

Politics, law and ritual in tribal society. Oxford, 1965.

Goody, Jack. 'Feudalism in Africa?' *Journal of African History*, 1963, **4**, no. 1.

'Fields of social control among the LoDagaba', Royal Anthropological Institute, *Journal*, 1957, **87-8**, pt. 1.

Gray, Robert, and P. H. Gulliver, eds. *The family estate in Africa: studies in the role of property in family structure and lineage continuity.* Boston University Press, 1964.

Gulliver, P. H. *Social control in an African society: a study of the Arusha, agricultural Masai of northern Tanganyika.* Boston University Press, 1963.

Gutkind, Peter. 'Note on the Kibuga of Buganda', *Uganda Journal*, 1960, **24**.

Hanna, A. J. *The beginnings of Nyasaland and north-eastern Rhodesia, 1859-95.* Oxford, Clarendon Press, 1956.

Herskovits, Melville J. *Dahomey, an ancient West African kingdom.* New York, 1938.

Hinde, S. *The fall of the Congo Arabs.* London, 1897.

International African Seminar, 2nd, Lovanium University, Leopoldville, Congo, 1960. *African agrarian systems: studies presented and discussed at the Second International African Seminar, Lovanium University, Leopoldville, Jan. 1960*, Daniel Biebuyck, ed. London, Oxford University Press, 1963.

International African Seminar, 3rd, Salisbury, Southern Rhodesia, 1960. *African systems of thought: studies presented and discussed at the Third International African Seminar in Salisbury, Dec. 1960.* London, Oxford University Press, 1965.

International African Seminar, 4th, Dakar, Senegal, 1961. *The historian in tropical Africa: studies presented and discussed at the Fourth International African Seminar at the University of Dakar, Senegal, 1961*, Jan Vansina,

Raymond Mauny and L. V. Thomas, eds. London, Oxford University Press, 1964.

Jones, G. I. *The trading states of the Oil Rivers: a study of the political development in Eastern Nigeria*. London, Oxford University Press, 1963.

Kirk-Greene, A. H. *Adamawa past and present: an historical approach to the development of a Northern Cameroons province*. London, Oxford University Press, 1958.

Kuper, Hilda. *An African aristocracy: rank among the Swazi*. London, Oxford University Press, 1947.

Lebeuf, A. 'The role of women in the political organization of African society', in *Women of tropical Africa*, Denise Paulme, ed. Berkeley, University of California Press, 1963.

Liebenow, J. G. 'The Sukuma', in *East African chiefs*, Audrey I. Richards, ed. London, 1960.

Little, Kenneth. 'The political function of the Poro', *Africa*, 1965, **35**, no. 4.

Lloyd, Peter C. 'The political structure of African kingdoms: an exploratory method', in Conference on New Approaches in Social Anthropology, Jesus College, Cambridge, 1963, *Political systems and the distribution of power*. New York, 1965.

'Sacred kingship and government among the Yoruba', *Africa*, 1960, **30**, no. 3.

Lombard, Jacques. 'La vie politique dans une ancienne société de type féodal: les Bariba du Dahomey', *Cahiers d'Etudes Africaines*, 1960, **I**, no. 3.

Low, D. Anthony. 'The northern interior, 1840–1884', in *History of East Africa*, vol. 1, Roland Oliver and Gervase Mathew, eds. Oxford, Clarendon Press, 1963.

Mair, Lucy. 'Clientship in East Africa', *Cahiers d'Etudes Africaines*, 1961, **2**, no. 6.

Primitive government. Baltimore, 1962.

Marshall, Lorna, ' !Kung Bushman bands', *Africa*, 1960, **30**, no. 4.

Meek, C. K. *Law and authority in a Nigerian tribe: a study in indirect rule*. London, Oxford University Press, 1950.

Middleton, John, and David Tait, eds. *Tribes without rulers: studies in African segmentary systems*. London, 1958.

Middleton, John, and Edward Winters, eds. *Witchcraft and sorcery in East Africa*. London, 1963.

Mitchell, J. Clyde. *The Yao village: a study in the social structure of a Nyasaland tribe*. Manchester University Press, 1956.

Morton-Williams, Peter. 'The Yoruba Ogoono cult in Oyo', *Africa*, 1960, **30**, no. 4.

Nadel, S. F. *A black Byzantium: the kingdom of Nupe in Nigeria*. London, Oxford University Press, 1942.

Namier, Sir Lewis Bernstein. *Vanished supremacies: essays on European history*. New York, 1963.

Newbury, Colin W. *The western Slave Coast and its rulers: European trade and administration among the Yoruba and Adja-speaking peoples of south-western Nigeria, southern Dahomey and Togo*. Oxford, Clarendon Press, 1961.

Oliver, Roland, and John D. Fage. *A short history of Africa*. Harmondsworth, Middlesex and Baltimore, 1962.

Oliver, Roland, and Gervase Mathew, eds. *History of East Africa*, vol. I. Oxford, Clarendon Press, 1963.

Omer-Cooper, J. D. *The Zulu aftermath: a nineteenth-century revolution in Bantu Africa*. Evanston, Northwestern University Press, 1966.

Ottenberg, Simon. 'Ibo oracles and inter-group relations', *Southwestern Journal of Anthropology*, 1958, **14**, no. 3.

Paulme, Denise, ed. *Women of Tropical Africa*, trans. from the French by H. M. Wright. Berkeley, University of California Press, 1963.

Radcliffe-Brown, A. R., and Daryll Forde, eds. *African systems of kinship and marriage*. London, Oxford University Press, 1950.

Read, M. *The Ngoni of Nyasaland*. London, Oxford University Press, 1956.

Reclus, Elisée. *The earth and its inhabitants: the universal geography*. London, 1876–94. 19 vols. Africa-related volumes, edited by A. H. Keane, are X-XIII.

Richards, Audrey I. *Land, labour and diet in Northern Rhodesia: an economic study of the Bemba tribe*. London, Oxford University Press, 1939.

' Social mechanisms of the transfer of political rights in some African tribes', Royal Anthropological Institute, *Journal*, 1960, **90**.

ed. *East African chiefs*. London, Oxford University Press, 1960.

Schapera, I. *Government and politics in tribal societies*. London, 1956.

Skinner, Elliott P. *The Mossi of the Upper Volta: the political development of a Sudanese people*. Stanford University Press, 1964.

Smith, Alison. 'The southern section of the interior, 1840–1884', in *History of East Africa*, vol. I, Roland Oliver and Gervase Mathew, eds. Oxford, Clarendon Press, 1963.

Smith, M. G. *Government in Zazzau, 1800–1950*. London, Oxford University Press, 1960.

Southall, Aidan. *Alur society: a study in processes and types of dominations*. Cambridge, 1956.

Stenning, Derrick J. *Savannah nomads: a study of the Wodaabe, pastoral Fulani of Western Bornu Province, Northern Region, Nigeria*. London, Oxford University Press, 1959.

Sundström, Lars. *The trade of Guinea*. Studia Ethnographica Upsaliensia, no. 24. Uppsala, 1965.

Tordoff, William. 'The Ashanti confederacy', *Journal of African History*, 1962, **3**, no. 3.

Uchendu, Victor, *The Igbo of southeast Nigeria*. New York, 1965.

Vansina, Jan. 'A comparison of African kingdoms', *Africa*, 1962, **32**, no. 4.

    'L'état Kuba dans le cadre des institutions politiques africaines', *Zaïre* (Brussels), 1957, no. 5.

    'The foundation of the kingdom of Kasanje', *Journal of African History*, 1963, **4**, no. 3.

    'Long-distance trade-routes in Central Africa', *Journal of African History*, 1962, **3**, no. 3.

Wolfson, Freda. *Pageant of Ghana*. London, Oxford University Press, 1958.

CHAPTER 2

TRADE AND AUTHORITY IN WEST AFRICA FROM 1850 TO 1880

by COLIN W. NEWBURY

The development of trade plays a dominant role in the imperial phase of Africa. We must make a clear distinction at the outset, however, between two separate aspects of this phenomenon: first, the commercial relations between buyer and seller in the African market; and, secondly, the underlying causes of European expansion. Few would now accept the proposition once formulated by Allan McPhee that 'the Scramble for Africa was nothing more than a visible token of the demand which had been gradually arising in Europe for the products of Africa'.[1] On the other hand, his general account of the 'revolutionary' exchange of tropical produce and manufactures in the nineteenth century remains the starting-point for subsequent surveys of the West African economy. By and large, these surveys agree that European trade inland followed the flag. Why the flag was planted at all is still a subject for research and debate in which the complex variables of European and African politics rule out simple equations of the 'economic imperialism' type. It seems useful at this stage, therefore, to look afresh at the conditions of trade in West Africa in the decade immediately before partition to see how European entrepôts on the coast operated in relation to the interior as a whole. The aim is one of perspective rather than of polemic; and this essay begins in the market-place, on neutral ground.

Whatever the origins of markets in West Africa, it is clear from nineteenth-century sources that they were more numerous than in any other region, except in the Mediterranean littoral; and that they varied in scale from the 'regular concourse' of a few hundred traders to large emporia with specialized techniques of wholesaling and manufacturing. Evidence from explorers and from more recent studies suggests, too, that population, migration and ecological zones were important factors determining the distribution of markets, although no precise correlation between systems of exchange, ethnic groups and methods of

[1] Allan McPhee, *The economic revolution in British West Africa* (London, 1926), p. 21.

66

agriculture has, as yet, been worked out. Consequently, it is impossible to present a satisfactory typology of markets for the pre-colonial period without more information on the regional conditions that influenced many centuries of location and growth.

But, broadly speaking, West African markets had two main functions: to move consumer goods through exchange cycles between areas that were not self-sufficient in their economy; and, more particularly, to serve as bulking and wholesale centres for professional long-distance traders dealing in rarer and more valuable commodities. The large and spectacular markets of the savannah and the forest cities are well enough known. For most of the population the purpose of the myriad of smaller periodic locations was to supplement diets short in protein or salt, to purchase clothing and elementary artifacts and to save a modicum of capital to meet ceremonial expenses or to serve as a basis for further exchange.

In this respect, the terms 'savannah' and 'forest', 'subsistence' and 'surplus', 'wholesale' and 'retail' must be used with reservations in descriptions of the ways in which internal trade worked. With the possible exception of the kola trade, it is hard to discover 'border' markets consistently arranged along ecological latitudes in West Africa; and in any case trade routes were lateral as well as vertical.[1] It is difficult to think of any West African community which relied solely on subsistence crops and lacked the simplest surplus for gifts, tribute and trade.[2] Finally, long-distance 'wholesale' caravans—from Kano to Gonja, for example—were 'in themselves a moving market, buying and selling everywhere along the road' and broke bulk as easily as urban pedlars.[3]

More significant than these kinds of analytical contrast are the degrees of professional specialization that distinguish routine produce markets from the transport and sale of long-distance staples. At the lowest level, periodicity may well have been the necessary result of a relative lack of specialization among women farmers and food processors. From the highest level of long-range specialized trade, caravans filtered through to the principal periodic markets small quantities of luxury

---

[1] E. W. Bovill, 'Jega market', *African Affairs*, 1922, **22**, no. 84, pp. 50–60.

[2] Cf. McPhee, *Economic revolution*, p. 7: 'There was also the revolution in agriculture, whereby natives were going over from subsistence agriculture to exchange cultures.'

[3] Capt. Lonsdale, report on his mission to Kumasi, Salaga and Yendi, Oct. 1881–Feb. 1882, in Great Britain, *Parliamentary papers*, vol. XLVI, C. 3386, *Further correspondence regarding the affairs of the Gold Coast* (London, 1882), p. 72.

goods, salt and livestock. These markets, in turn, served as collection centres for palm-oil, kolas, cotton and other agricultural produce exported through long-distance trade. Yoruba markets in the 1850s, for example, offered many types of goods for sale, including:

Various kinds of meat, fowls, sheep, goats, dogs, rats, tortoises, eggs, fish, snails, yams, Indian corn, Guinea corn, sweet potatoes, sugar cane, ground peas, onions, pepper, various vegetables, palm nuts, oil, tree butter, seeds, fruit, fire-wood, cotton in the seed, spun cotton, domestic cloth, imported cloth, as calico, as shirting, velvets, etc., gunpowder, guns, flints, knives, swords, paper, raw silk, Turkeyred thread, beads, needles, ready made clothing, as trowsers, breeches, caps, shirts without sleeves, baskets, brooms.[1]

Important items are missing from the list, but the bulk of it would be common to most medium or small West African markets of which we have descriptions for the period. And at all of these, the specialized products—cloth, cattle, ivory, gold, slaves or salt—are only a small proportion of the consumer goods available for sale. Barth, who recorded in great detail the processes of long-distance trade, did not fail to notice the important grain and rice-trade of Bornu, or the intense speculation in millet at Agades, where the crop had replaced gold as 'the real standard of the market'; and later travellers confirm his picture of grain and cattle (not arms or slaves) as major staples passing between the Niger markets of Djenne, Sansanding and Timbuctu.[2] Everywhere the preoccupation with edible surplus formed the background for the passage of more exotic items of exchange. Both Baikie and Whitford singled out the slave and ivory market of Igbegbe at the Niger–Benue confluence for its grain, salt, beans, seeds, butter, oil, honey, livestock and country cloth.[3] Benjamin Anderson on his trip to

[1] T. J. Bowen, *Central Africa: adventures and missionary labours in several countries in the interior of Africa from 1849 to 1856* (London, 1857), p. 297.
[2] Henry Barth, *Travels and discoveries in North and Central Africa* (London, 1890), I, 179; and for similar observations on Kano, Timbuktu, Jega, Juka, Yola and Say, 175, 178, 369; II, 180, 355; for Salaga and the central Mande markets, see L. G. Binger, *Du Niger au Golfe de Guinée...1887–1889* (Paris, 1892), 2 vols.; and his valuable articles: 'Transactions, objets de commerce, monnaie des contrées d'entre le Niger et la Côte d'Or', Société de Géographie commerciale de Paris, *Bulletin*, 1889–90, 12, 77–90; 'Les routes commerciales du Soudan occidental', *La Gazette Géographique*, 1886, n.s., 12, no. 1, pp. 201–6; and 'Tombouctou', *Société Normande de Géographie*, 1879, I, 161–4 (report by a Moroccan Jew); Charles Monteil, *Une cité soudanaise: Djénné, métropole du delta central du Niger* (Paris, 1932), pp. 199–280.
[3] W. B. Baikie, *Narrative of an exploring voyage up the rivers Kwora and Bínue (commonly known as the Niger and Tsadda) in 1874* (London, 1856), p. 219; S. Whitford, *Trading life in west and central Africa* (Liverpool, 1877), p. 194.

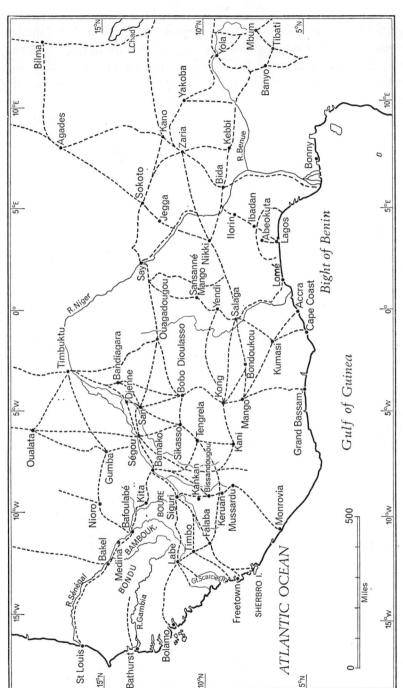

Fig. 2. Western Sudan trade routes.

Musadugu passed through four periodic markets in the Liberian interior, all full of women traders selling oil, rice, meat, root crops and fish, gradually infiltrated by Mandinka traders bringing cloth and cattle from the north.[1] At Musardu itself there was still further specialization in gold, horses, slaves, ostrich plumes, leather goods, together with the usual foodstuffs common from the savannah to the coast.

The general picture, then, of internal trade in the decades before partition is one of a complex series of produce markets the largest of which were connected by caravans bringing dietary supplements, cloth, arms and lesser items of European manufacture from the Mediterranean and Atlantic seaboards. The main trade routes, as shown in Fig. 2, lay along three major axes, each with subsidiary complexes between the Sahara and the coast.[2] The first—the Niger–Guinea route—was connected with Morocco through the entrepôts of Timbuctu, Gumba and Nioro on the edge of the desert. To the south a chain of markets stretched from the upper Niger, Bambuka and Bouré towards French posts on the Senegal and passed either through the Fouta Djallon and Sierra Leone to the coastal rivers or to the Diula markets along the kola belt to Kong. A second complex of central routes connected Timbuctu and Djenne through Bobo Dioulasso and Kong with the kola and gold markets of the Ivory Coast interior and Ashanti, linking the upper Niger, too, with the Mossi states and the entrepôt at Salaga. A third complex of Hausa–Benin–Delta trade routes joined up Bornu and Kano, at the end of the trans-Saharan roads, with trans-Niger trade through Borgou and Yoruba in the west and with Benue and Grassfields trade to the east. In addition, merchants travelled from Kumasi to Salaga and beyond, into what is now northern and north-western Nigeria.

To some extent these ancient links between markets were avenues for migration as well as for trade. From another point of view they were extensions of Mediterranean trade into the western Sudan. By the latter half of the nineteenth century both of these aspects of inter-regional communication were influenced by changing political conditions in the savannah and forest states and by the French occupation of Algeria, which split the long-distance routes to Morocco and the Turkish provinces of Tunisia and Tripoli.

---

[1] Narrative of a journey to Musardu, the capital of the Western Mandingoes (New York, 1870), pp. 44–79, 104–5.

[2] Binger, Du Niger, II, appendix; Great Britain, War Office, Intelligence Division, 'Western Sudan', no. 1290, 1897; Major A. M. Festing, 'Caravan routes from Sego-Sikoro, Timbo, etc. to Sierra Leone, W. Africa', 23 Nov. 1885 (Sierra Leone Archives).

Imported goods from the north were mainly fabrics and cotton stuffs, glass beads, perfumes, needles, cloves, paper, swords and mirrors, in exchange for indigo, ivory, gold dust, gums, hides, plumes and slaves.[1] The trading principals were Tripoli, Tuat and Ghadames Arabs, with a sprinkling of Moroccans and Moroccan Jews. Few settled south of Timbuctu. For in the savannah itself long-distance trade was very much in the hands of a variety of Mande-speaking groups, in the north and west, who commingled in the central markets with the Mossi and Hausa from the east. The Mandinka, Sarakole and Diula traders (or 'Wangarawa') were probably more widespread than the Hausa ('Marraba'), though the explorer L. G. Binger encountered two of these west of Kong in the late eighties; and there was a considerable colony of Hausa established as weavers and dyers at that Diula market itself.[2] The Sarakole of Kaarta and Ségou were to be found engaged in the salt, slave and gold trade along the Niger–Guinea routes. The Diula proper, as colonists of earlier Mande dispersal, were settled in islamized trading corporations in markets stretching from Djenne to Begho and from Kankan to Bondoukou and dominated the cattle, cloth and kola trade from the Guinea forests to the Niger bend. Mossi and Hausa traders played a similar role as brokers, carriers and principals between Timbuctu, Kintampo, Salaga and the Hausa states. Farther east, Hausa traders had by the seventies begun to probe south of the Benue into Bamum.

What was the value of internal trade? Much depended on the relative price of goods and units of currency in different areas through which the caravans passed. Although the export of gold dust from the Atlantic ports and across the Sahara declined in the nineteenth century, this commodity was still in widespread use as a staple of trade and as a unit of account. The gold standard was basic to many commercial operations in the western Sudan markets and was particularly valuable in a period when both the cowrie and the silver dollar were depreciating fast. Gold entered market operations direct from the alluvial deposits and mines of Bouré, Bambuka, Lobi and Ashanti in very small amounts and at a low price—less than 8 s. a 'heavy' *mithqal* of slightly over four grammes. It was sold at progressively higher prices for smaller *mithqal* in markets farther away from the source, roughly doubling in value

---

[1] See Mircher to the Duke de Malakoff, 23 Jan. 1862, F[12] 7211 (Paris, Archives Nationales), for the MSS. reports of a French expedition to Ghadames.
[2] Binger, *Du Niger*, I, 188, 294.

by the time it had reached Morocco or Tripoli.[1] Differences in value through the movement of gold over the long trade routes of the western Sudan gave commercial exchanges there much of their profit. Barth describes a Ghadamsi merchant who traded Kano cloth against salt at the Arawan market for a rate of 6 *turkedi* to 9 bars. The salt bars could then be sold at Sansanding on the Niger for 2 *mithqal* a bar— roughly six times the cost of a cloth *turkedi* at Kano. There was, of course, a considerable cost factor (transport, taxes, etc.) which reduced the gross profit to the extent of one-third of the salt bars on the passage through Macina to the gold market.[2] On the other hand, very little incentive was needed to attract brokers and carriers. In a hypothetical example of a salt and kola transaction between the markets of Kong, Kintampo and Bobo Dioulasso, Binger estimated that a Diula might make only about £8–9 gross profit for a journey of a hundred days.[3] At Sokoto, Barth noticed a 'mercantile speculation' in grain and live-stock brought only a short distance to the capital, where sheep sold for 300 cowries (6d.) profit, or 100 cowries (2d.), 'when on credit'.[4] Later examples of trading profit in the pre-colonial period concern the sale of Mossi cattle at Salaga for 10,000 kolas (£4) a head, which, in turn, were worth £20 back in Mossi markets; and, finally, there is the case of a Sarakole Diula from Kaarta who traded cloth, salt bars and gold between Bakel and Bouré for an estimated return of about £14 (gross) on an outlay of 12s. at the beginning of his tour.[5]

Other estimates of value are limited to the total trade of Kano and Kong. Barth reckoned Kano cloth production in 1851 at about 300 million cowries, or £25,000. The value of selected exports and imports —slaves, kolas, hides, sandals, natron, salt and European goods—he set at 588 million cowries (£49,000), making a total foreign trade

---

[1] For the decline and revival of gold exports on the Gold Coast, see David Kimble, *A political history of Ghana: the rise of Gold Coast nationalism* (Oxford, Clarendon Press, 1963), pp. 15–25; George Macdonall, 'Gold in West Africa', *African Affairs*, 1902, no. 4, pp. 416–28; Henri Labouret, 'L'or du Lobi', *Renseignements Coloniaux*, 1925, no. 3, pp. 69–73; Mircher to the Duke de Malakoff, 28 Jan. 1862, F12, 7211 (Paris, Archives Nationales); Binger, 'Transactions', pp. 77–90; Barth, *Travels*, II, 351.

[2] Barth, *Travels*, II, 353.

[3] *Du Niger*, I, 313.

[4] Barth, *Travels*, II, 180.

[5] Louis Tauxier, *Le noir du Yatenga: Nioniosses, Samos, Yarsés, Silmi-Mossis, Peuls* (Paris, 1917), pp. 220–1; R. Chudeau, 'Le grand commerce indigène de l'Afrique occidentale', Société de Géographie commerciale de Paris, *Bulletin*, 1910, 23, 398– 412; Paul Soleillet, *Voyage à Ségou, 1878–1879, rédigé d'après les notes et journaux de voyage de Soleillet par Gabriel Gravier* (Paris, 1887), pp. 222–3.

(excluding grain and livestock) of some £74,000 annually—a figure equal to about half the total foreign trade of Lagos in 1862.[1] In the late eighties Binger calculated that the small caravans bringing salt, iron ore and cloth from Bobo Dioulasso to Kong during a period of twenty days were worth £4,000 (Kong prices), or a total trade of £96,000 a year for this route alone.[2]

At this stage in the study of African economic history too much weight should not be placed upon illustrations of the value of internal trade advanced by Europeans at different places and times. Barth was an experienced observer, but he does not tell us how he arrived at his figures; and Binger was arguing a case for imperial expansion from the Ivory Coast. These examples merely serve to show that African organization of periodic markets and long-distance trade in the western sector of the continent was not a negligible factor in the West African economy as a whole. But given the immense distances and the slow means of transport, this internal trade does not seem to have produced a class of merchant princes. Barth did not find any men of great substance among the traders at Timbuctu—'the actual property of none of them exceeding probably 10,000 dollars [£2,000?], and even that being rather an exceptional case'.[3]

One of the side-effects of the limited scale of internal trade was the relatively low contribution made by tolls to the revenues of African government. For example, in 1863 the cost of transport on goods between Ghadames and Kano was about three times the transit duties paid at Agades, Tessaoua, Katsina and Kano—some 16,000 cowries (just over 16s.)—on cloth valued at £312 in the Kano market. The highest proportion of these tolls was levied at Agades, where there was also a heavy duty of 10 *mithqal* on every camel load. This seems to have been normal for a small entrepôt that had no agriculture. Larger markets such as Kano were more moderate in their tolls; and, in general, duties from trade were not of primary importance in the long list of emirate revenues. It must be remembered, too, that the collection of tolls and licences was often a specialized occupation of hereditary officials who paid over only a fraction of such revenues to a political superior.

Elsewhere in the savannah states taxes on crop lands and markets

[1] *Travels*, I, 303–9; A. Adu Boahen, *Britain, the Sahara and the Western Sudan, 1788–1841* (Oxford, Clarendon Press, 1964), p. 119.
[2] 'Transactions', p. 86.   [3] *Travels*, II, 356.

seem to have been commonplace but less detailed than in the Hausa states. Gallieni and Soleillet found the usual tithes and head taxes in Ségou. But, although the confederation of states left by El Hadj Omar to his sons lay across some of the busiest trade routes in the western Sudan, little was derived from direct imposts on goods or traders. At least one market was deliberately created by Sultan Ahmadu at Guigué in 1874 with the object of rivalling Nioro. But it was not a rich source of revenue compared with the gold-producing tributary of Bouré, which had once paid El Hadj Omar £3,600 a year. Tribute was the result of conquest, not of the administration of trade. In the Fouta Djallon, provincial chiefs and Almamys claimed regular amounts from coastal tribes to supplement revenue from war booty, inheritances and land tax. Caravan and trade duties do not figure at all. Among the Egba Yoruba, tolls were certainly levied on caravans passing through Abeokuta, though it is doubtful whether the *parakoyi* trade chiefs paid very much towards the Basorun's government in the 1860s; and they vigorously opposed an attempt to extend the fiscal system in 1867. In Yoruba, as in Hausa and Ségou, 'the basic ingredients of power were land and taxable peasants. Each state sought to win control over as many towns and villages as possible, and to tax them...to capture slaves in war who were valuable both for work on the farms and service in the ranks of the armies'.[1] In this scheme of things indirect taxes had little place.

On the coast, however, the trading states of Dahomey or the Niger Delta (also known as the Oil Rivers) would seem to provide better examples of African rulers supported by income from trade. Revenues in cash or in kind were derived from payments to brokers, from presents and from shipping charges based on the size of vessels or on their holding capacity in slaves and palm-oil. For Dahomey the royal income from duties and the sale of slaves at Ouidah (Whydah) in the late forties has been estimated at about £60,000 annually. With the expansion of the palm-oil trade, toll posts were set up on the main village paths, tonnage duties were raised and fixed sums were levied from licensed brokers, who were allowed a monopoly of supply to European exporters. In the Delta ports the traditional 'comey' which fell on palm-oil exports was supplemented by minor handling charges and a multitude of 'dashes' to all concerned. In both areas the king's

[1] J. F. A. Ajayi and Robert S. Smith, *Yoruba warfare in the nineteenth century* (Cambridge University Press, 1964), p. 125.

wealth was a fundamental (but not unique) source of political power. It is possible to suggest, however, that perhaps more of this wealth came from trading operations than from duties. Rulers such as Ja Ja of Opobo or Nana of Warri were astute merchants, rather than African bureaucrats milching traders. In Ashanti, too, it was not tolls on trade, but royal monopolies in the export of kolas and gold to the north and the import of 'gin, powder and lead bars' from the coast which provided some of the Asantehene's wealth.[1] The Emir of Nupe, who conquered Kakanda on the Niger to obtain free access to trade below Egga, obtained little or no fiscal benefit from the export or import of goods by this route. His kingdom was itself a great market, not a customs house.

Furthermore, it must be remembered that much of the accumulated wealth of West African states was disbursed in hospitality, ceremonial and rewards. In Ashanti, capital could not be accumulated with the Stool. The royal monopoly of ivory in the Bamenda Grassfields was used to extend the king's clientage relations by 'gift-exchanges or royal favours' (though some of it did enter into external trade through officials).[2] Much of the point of acquiring surplus was its effect in cementing social relations for political ends. Nowhere was indirect taxation highly enough developed to permit the gathering of revenue on the scale of the seaboard colonial states. Many polities, therefore, were significant in terms of area and political organization, but 'structurally weak' because their 'economic base was never strong enough to support a higher degree of centralization'.[3] With fuller investigation this statement about the Mossi kingdoms might perhaps be applied to Macina, Ségou, Fouta Djallon, the smaller Hausa emirates and the Yoruba states. In the meantime, it is safer to conclude that internal and external trade was for the most part less valuable to African rulers than land, crops, shares of inheritance, war booty and slaves.

Barriers to trade in West Africa, then, were not geographical nor fiscal, but human. McPhee's famous 'Jungle Forest', which is supposed to have constituted an impenetrable obstacle to intercourse between Europeans and 'the civilised peoples of the Savannah Country', did not stop Mandinka, Hausa, Susu and others trading to the coast.[4] A more

[1] R. S. Rattray, *Ashanti law and constitution* (Oxford, Clarendon Press, 1929), pp. 109–11.
[2] E. M. Chilver, 'Nineteenth century trade in the Bamenda Grassfields, Southern Cameroons', *Afrika und Übersee*, 1961, **45**, no. 4.
[3] Elliott P. Skinner, *The Mossi of the Upper Volta: the political development of a Sudanese people* (Stanford University Press, 1964), p. 125.
[4] McPhee, *Economic revolution*, p. 25.

important consideration than physical distance was the need to respect the political convention which required middlemen to purchase goods at stated places, rather than moving behind a market to its source of supply. For example, the traveller Winwood Reade noted in 1869 that Susu, Temne and Limba traders north-west of Sierra Leone were not allowed to pass through to markets on the upper Niger, but were 'compelled to stop at Falaba and buy their hides and Gold in the Town'.[1] On the great desert route from Morocco to the Niger there was a complete change of caravan ownership at Oualata (Walata), where a new set of traders took over to deal with buyers farther south. Such examples could be multiplied—from the Tuareg of Agades, who monopolized the Bilma salt trade, to the Moors of Senegal, who supplied gum, or from Brassmen on the lower Niger with a stake in palm-oil, to the Ijebu Yoruba, who prohibited access to markets north-east of Lagos. The King of Ijebu summed up the general rule: 'The Lagos people sell to the Jebus, and Jebus to their neighbour & the neighbour to the interior & vice versa to the Coast. This is the custom of whole countries in the interior and the Governor [of Lagos] must not interfere.'[2] In West Africa goods passed through many hands. The feeling that somehow Europeans were being denied 'freedom' to trade because of controlled markets was one of the most powerful springs of official policy after 1850.

There is no shortage of material on European speculations about the value of West African trade. But if one wishes to know the exact state of commercial operations on the coast at any particular time, major difficulties over evidence arise. It is easier to describe the aspirations of humanitarians or market-minded administrators, the minutiae of cowrie prices or the coming of the steamer, than to provide an accurate estimate of the commercial stake of France, Britain, Germany and the United States in West Africa. The tall columns of statistics from the Blue Books look less convincing when it is remembered that they are based on customs returns collected by notoriously unreliable departments only at official ports; that interior and transit trade in goods and livestock are mostly unrecorded; and, finally, that a variety of ways for calculating values makes comparisons hazardous. As a French consul at Freetown pointed out a century ago, in the local British official returns of trade:

[1] Reade to Kennedy, 20 June 1869, C.O. 267/301.
[2] In Kimberley, minute, 6 Aug. 1872, C.O. 147/23.

Import values are increased by about two-thirds of their real value and export products are given at the same prices as in the Sierra Leone market, which are about half the value adopted for the publication of our Customs records in France. Thus, for example, for groundnuts the value in the Blue Book is 20 centimes a kilogramme, valued at 40 centimes in the general table of French trade.[1]

Nevertheless, the attempt must be made. The returns of total external trade calculated here are useful as an indication of long-term trends, rather than as absolute indices of value.[2] They suggest that throughout the decades of the 'economic revolution' in the palm-oil and ground-nut trade there was an erratic upward progression in the value of exports between 1850 and 1880, as shown in Fig. 3, with two serious crises (partly related to political crises in Ashanti) in the early sixties and seventies. A conservative evaluation of the total trade of the British West African settlements together with United Kingdom trade with 'foreign' ports and the total trade of Senegal would indicate that the general rise was in the order of £3½ million to £8 million. In other words, between the fifties and the eighties the value of West Africa's import and export trade on the coast roughly doubled, assisted by the occupation of Lagos and the development of Senegal in the sixties, both of which offset a bad period for the Gold Coast. Thereafter, in the next decade Senegal trade seems to have declined slightly and levelled off, before rising again after railway investments in the early eighties. In the same decade United Kingdom trade with areas outside the

[1] Braouezec to Ministry of Foreign Affairs, 16 April 1867, *Correspondance commerciale, Sierra Léone*, II (Ministère des Affaires Etrangères).
[2] Sources for the value of total trade are William Page, *Commerce and industry: a historical review of the economic conditions of the British Empire from the Peace of Paris in 1815 to the declaration of war in 1914*: vol. II, *Tables of statistics for the British Empire from 1815* (London, 1919), 108–9; Great Britain, *Parliamentary papers*, vol. LXXXIII, C. 4520, *Statistical abstract for the several colonial and other possessions of the United Kingdom in each year from 1870–1884* (London, 1884–5); Great Britain, *Parliamentary papers*, vol. XXIX, C. 941, *Return of revenue and expenditure and imports and exports of the British possessions in West Africa for twenty years: also, comparative statement of the trade of Great Britain with the British and non-British ports in Africa for twenty years* (London, 1874); *Sénégal et dépendances*, XIII, IX (Archives des Colonies); G. Hervet, *Le commerce extérieur de l'Afrique occidentale française* (Paris, 1911); Ernest Fallot, *Histoire de la colonie française du Sénégal* (Paris, 1884). All these require revision from unpublished returns in the P.R.O. Customs series, and with due regard for changes in values, measures and geographical origins. Page, in particular, must be used with caution. It is likely that there is some United Kingdom 'foreign' West African trade repeated in the total trade of Senegal. British values are declared or 'real' for U.K. imports and exports.

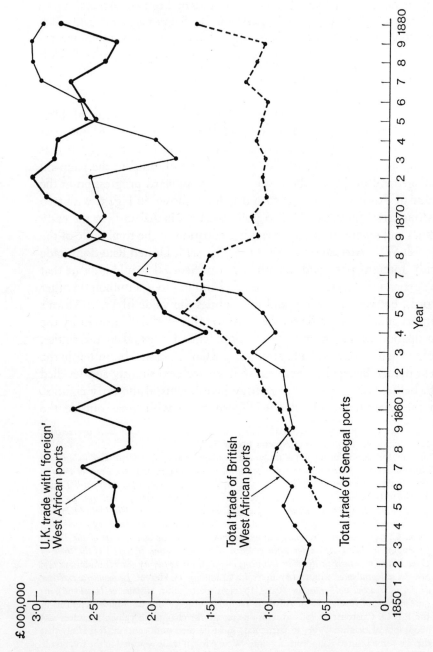

£ 000,000

3·0 —

2·5 —

2·0 —

1·5 —

1·0 —

0·5 —

0 —

U.K. trade with 'foreign' West African ports

Total trade of British West African ports

Total trade of Senegal ports

1850 1 2 3 4 5 6 7 8 9 1860 1 2 3 4 5 6 7 8 9 1870 1 2 3 4 5 6 7 8 9 1880

Year

Fig. 3. West African external trade, 1850–80.

settlements and the total trade of the settlements themselves increased by about £1 million.

A second feature of the pre-partition period is the general predominance of British trade and the relative importance of British relations with markets outside colonial control. In 1868 a French consul calculated that Britain and France shared about four-fifths of the total trade of the coast between them; and, of this, roughly two-thirds was with the United Kingdom.[1] The British share for different periods was as follows:

Total External Trade[2] (£ million)

	1853–62	1863–72	1873–82
Total trade of British West Africa	8·9	19·0	27·3
Great Britain's share of total trade with British West Africa	5·7 (64%)	10·7 (50%)	13·9 (50%)
Trade between Great Britain and other West African ports	25·8	26·2	20·1

Expressed as a percentage, the United Kingdom share with British possessions on the coast declined between the fifties and sixties to about half of their total trade, as German, French and American agents took advantage of the lack of restrictions at Bathurst, Freetown, Cape Coast and Lagos. This is confirmed by evidence of the strong position of American imports in British West African ports between 1840 and 1860.[3] British trade with other parts of the coast (though still much greater than Britain's stake in her own West African colonies) also declined. By contrast, France's trade was predominantly with Senegal, where her share of the total varied between 62 per cent and 76 per cent. For Americans or Germans not enough data are available to make a comparative estimate. If the statistics for the next decade of the eighties are examined, a considerable downturn in British West African trade is evident at the beginning of the scramble for the interior. In 1887 the value of total trade for British West Africa fell off to £2,477,000—the lowest figure for over a decade—as a result of a sharp decline in European palm-oil prices. Recovery from this period of depression may be

[1] Braouezec, 'La Côte occidentale d'Afrique & son commerce' (Memorandum, n.d. [1869?]), Correspondance commerciale, Sierra Léone (Ministère des Affaires Etrangères).
[2] Great Britain, Parliamentary papers, Return of revenue; Great Britain, Parliamentary papers, Statistical abstract.
[3] George Brooks, 'American legitimate trade with West Africa, 1789–1914' (Ph.D. thesis, Boston University, 1962), p. 243.

dated from 1891. At the same time there was a drop in the value of British trade with foreign (non-British) West African ports. This trade did not recover, but declined still further in the nineties, as British merchants were excluded from French and German areas and concentrated on British possessions—particularly the Niger Coast Protectorate.

On the face of these general observations, then, it would seem that British predominance was gradually being challenged in a variety of ways by other European competitors, at a period when palm-oil prices were in decline and the valuable, though smaller, ground-nut trade was very much in French hands.

Not all sectors of the coast were affected in the same way. The fall in European market prices was to some extent compensated by cheaper freight rates with the coming of regular shipping lines after 1852, though not all coast markets were points of call; and in the early eighties it was still easier to freight produce from Cotonou to Marseille by sail at 35 fr. a ton than from Lagos at 80 fr.[1] Local prices for palm-oil varied, too (as did the margin of profit) from £15 to £20 in the Delta to as low as £10 a ton on the Ivory Coast. The West African price for ground-nuts rose to 20 fr. a quintal in Senegal by 1867 (25 fr. in the Gambia), and then to 27 fr. by 1877, compared with Marseille prices, which rose from 35 fr. to 43 fr. over the same period.[2] With a slightly better profit margin, ground-nuts were less accessible, as yet, than palm-oil—a difference further increased by German exploitation of palm-kernels in the sixties. Both staples were subject to great fluctuation in supply arising from climatic factors and political unrest.

Much depended, too, on merchants' agents, on African brokers and on the thousands of middlemen, carriers and canoemen who lived off

[1] Dorat to the Ministry of Marine and Colonies, 6 Oct. 1884, *Gabon*, XIII/2 (Archives des Colonies). On the other hand, freight rates at Senegal ports were also as high as 80 fr. before the opening of Dakar as a steamer port in 1866. See Jacques Charpy, ed., *La fondation de Dakar* (Paris, 1958), p. 240.

[2] McPhee, *Economic revolution*, p. 33 n.; Paul Atger, *La France en Côte d'Ivoire de 1843 à 1893: cinquante ans d'hésitations politiques et commerciales* (University of Dakar, 1962), p. 50; Burton to Russell (private), 15 April 1864, F.O. 84/1221; H. L. Muller, *Le commerce du globe...* (Le Havre, 1865-[6]), p. 644 (wholesale and retail prices for Senegal); Marseille, Chambre de Commerce, *Compte-rendu de la situation commerciale et industrielle de la circonscription de Marseille pendant les années 1853-1888*, especially valuable for local palm-oil and ground-nut imports; Ministry of Agriculture and Commerce to Marseille Chamber of Commerce, 29 May 1860 (enclosing traders' reports from Bathurst, 31 Dec. 1859), Chamber of Commerce Archives, Marseille, Series *OK*.

the commercial operations of the shore factories and the hulks. Coast trade was still, in the years before partition, a mixture of cash sale and barter in which traditional currency and units of account—cowries, gold, dollars, manillas, bars, puncheons, cloths, etc.—were used along-side francs and copper coin. In the absence of large accumulations of capital on the part of the middlemen, the basis of trade nearly every-where was extended credit, or 'trust', by which European imports were marked up from 50 to 100 per cent of cost price and distributed against future supplies of produce. The risk of loss had to be balanced finely against appreciations of character and inability on the part of the exporters to contact interior markets directly. Inflated wholesale prices of imports were some insurance. But from the Senegal to the Niger Delta a great part of merchants' capital was tied up every year in the hands of an army of royal brokers, independent creole and African traders and fully or part-paid commission agents of African origin.

Thus, the price and credit structure of West African trade was a source of wonder and dismay. The sixty or so Mandinka, Wolof and Serer traders in the Medina and Bakel gum markets in the late seventies, for example, all had goods on credit from importers at St Louis. With these goods gum was purchased at 50–80 centimes a kilo; and a trader who left with £6,000 of cloth from St Louis might return with only £4,000 of produce. But the cloth he carried had been marked up by at least 100 per cent, leaving the importer with a gross profit of about £1,000 on this transaction. 'Thus is explained the inexplicable pheno-menon', commented a French observer, 'that the traders always have enormous debts with the firms which supply them, and yet, however, these firms continue to give them credit and make a fortune.'[1]

The scale of trust was very high. Gambia merchants stated in 1860 that the amount of credit given to the eight or ten agents of each firm in the river varied from £200 to £2,000, according to the reputation of the middleman concerned.[2] At the beginning of the trading season a firm might have as much as £16,000 'in trust' at marked-up prices. This figure may have been exceptional for the Gambia, but it was close enough to the case of New Calabar in 1856, when supercargoes claimed to have purchased palm-oil 'for $2\frac{1}{2}$ years in advance' by giving out

[1] Georges-Charles-Emile Colin, 'Le commerce sur le Haut Sénégal: conditions de son développement', Société de Géographie commerciale de Paris, *Bulletin*, 1882–3, 5, 165.
[2] Ministry of Agriculture and Commerce to Marseille Chamber of Commerce, 29 May 1860, Chamber of Commerce Archives, Marseille, Series *OK*.

trust on some 9,000 tons of the product, worth perhaps £18,000 at local prices. Condemned by consuls, naval officers and Foreign Office under-secretaries, the credit system flourished in the absence of banking institutions and in the presence of a produce export trade valued at nearly £1 million annually in the Oil Rivers alone.

At the same time as well-tried and archaic methods kept trade expanding, the 'race of native capitalists' demanded by the *African Times* in 1868 also grew in numbers, as more local agents entered the import trade. With their origins in the centuries of the slave trade, encouraged by philanthropy and commerce alike, the literate creoles, mulattoes and liberated Africans were important links between the Atlantic entrepôts and interior markets. Closer study of their role would be necessary to determine how much they benefited from the steamer lines or the commission houses and how they operated as middlemen and correspondents. Of their ability to amass small amounts of capital, to reinvest in property, and to found professional families there is already ample record.

The one branch of trade they found it difficult to enter, however, was the export of produce overseas; and even for those who wished to import European goods there were limitations. In Senegal, for example, by the end of the seventies, the 102 African gum traders and carriers were definitely excluded by European merchants and by administrative regulation from ordering goods on their own account, without paying prohibitive licences and leaving the list of approved middlemen. They protested when merchants from St Louis began to employ paid agents on a commission basis to undercut them in the river markets, and summed up the difficulty of hundreds of small African traders on the coast, where 'the struggle between the traders and the importer who has supplied his goods...must inevitably lead to a monopoly in the importer's favour'.[1]

In the rivers between Senegal and Sierra Leone, for the most part outside European administrative control, a series of working agreements between foreign and African factors recognized both the competition and the services of the latter group. From the Casamance to the Scarcies

[1] African traders to Brière de l'Isle (1878), *Sénégal*, XIII/31/b (Paris, Archives Nationales); Procès-verbal du conseil d'administration, 14 Oct. 1880; Brière de l'Isle to Ministry of Marine and Colonies, 23 Feb. 1880, 8 Nov. 1880; Genouille to Ministry of Marine and Colonies, 20 Dec. 1886, *Sénégal*, XIII/32; *Moniteur du Sénégal*, 24 Feb. 1885 (for closure of gum markets). The average export of gum from the river in the late seventies was about 2,500 tons a year, worth £120,000.

there were some 64 European agents together with 180 African traders operating in the early eighties.[1] The Europeans were employees of half a dozen firms; the Africans were mainly independent middlemen or small partnerships from Sierra Leone, importing on their own account. Many supplied direct to the European exporters, enjoying credit facilities in return. In the Gambia, too, by 1870, eight European and six British African houses worked through 200 African agents in the ground-nut trade below MacCarthy Island.[2] In and around Freetown, creoles began to expand into the interior markets, looking on the Sherbro hinterland, for example, as 'a kind of Australia' wide open to their enterprise.[3] By the seventies almost all of Sherbro trade was done by small literate African traders beyond the colonial boundary in competition with Temne suppliers.

For the African suppliers there were many ways of operating, according to the structure of local society. On the Ivory Coast, within a stretch of 150 miles there were at least three trading systems. At Assinie brokers dealing in gold and ivory were strictly controlled by the Sanwi kingdom of Krinjabo; at Grand Bassam the 'king' was one middleman among many; and on the Ebrié lagoon a dozen African brokers (Jack Jacks) had built up small dynasties of monopoly suppliers. In the seventies the firms of Verdier and Swanzy, which traded with this part of the coast, saw their own form of monopoly cut into at Grand Bassam by the 'esquires'—English-speaking Africans from Liberia, Sierra Leone and the Gold Coast—to the extent of losing to them one-fifth of the import and export trade. In southern Dahomey the king's brokers continued to regulate legitimate trade as they had the slave-trade, though there were signs by the late seventies that alternative sources of supply were building up at Porto Novo. At Lagos membership of particular ethnic groups, or even religious affiliations, were important criteria for determining sources of supply. In the Delta the trading corporations of canoe Houses held sway.

Colonial capitals were populated by similar immigrant communities. Lagos, which grew out of the ruins of a slave-market, or Dakar, which was founded to provide a wharf for Messageries Impériales, attracted traders and liberated slaves from the coast and the interior. The former

[1] 'Côtes occidentales d'Afrique. Etat nominatif des négociants commerçants et traitants établis dans les Rivières du Sud du Sénégal', 1886, Sénégal, XIII/II.
[2] British Jurisdiction in the River Gambia, 1876–1878, C.O. 879/13, Conf. Print no. 152.
[3] Christopher A. Fyfe, A history of Sierra Leone (London, Oxford University Press, 1962), pp. 400, 411.

port had a population of 50,000 by 1881, having nearly doubled in the previous twenty years. Dakar, with only about 7,000 by 1882 had rapidly overtaken Gorée, but remained much smaller than St Louis (15,000). At least one-third of the occupational structure of the population of Lagos Colony and Protectorate was devoted to commerce in all its forms, with a solid sub-stratum of agriculturalists and fishermen underneath and a small élite of twelve European firms and thirty African merchants on top. All depended for sources of supply on several thousand African traders who bought at lagoon markets and disposed of imported goods.

From the Senegal to the Niger, then, one may discern a 'traders' frontier' (in Professor Hancock's phrase) whose 'spontaneous advance' was the mainspring of British West African policy before Chamberlain. But it should be remembered, before this imaginary demarcation is accepted too readily, that the coastal and river markets interlocked with the network of suppliers who exported staples from deep in the palm-oil and ground-nut zones. And this network of internal traders included other economic complexes based on the exchange of cattle, kolas, grain, salt and cloth along the 'frontiers' of the savannah and the *sahel*.

The coastal trading markets, however, differed in at least one vital aspect from the periodic markets of the interior, namely, in the competition between European and African jurisdiction over the traders. In the mutually antagonistic methods of bringing sanctions to bear against thieves and debtors, in the struggle between the rough justice of the 'palm oil ruffians' and the attempt to extend the powers of colonial courts, in the sanctions of African boycott and European naval blockade lay a search for authority which transcended the search for trade.

By the seventies this quest for commercial security and political control of the coastal markets had produced a variety of solutions and compromises between Africans and Europeans. These ranged all the way from outright acceptance of controls enforced by African rulers to outright annexation and the introduction of alien laws. At one end of the scale were the European settlements, many the legacy of the slave-trade, a few founded and expanded slightly in the fifties and sixties, all increasingly expensive to administer, all in a state of armed truce with African neighbours. At the other end were long stretches and pockets of African independence, either too insignificant to attract attention, or too formidable in reputation to invite conquest. Gradually this broad distinction diminished as the informal controls of naval and consular supervision made many of the independent areas into satellite economic dependencies of the colonial capitals. By the late seventies the only substantial pieces of coast outside European control were from Bulama to Dubreka, Liberia to Grand Bassam, Lome Beach, Dahomey, Benin and the more powerful of the Oil Rivers states. Among the latter there were already considerable inroads into the authority of the rulers of Bonny and Calabar, partly because of structural change in their constitutions, and partly from the operation of consular jurisdiction and the courts of equity after 1872. More astute rulers might arise, such as Ja Ja, with whom traders had to come to terms. But the generality of Niger Delta chiefs (and eventually Ja Ja himself) were open to coercion. Even prudent diplomats farther from the sea, like King Gelele of Dahomey, laid in a store of future trouble by 'ceding' Cotonou and allowing it to be annexed in 1878. And where the most independent were compromised, the chiefs of lesser polities in the Popos or the Scarcies could not long survive the exercise of rival authority.

But, despite these incursions into the affairs of the coast, the internal political history of West Africa was little influenced by Europeans before the Ashanti war, 1873–4. It was only in lower Senegal, the Gambia, the Gold Coast or in southern Yoruba that colonial administrations were made aware that much of the disunity and civil unrest on their boundaries was evidence of greater historical disturbances well outside their control. French conflicts with Ma Ba in the Salum, the brief clash with the Tukulor, the seemingly inexplicable continuation of the Gambia 'Marabout' wars—all these were local eddies and currents of the Islamic groundswell of the late eighteenth and early nineteenth centuries. To the east, the discord in the Fon and Yoruba interior had resulted from the decline of Oyo hegemony about the same time. These themes are beyond the scope of this essay. But the more local manifestations of religious and political change were not always considered by governors to be beyond their power to guide and correct. For this reason there was a long tradition of diplomatic and exploring missions to the Niger, Timbo, Ashanti, Abomey, Abeokuta, Ibadan and Bida which had resulted in stipends for Temne and Mende chiefs, treaties ending the slave-trade and promising to keep open paths, and between 1863 and 1874 a few costly expeditions to Cayor, Salum and Kumasi. Such efforts were probably most successful in Senegal where a *modus vivendi* was reached with the Moors and the empire of El Hadj Omar, in Sierra Leone where the caravan traffic expanded fruitfully during the seventies, and on the Niger where excellent relations were established with the emirs of Nupe by Baikie and Crowther.[1] The benefits were less obvious in Ashanti; and they were nullified in Yorubaland by suspicion and hostility between the Egba and Lagos and the difficulty of communications with Ibadan during civil wars. In the name of trade, use was made of money, diplomacy and force according to the lights of officials on the spot and to the anxiety or indifference of their superiors at home.

With what results? The points of European penetration through the great complex of internal markets to the savannah were relatively few—the Senegal, as far as Medina, the Gambia to MacCarthy Island, the Salum to Kaolack, the lower Volta, and the Niger as far as Egga. The most promising and recent of these—the Niger—seemed slow to bring returns for the investment in men and money begun in the early fifties. Exports of produce below Lokoja, 1870–1, were valued at only £54,000—less than half a good year's exports in the Senegal gum-trade.[2] Attacks by enraged middlemen down-river and the complete loss of a trading steamer postponed the exploitation of this 'Channel in Central Africa', which had excited the imagination of religious societies and of the Foreign Office.[3] A pessimistic government commissioner summed up the Niger case:

What was originally 'exploration' became 'expedition', and 'expedition' shorn of its [fictitious?] importance, became 'trade'; and then, and then only, when tried by the vulgar test of facts and figures, it became apparent how exaggerated were the expectations that had been formed, and a natural disappointment ensued. Probably with the exception of the Arctic regions in no portion of the globe has the British Government and British enterprise devoted so much persistent energy, and expended so much life and treasure hitherto, to little advantage.[4]

Only ten years before the decade of the scramble this was a poor start. Yet trading activities on the river expanded rapidly after 1871 among five firms, each with a steam vessel plying some 200 miles inland

[1] For the expansion of Sierra Leone trade from about 3,000 to 10,000 caravans passing through to Freetown or Port Loko annually in the seventies, see Lawson to Rowe, 4 July 1878, C.O. 267/335; and C.O. 879/15, no. 175. A 'caravan' might be only one or two traders. For diplomacy with Nupe, see emir of Nupe to Granville, 22 Sep. 1871, F.O. 84/1351.
[2] Simpson to Granville, 21 Nov. 1871, F.O. 84/1351.
[3] Wylde, minute, 8 Jan. 1862, F.O. 97/434.
[4] Simpson to Granville, 21 Nov. 1871, F.O. 84/1351.

between the Delta and Lokoja. The reasons for this improvement are not fully understood. But one reason at least was the acceptance of the cost of protection by the British government, which sent expeditions to punish the Brassmen in 1877 and to bombard Onitsha in 1879. By then there were fourteen trading stations, six steamers and six launches on the river.[1] The export of produce for 1878 was valued at £309,700, or slightly more than the Senegal gum-trade, but less than half of Lagos exports for the same year. With the incorporation of the United African Company in 1879 and the consequent pooling of assets among the river firms, a new stage in the consolidation of British interests began. The trend was set firm towards monopoly, irksome to Brassmen and Delta supercargoes alike and a source of international discord in the early eighties. But however much Liverpool or foreign traders might complain, the initial expansion of the Niger trade was at the expense of the African carriers at Brass, whose chiefs petitioned in 1877 that European competition had ruined them by cutting their annual export of 5,000 tons of oil by some two-thirds.[2] One middleman's wall had been breached to the profit of other middlemen up-river. Brass languished and Nupe thrived as the traditional position of the kingdom as broker to the Hausa and forest markets was reinforced by new suppliers from the south.

The Niger is perhaps a special case (the bulk of palm-oil trade was still done in the Delta ports). Traders were often less anxious than officials to risk their capital in the interior in this way. With the exception of the ubiquitous Frenchman Bonnat none of the Gold Coast firms sent agents to Kumasi or Salaga or moved up the Volta in the late seventies, after the defeat of Ashanti. At Lagos they were kept firmly out of the Ogun or the Ondo trade routes. In the Casamance they did not venture beyond Sedhiou, in the Salum beyond Kaolack. And for Senegal, as a whole, the idea that St Louis was destined to replace Mogador as a port of entry to the Western Sudan was inspired by Faidherbe in 1863, not by Bordeaux.[3]

The role of the administration became even more decisive in the seventies. In Senegal official policy was responsible for the plan to establish 'free trade' in the gum markets by ending African traders' payments to the Moors in favour of stipends from an export duty at

[1] Hopkins to Foreign Office, 18 Nov. 1878, F.O. 84/1508.
[2] King Ockai and chiefs of Brass, petition, 21 Feb. 1877, F.O. 84/1498.
[3] *Moniteur du Sénégal*, 22 Sep. 1863, in Charpy, *Fondation*, p. 333.

4-2

St Louis. The river-trade was so disrupted by this that it came to a stop in 1886 and the old system of fixed *escales* was revived. Elsewhere, too, in French and British enclaves, there were new responsibilities for roads, ports, mineral concessions, the transfer of land rights, demonetization of silver dollars, as well as the accumulation of older problems concerning debt-collection, jurisdiction, the supply of foodstuffs, the adulteration of produce, all of which encouraged administrative interference in the working of the coastal markets. On the other hand, merchants and their pressure groups in the colonial capitals and at home were by no means unanimously insistent as yet for the acquisition of territory as an answer to complaints about trade with African states. For example, the minute books of the Bordeaux and Marseille chambers in the seventies and early eighties do not reveal any burning desire for expansion in Africa; and the record of specific grievances against French, British or Portuguese interference with French trade depended greatly on the interests at stake on the part of particular members of the chambers' governing councils, such as Cyprien Fabre, who became president of the Marseille chamber in 1881, or Marc Maurel at Bordeaux.[1] Similarly, Manchester, Liverpool and London merchants with a stake in the West African market were more anxious about competition with the United (National) African Company or the separation of Lagos from the Gold Coast than about new annexations inland. Their agents in the Delta maintained the traditional trading structure, as modified by their own conception of regulation and contract enforced on African middlemen by consuls and courts of equity. On the whole, they did not need to control a hinterland as well.

But there were other factors arising from colonial fiscal controls that kept alive fears of excessive competition among Europeans themselves and strengthened the position of the administrator as adviser on the limits of colonial rule. The expanded administrations of the sixties and seventies had to be paid for by metropolitan subsidies and taxes on trade. In Senegal subsidies dwindled and came to an end in 1874. In the British settlements, British merchants had traditionally looked askance at trade restrictions. During the first three decades of the nineteenth century, trade was liberalized; in 1834 a local enactment ended the remaining discriminatory tariffs and opened the British ports to foreign

[1] Bordeaux, Chambre de Commerce, *Extraits des procès-verbaux, lettres et mémoires de la Chambre de Commerce de Bordeaux* (1860–80), vols. 11–31; Marseille, series *MA*, *Délibérations de la Chambre de Commerce* (1871–86), vols. 66–84.

goods. Only Sierra Leone and Lagos retained both *ad valorem* and specific duties. The expanded administrations all required additional revenue. Financial ineptitude during Pope Hennessy's governorship of Sierra Leone and ambitious public work programmes at Lagos and the Gold Coast placed local treasuries in a similar dependence on customs. In addition, Sierra Leone and Lagos were forced to rely on the imperial government to an extent unforeseen a decade earlier. The Colonial Office disliked but tolerated Pope Hennessy's abolition of the *ad valorem* duties and other local imposts, which left only specific duties as the mainstay of the local budget. The Office fought successfully to retain a subsidy from the Treasury for steamers carrying African mail, and in 1873 Lord Kimberley secured for Lagos a loan of £20,000. Both French and British colonial governments had to raise additional duties to cover their administrative expenditure; both governments justified their policy to traders in similar terms, and the French Colonial Department indeed cited British precedents in support of its actions.

There were some differences, however, between the two fiscal systems on the coast. St Louis had *ad valorem* duties of 5 per cent on imports after 1872, like British ports. Gorée and Dakar remained free ports. Dependencies south of Dakar had only low duties on exports at the general level of 4 per cent *ad valorem*, and 2 per cent for the Melakori. In the seventies the Senegal administration began to have second thoughts about 'free trade'. Despite the removal of all discriminatory duties by the decree of 1864, which brought French African colonies into line with their neighbours, French traders never accepted that the Senegal was open to foreign trade. Surtaxes on foreign tonnage were levied at all French West African ports from 1868 to 1872 and again after 1880. A differential tariff was applied to imported foreign 'Guinea' cloths in 1877 to protect French India manufactures.[1] Small steps in themselves, they complemented the turn of the protectionist tide manifest in the revision of the French General Tariff in 1881. Indeed, the Senegal administration under L. A. E. G. Brière de l'Isle would have gone a good deal farther in 1877, when the governor submitted a draft project for high duties on all foreign imports.[2] Approved by both the Ministry for Marine and Colonies and by the Ministry for Agriculture and

---

[1] *Sénégal*, IX/22/c (administration of customs).

[2] Brière de l'Isle to Roussin, 2 April 1877, *Sénégal*, IX/21/b; Pothuau to Ministry of Agriculture and Commerce, 8 April 1878; Teisserène de Bort to Pothuau, 24 July 1878. According to this project a 15 per cent differential would have been raised against imports of British manufacture by specific duties.

Commerce, its implementation was delayed only by the necessity of providing Senegal with local representation in the form of a *conseil général*. The delay was long enough for the Bordeaux, Marseille and Manchester Chambers of Commerce to muster opposition. In 1880, in a series of local and metropolitan commissions, the tariff project was lost in general debate on Senegal customs. But the special duties on foreign Guinea cloths remained, after French Chambers of Commerce voted narrowly in favour of the 1877 decree. Le Havre and Marseille voted against the 1877 decree; Nantes and Rouen voted for a continuation of protection; Bordeaux was split in the Council of the Chamber of Commerce, and by one voice sided with the protectionists. The Senegal *conseil général* voted against the decree, but by its constitution it did not have a decisive voice in local administration of tariffs (unlike such councils in other French colonies).[1] By this time the whole concept of West African 'free trade' as it had evolved since the thirties had been dealt a blow. The impact of the French example in Senegal was increased, moreover, by monopoly of navigation in the Salum, Casamance and Melakori rivers and by high differential duties applied in the Congo after 1881.

For their part, French traders had much to complain about, too. High specific duties on wines and brandies at British ports and general import tariffs tended to operate differentially against major items of French manufacture and trade. This long-standing discontent with British customs was aggravated by extension of fiscal jurisdiction near Lagos in 1861 and at Bendu, Sherbro, Bulama, and the Iles de Los from 1873 to 1875, by the blockade of Dahomey in 1877, and by British claims to Matacong, the eastern Gold Coast and a strip of territory from Sierra Leone to the Melakori in 1879. Behind all these minor annoyances lay the fear of competition from British trade. Plans for the equalization of customs were refused by the Colonial Office.[2] The balance of commercial interests in the region of the coastal ports became the subject of diplomatic partition and national control; from the unratified Anglo-French Convention of 1882, through the Berlin Act to the Anglo-French Agreement of 1898, problems of 'free trade' and the fear of exclusion from West African markets provide a key to an understanding of the motives for the scramble.

[1] *Sénégal*, IX/27.
[2] Rowe to Hicks Beach, 14 July 1879, C.O. 879/15, Conf. Print no. 175; Hemming, minute, 17 Nov. 1879, C.O. 267/338.

The history of European trade with West Africa up till partition is a long series of attempts to encourage traditional methods of supply to meet new and changing demands. By contrast with East Africa, the lines of supply from the interior markets had existed for centuries and were ramified in complex patterns of internal trade in consumer goods. A number of these supply lines linked the western Sudan with North Africa, where the sale of a few staples expanded total trade in this direction during the sixties and seventies, even as new markets grew up on the Atlantic coast. In both areas of long-distance trade the choice of products for export was designed ultimately to meet European needs.

Consequently, the scale of such external trade depended greatly on market prices abroad—in particular for vegetable oils, ivory, timber and a little cotton and gold. Encouraged by the palm produce and ground-nut 'revolution', total West African trade grew in value after 1850, gradually encountering narrower margins of profit and increased competition for available supplies. In the sum of Europe's trade with Africa, it was less by 1880 than Cape Colony's $\pounds 12\frac{1}{2}$ million (a gap that was not to close), but more than Natal, or the $\pounds 2$ million total trade of Zanzibar.[1] For Europeans the stakes were not insignificant; and for Africans the structure of economic dependency was taking shape.

This process must not be exaggerated. The bulk of West African trade was still in the periodic markets and along the caravan routes of the forest and savannah zones, where foodstuffs and cloth were the staples of exchange. The cultivation of ground-nuts or the gathering of palm-kernels did not change the fundamental interdependence of pastoralists, grain-growers, fishermen and root-croppers. Indeed, in southern Togo a promising export of ground-nuts from the interior was halted in the eighties by the lagoon population, when it caused a decrease in their supplies of maize and yams.[2] Manchester prints and India guineas might work their way into the Niger and Senegal markets in the seventies, but cloth from Kano and Bida was still exported down-river to the coast; and the woven manufactures of Kaarta and Ségou were still needed to pay local tax. With slow communications and low purchasing power the West African interior was not wide open to European trade.

---

[1] Great Britain, *Parliamentary papers, Statistical Abstracts*; J. M. Gray, 'Zanzibar and the coastal belt, 1840–1884', in *History of East Africa*, vol. I, Roland Oliver and Gervase Mathew, eds. (Oxford, Clarendon Press, 1963), 241.

[2] Lieut. Martin, 'Commerce sur la côte de Guinée', 20 March 1872, *Sénégal*, XX, 8.

Failure to appreciate this situation encouraged undue optimism on the part of colonial administrations about the economic possibilities of political change. To some extent the substitution of European for African authority along the coast had worked to the advantage of the European merchant, though a closer examination of the conditions of trade revealed how much he was still dependent on African middlemen and markets outside colonial control. Diplomatic and military incursions into the interior were not conclusive in their results. As administrators were listened to more closely in the years of uncertain revenue from trade, however, the idea that there might be administrative solutions for the problems of supply gained ground.

Two main solutions were proposed: increased jurisdiction over the unclaimed portions of the coast and improved communications with the interior through the relays of middlemen 'blocking' the way. Fiscal jurisdiction, unfortunately, served only to exacerbate the latent international rivalry between Britain and France, whose protectionist policy in Senegal did not help either. Better communications up the Niger paved the way· to chartered company administration and a monopoly of grand design. Up the Senegal the projection of a railway beyond Medina to Kita and Bafoulabé in 1878 led inevitably to a political crisis in relations with the Tukulor, to confrontation with Samory and to a long series of military promenades in the western Sudan. It is, therefore, to the period 1871–80 we should look for the immediate causes of partition during the next two decades. These are to be found in Europe—more particularly in French plans for a public works programme to link North Africa and Senegal to the Niger and in the capital formation and policy of the National African Company. In Africa the causes stem from the trade and tariff policies of the Senegal administration and the Sierra Leone government, and from the increasing interference of the Gold Coast and Lagos administrations in the politics of interior states.

Once begun, however, partition did not proceed at a steady pace. There were many factors to be weighed in a decision about the Popos or Portuguese tariffs or the price of a protection treaty in the Cameroons. 'Rival' powers did not always feel particularly competitive during the opening manoeuvres. Lord Kimberley looked on the French Senegal–Niger railway scheme with favour, hoping the Gambia might be roused out of economic lethargy to profit, too. By 1880 official French interest in the lower Niger had become resigned to British hegemony on the right bank, and apart from a brief enthusiasm for a route through the Benue valley to Chad in 1883 desired only unrestricted access for trade. Neither the Colonial Office nor the Colonial Department of the Ministry of Marine fully appreciated, as yet, the impetus given to colonial expansion in West Africa by responsible administrators and irresponsible soldiers in the name of national commerce. In a real sense it was Brière de l'Isle at St Louis, not ministers at home, who set the pace in 1880 by rejecting for Senegal the economic liberalism favoured by France and Britain since the sixties.

In such a country the theory of free trade cannot be put into practice, and those who use it to have trade goods at low prices would certainly be the first to reject it, if it were proposed to extend it to the business of trading manufactured goods for natural products in Senegambia. At a time when France is trying to increase her volume of business with Senegal, to develop the resources of her colony and to create new outlets in the very center of Africa, it does not seem to me possible that all this effort should be made for the profit of foreign industry, while French industry would be in a way excluded from the Senegal market by a few Bordeaux firms.[1]

The French governor's reference to the safe position already won by Bordeaux in the gum markets—to the detriment of French as well as of foreign rivals—draws attention to a situation which is not dissimilar to the case of the Niger. Within the framework of protected national interests in any area of European authority there was room for considerable antagonism between rival firms, backed by influential corporations at home. Once administrative action had been taken to expand the market, these interests—at Lagos or on the Niger, at Dakar or in St Louis—could hardly remain indifferent to the form and extent of internal partition.

The last word in deciding expansion had never rested solely with the traders; and their voices in the early eighties were confused by internal debate about the desirability and ultimate cost of increased European control. A more sharply defined competition for authority in the African hinterland lay between rival administrations with inflated conceptions of the prospects offering for trade. While the traders hesitated, local colonial officials were never free from the urge 'to make their mark'. Brière de l'Isle in Senegal or Sir Samuel Rowe farther along the coast were the forerunners of Carter and Denton in southern Nigeria, Cardew in Sierra Leone, Griffith on the Gold Coast and

[1] Brière de l'Isle to Ministry of Marine and Colonies, 7 Jan. 1880, *Sénégal*, IX/27.

Macdonald on the Niger. We do not know enough about these men, their ambitions and their conception of their role in Africa. Although they worked in different contexts, they do seem to have held in common a belief that economic expansion was a consequence of a European *pax*; and that if they did not establish 'order and good government', other rivals would. They stood in the tradition of Beecroft, Glover and Faidherbe. How they persuaded or failed to persuade their superiors at home to accept their ideas is one of the themes of imperial history in West Africa and fundamental to an understanding of the partition of the eighties and nineties.

The most important aspect, then, of the interlocking coastal and interior markets that had expanded from the middle of the nineteenth century was the question of their control. By the end of the seventies, limited colonial enclaves and consular jurisdiction were no longer felt to be enough where relations with African rulers were concerned. And because these enclaves were vulnerable to disruptions of trade and increasingly expensive to run, the responsibility for improving the conditions of European trade was accepted by local officials in terms of increased customs posts and extended systems of river and rail communication. Indeed, it was precisely because the small European coastal territories set greater store by revenue from trade than did their African neighbours, that the rather facile argument concerning the need for markets to offset rising administrative costs gained support. Once this had been accepted, it followed that every coastal colony needed as large a hinterland as possible—at the expense of its neighbours. The political and international implications of this correlation of authority with trade occupied Africans and Europeans for the remainder of the century; and their decisions were to restructure the government and the economy of West Africa in the years to come.

BIBLIOGRAPHY

Ajayi, J. F. A. *Christian missions in Nigeria, 1841–1891: the making of a new élite.* London, 1965.

Ajayi, J. F. A., and Robert S. Smith. *Yoruba warfare in the nineteenth century.* Cambridge University Press, 1964.

Anderson, Benjamin. *Narrative of a journey to Musardu, the capital of the Western Mandingoes.* New York, 1870.

Atger, Paul. *La France en Côte d'Ivoire de 1843 à 1893: cinquante ans d'hésitations politiques et commerciales.* University of Dakar, 1962.

Baikie, W. B. *Narrative of an exploring voyage up the rivers Kwora and Bínue (commonly known as the Niger and Tsadda) in 1854.* London, 1856.

Baltzer, F. *Die Kolonialbahnen, mit besonderer Berücksichtigung Afrikas.* Berlin and Leipzig, 1916.

Barth, Henry. *Travels and discoveries in North and Central Africa.* 2 vols. London, 1890.

Bauer, P. T. *West African trade.* Cambridge University Press, 1954.

Bevin, H. J. 'The Gold Coast economy about 1880', Gold Coast and Togoland Historical Society (superseded by Historical Society of Ghana), *Transactions*, 1956, **2**, pt. 2.

Binger, L. G. *Du Niger au Golfe de Guinée par le pays de Kong et le Mossi, 1887–1889.* 2 vols. Paris, 1892.

'Les routes commerciales du Soudan occidentale', *La Gazette Géographique*, 1886, n.s. **12**, nos. 1–2.

'Tombouctou', *Société Normande de Géographie*, 1879, vol. **I**.

'Transactions, objets de commerce, monnaie des contrées d'entre le Niger et la Côte d'Or', Société de Géographie commerciale de Paris, *Bulletin*, 1889–90, **12**.

Biobaku, S. O. *The Egba and their neighbours, 1842–1872.* Oxford, Clarendon Press, 1957.

Boahen, A. Adu. *Britain, the Sahara and the Western Sudan, 1788–1861.* Oxford, Clarendon Press, 1964.

Bohannan, Paul, and George Dalton, eds. *Markets in Africa*, Evanston, Northwestern University Press, 1962.

Bovill, E. W. *The golden trade of the Moors.* London, Oxford University Press, 1958.

'Jega market', *African Affairs*, 1922, **22**, no. 84.

Bowen, T. J. *Central Africa: adventures and missionary labors in several countries in the interior of Africa from 1849 to 1956.* Charleston, S.C., 1857.

Brooks, George. 'American legitimate trade with West Africa, 1789–1914'. Ph.D. thesis, Boston University, 1962.

Buonfanti. 'Le Sahara et le Soudan occidental, relation de voyage de M. Buonfanti', Société Royale Belge de Géographie, *Bulletin*, 1884, **8**.

Charpy, Jacques, ed. *La fondation de Dakar (1845–1857–1869).* Paris, 1958.

Chilver, E. M. 'Nineteenth century trade in the Bamenda Grassfields, Southern Cameroons', *Afrika und Übersee*, 1961, **45**, no. 4.

Chudeau, R. 'Le grand commerce indigène de l'Afrique occidentale', Société de Géographie Commerciale de Paris, *Bulletin*, 1910, **32**.

Clough, S. B. *France: a history of national economics, 1789–1939.* New York, 1939.

Colin, Georges-Charles-Emile. 'Le commerce sur le Haut Sénégal: conditions de son développement', Société de Géographie commerciale de Paris, *Bulletin*, 1882–3, **5**.

Cox-George, N. A. *Finance and development in West Africa: the Sierra Leone experience*. London, 1961.

Croft, J. A. 'Exploration of the River Volta, West Africa', Royal Geographical Society, *Proceedings*, 1873–4, **18**.

Demougeot, Antoine M. J. *Notes sur l'organisation politique et administrative du Labé avant et depuis l'occupation française* (Mémoires de l'Institut Français d'Afrique Noire, no. 6). Paris, 1944.

Dike, Kenneth O. *Trade and politics in the Niger Delta, 1830–1885: an introduction to the economic and political history of Nigeria*. Oxford, Clarendon Press, 1956.

Duché de Bricourt, J. *L'évolution de la question douanière au Sénégal et dans ses anciennes dépendances (Guinée française, Côte d'Ivoire, Dahomey et dépendances)*. Paris, 1902.

Fallot, Ernest. *Histoire de la colonie française du Sénégal*. Paris, 1884.

Flint, John E. *Sir George Goldie and the making of Nigeria*. London, Oxford University Press, 1960.

Forde, Daryll. 'The cultural map of West Africa: successive adaptations to tropical forests and grasslands', New York Academy of Sciences, *Transactions*, April 1953, ser. 2, **15**, no. 6.

Frey, H. *Campagne dans le Haut Sénégal et dans le Haut Niger*. Paris, 1888.

Fyfe, Christopher A. *A History of Sierra Leone*. London, Oxford University Press, 1962.

Gallieni, J. S. *Mission d'exploration du Haut-Niger: voyage au Soudan français (Haut-Niger et pays du Ségou), 1879–1881*. Paris, 1885.

Gray, J. M. 'Zanzibar and the coast belt, 1840–1884', in *History of East Africa*, vol. I, Roland Oliver and Gervase Mathew, eds. Oxford, Clarendon Press, 1963.

Great Britain. *Parliamentary papers*. vol. XXIX, C.941. *Return of revenue and expenditure and imports and exports of the British possessions in West Africa for twenty years: also, comparative statement of the trade of Great Britain with the British and non-British ports in Africa for twenty years*. London, 1874.

Great Britain. *Parliamentary papers*. vol. XLVI, C.3386. *Further correspondence regarding the affairs of the Gold Coast*. London, 1882.

Great Britain. *Parliamentary papers*. vol. LXXXIII, C.4520. *Statistical abstract for the several colonial and other possessions of the United Kingdom in each year from 1870–1884*. London, 1884–5.

Great Britain. War Office. Intelligence Division. 'Western Sudan', no. 1290, 1897.

Hancock, Sir William Keith. *Survey of British Commonwealth affairs*. 2 vols. in 3. London, Oxford University Press, 1937–42.

Hargreaves, John D. *Prelude to the partition of West Africa*. London, 1963.

Hecquard, H. *Voyage sur la côte et dans l'intérieur de l'Afrique occidentale*. Paris, 1855.

Herskovits, Melville J., and Mitchell Harwitz, eds. *Economic transition in Africa*. London, 1964.

Hervet, G. *Commerce extérieur de l'Afrique occidentale française*. Paris, 1911.

Hieke, E. *G. L. Gaiser: Hamburg-Westafrika: 100 Jahre Handel mit Nigeria*. Hamburg, 1949.

Hill, Polly. 'Notes on traditional market authority and market periodicity in West Africa', *Journal of African History*, 1966, **7**, no. 2.

Hodder, B. W. 'Distribution of markets in Yorubaland', *Scottish Geographical Magazine*, 1865, **81**, no. 1.

Hopkins, A. G. 'An economic history of Lagos, 1880–1914.' Ph.D. thesis, University of London, 1964.

Jones, G. I. *The trading states of the Oil Rivers: a study of political development in Eastern Nigeria*. London, Oxford University Press, 1963.

Kimble, David. *A political history of Ghana: the rise of Gold Coast nationalism, 1850–1928*. Oxford, Clarendon Press, 1963.

Kopytoff, Jean Herskovits. *A preface to modern Nigeria: the 'Sierra Leonians' in Yoruba, 1830–1890*. Madison, University of Wisconsin Press, 1965.

Labouret, Henri. 'L'or du Lobi', *Renseignements Coloniaux* (supplement to the series of *L'Afrique Française*), 1925, no. 3.

Lambert, M. 'Voyage dans le Fouta-Djalon, exécuté d'après les ordres du Colonel Faidherbe, Gouverneur du Sénégal', *Le Tour du Monde*, 1861, **3**, no. 1.

Macdonnall, George. 'Gold in West Africa', *African Affairs*, 1902, no. 4.

McPhee, Allan, *The economic revolution in British West Africa*, London. 1926.

Mage, A. E. *Voyage dans le Soudan occidental (Sénégambie-Niger), 1863–1866*. Paris, 1868.

Marseille. Chambre de Commerce. *Compte-rendu de la situation commerciale et industrielle de la circonscription de Marseille pendant les années 1853–88*.

Mauny, R. 'Une route préhistorique à travers le Sahara', Institut Français d'Afrique Noire, *Bulletin*, 1947, **9**.

Meillassoux, Claude. *Anthropologie économique des Gouro de Côte d'Ivoire: de l'économie de subsistance à l'agriculture commerciale*. Paris, 1964.

Miège, Jean-Louis. *Le Maroc et l'Europe, 1830–1894*. 4 vols. Paris, Presses Universitaires de France, 1961–3.

Monteil, Charles. *Une cité soudanaise: Djénné, métropole du delta central du Niger*. Paris, 1932.

Morgan, W. B., and R. P. Moss. 'Savanna and forest in Western Nigeria', *Africa*, 1965, **35**, no. 3.

Muller, H. L. *Le commerce du globe: comptes de revient de marchandises échangées entre toutes les principales places de commerce du monde.* Le Havre, 1865–[6].

Nadel, S. F. *A black Byzantium: the kingdom of Nupe in Nigeria.* London, Oxford University Press, 1942.

Neumark, S. Daniel. *Foreign trade and economic development in Africa: a historical perspective.* Stanford, California, Food Research Institute, Stanford University, 1964.

Newbury, Colin W. 'The development of French policy on the Lower and Upper Niger, 1880–98', *Journal of Modern History*, March–Dec. 1959, **31**.

'North African and Western Sudan trade in the nineteenth century: a re-evaluation', *Journal of African History*, 1966, **7**, no. 2.

The western Slave Coast and its rulers: European trade and administration among the Yoruba and Adja-speaking peoples of south-western Nigeria, southern Dahomey and Togo. Oxford, Clarendon Press, 1961.

ed. *British policy towards West Africa: select documents, 1786–1874.* Oxford, Clarendon Press, 1965.

Oliver, Roland, and Gervase Mathew, eds. *History of East Africa*, vol. I. Oxford, Clarendon Press, 1963.

Page, William. *Commerce and industry: a historical review of the economic conditions of the British Empire from the Peace of Paris in 1815 to the declaration of war in 1914.* 2 vols. London, 1919.

Person, Yves. 'La jeunesse de Samori', *Revue Française d'Histoire d'Outre-Mer*, 1962, **49**, no. 175.

Polanyi, K., C. W. Arensberg and H. W. Pearson, eds. *Trade and market in the early empires: economies in history and theory.* Glencoe, Illinois, 1957.

Rattray, R. S. *Ashanti law and constitution.* Oxford, Clarendon Press, 1929.

Reader, D. H. 'A survey of categories of economic activities among the peoples of Africa', *Africa*, 1964, **34**, no. 1.

Redford, A. *Manchester merchants and foreign trade.* Manchester University Press, 1956.

Schnapper, Bernard, 'La fin du régime de l'exclusif: le commerce étranger dans les possessions françaises d'Afrique tropicale (1817–1870)', *Annales Africaines*, 1959.

La politique et le commerce français dans le Golfe de Guinée de 1838 à 1851. Paris, Ecole Pratique des Hautes Etudes, 1961.

Skinner, Elliott P. *The Mossi of the Upper Volta: the political development of a Sudanese people.* Stanford University Press, 1964.

'West African economic systems', in *Economic transition in Africa*, Melville J. Herskovits and Mitchell Harwitz, eds. London, 1964.

Smith, M. G. *Government in Zazzau, 1800–1950.* London, Oxford University Press, 1960.

Soleillet, Paul. *Voyage à Ségou, 1878–1879, rédigé d'après les notes et journaux de voyage de Soleillet par Gabriel Gravier.* Paris, 1887.

Tauxier, Louis. *Le noir du Yatenga: Mossis, Nioniossés, Samos, Yarsés, Silmi-Mossis, Peuls.* Paris, 1917.

Whitford, John. *Trading life in western and central Africa.* Liverpool, 1877.

Wilks, Ivor. *The northern factor in Ashanti history.* Accra, Institute of African Studies, University College of Ghana, 1951.

CHAPTER 3

REFLECTIONS ON IMPERIALISM AND THE SCRAMBLE FOR AFRICA

by L. H. GANN *and* PETER DUIGNAN

In the 1860s Karl Mauch, an adventurous German schoolmaster, discovered gold in Rhodesia. He described his finds in the most lyrical strains and made a profound impression in South Africa. The *Natal Witness*, to give but one example, burst into an article headed 'I speak of Africa and Golden Joys', and explained that the desire to prospect was perhaps part of God's great plan to replenish the earth. The editor, writing like Karl Marx turned company promoter, insisted that 'the power of the precious metal...has transcended the influence of all systems of morality, philosophy, jurisprudence, legislation or government ever known', and anticipated that new cities would spring forth in the wilderness at the yellow metal's magic touch. Biblical tales of Ophir, of King Solomon's supposed trading ventures in Central Africa and of his love for the fabulously wealthy Queen of Sheba added a touch of romance to the desire for riches; and some enthusiasts began to think of the Far Interior in terms as fantastic as those that had filled the minds of Spanish *conquistadores* in sixteenth-century America. The news reached England in 1868 and caused almost as much of a stir as in South Africa. The Central African gold deposits were described in newspapers, were discussed by learned societies, and were glowingly extolled by pamphleteers who used alluring titles such as 'To Ophir Direct'.

This interpretation might be called the 'tropical treasure house' theory of Africa. In Rhodesia, as in most other instances, it had little relation to reality. The white pioneers who trekked to Mashonaland in 1890 hoped to find a 'Second Rand' beyond the Limpopo. But there was little gold in Rhodesia, and few Rhodesian frontiersmen made money. The myth of Africa as a land of Cockaigne, however, was hard to dispel. The tropical treasure house theory received further support from erroneous assumptions concerning the fantastic fertility of Africa's tropical soils and verdant forests. Here again the planter's

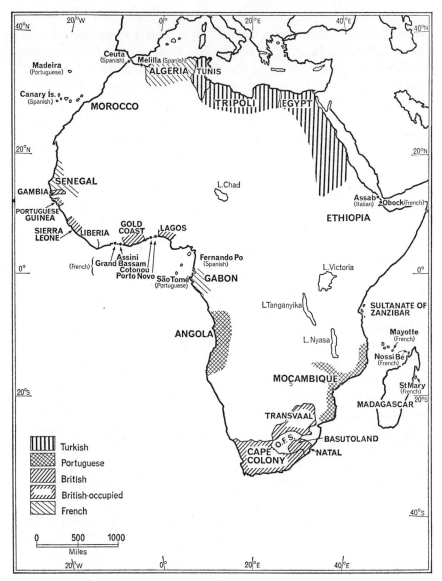

Fig. 4. Africa in 1879.

optimism fitted the facts no better than had the description of Rhodesia as an El Dorado. Europeans, like African farmers, had to contend with plant disease, floods, droughts and sickness, with poor communications; and high transport costs ate up the farmers' profits. Alien cash crops or imported pedigreed beasts might be struck down by strange sicknesses; pioneers moreover often had to cope with the unfamiliar properties of African soils. Many early white planters accordingly lost their capital, and plantation agriculture long remained a risky undertaking.

The myth of the tropical treasure house nevertheless made a deep impact on many political thinkers and statesmen of the Victorian era. Paul Leroy-Beaulieu, a noted French economist, deplored the reluctance of French investors to risk their savings in the colonies. Capital exports, he argued, would not only add to the world's wealth; they would also provide some kind of financial reinsurance, an argument designed to appeal to a nation that had not yet forgotten the disasters of 1871. Investments placed overseas would be immune from domestic upheavals, and were accordingly desirable from the national point of view as an emergency reserve. Leroy-Beaulieu accepted the views of John Stuart Mill, later elaborated for different purposes by critics of imperialism, that funds invested in the colonies would yield better returns than at home. Leroy-Beaulieu did not substantiate this essentially *a priori* contention, but insisted that French investors should show more daring and should lend their money in pursuit of *la grandeur nationale* as well as of profits.

Cecil Rhodes, one of the greatest imperialist-financiers of the nineteenth century, practised what Leroy-Beaulieu preached. Rhodes was firmly convinced that empire, investment and profits would go together; but he often had to use the strangest expedients to get his partners and stockholders to put more money into his chosen instrument in Rhodesia, the British South Africa Company, which from 1890 to 1923 never paid a single penny to its shareholders and was generally unprofitable.

The tropical treasure house theory was taken over later on by radical and socialist critics of imperialism, whose assumptions in some way exactly paralleled those of the most optimistic promoters of gold and other exotic shares. Financiers seeking capital for colonial investments argued that greater profits could be made in Europe's transmaritime possessions than at home; they felt convinced also that there was a good deal of idle capital in the metropolitan countries that ought to be mobilized for use overseas. European socialists soon began to employ similar arguments; but they drew very different conclusions from their premises. In 1898 Alexander Helphand, who was later to become a prominent revolutionary in Russia, published a pamphlet in which he attacked both German imperial expansion and naval armaments, and instead pleaded for an Anglo-German alliance abroad and social reforms at home. Helphand, writing under the pseudonym of 'Parvus', interpreted imperial expansion in terms of an under-consumptionist theory. Under the existing capitalist system the exploited masses in the metropolitan countries could consume only a small fraction of what they produced. The landlords and capitalists made exorbitant returns on their investments. But their vast surplus of capital could no longer be profitably used in the more developed countries. Financiers accordingly looked for investment opportunities in backward regions of the world where they employed their cash to build railways, sink mines and develop plantations. Capital exports allowed the capitalists to increase their gains overseas, but further impoverished the poor at home, and also led to increased armaments, wars of imperial conquests and a general world crisis. Capital should therefore be invested at home rather than abroad. The Europeans should get rid of the tariff shackles on international trade and should embark on a revolutionary policy of social reform. The contradictions of capitalism had developed to such a point that there were only two alternatives: either social reform and social revolution, or world crisis and social revolution.[1]

The South African War seemed to give further substance to what might be called the 'financial conspiracy' school. In the earliest stages of this war British public opinion was aroused by the Boer ultimatum and the disasters of the Black Week. But wartime chauvinism soon evaporated. The British moreover became increasingly preoccupied with social questions at home. There were strikes; there was syndicalist and suffragette agitation. The British had to contend with the intractable Irish issue that profoundly affected imperial policies in a wider sense. In addition, they faced German industrial competition and the growing German High Seas Fleet. There was a mood of disillusionment, and criticisms of social conditions at home easily blended with denunciations of imperialism abroad.

One of the most influential British writers in this tradition was John A. Hobson, whose theories of underconsumption foreshadowed

[1] 'Parvus' (pseud. of Alexander Helphand), *Marineforderungen, Kolonialpolitik und Arbeiterinteressen* (Dresden, 1898).

those of Keynes and shaped his thought on imperialism. Hobson, in his well-known book *Imperialism: a study* (1902) explained imperialism in terms comparable to those of Helphand. The scramble for Africa and similar forms of imperialism, according to Hobson, were occasioned by the superabundance of capital in the metropolitan countries looking for higher profits overseas. Foreign investment led to conquest. Empire led to wars that profited none but a privileged group of financiers who were abetted in their machinations by a great horde of political, military, ecclesiastical and literary hangers-on.

Ideas such as those of Hobson could be put to many different uses. Many German advocates of *Weltpolitik*, for instance, analysed Britain's world position in terms comparable to those adopted by Hobson. Foreign powers, headed by jealous Albion, had supposedly tried to prevent the emergence of a united Reich. By the time Germany had united, foreign powers had pre-empted the best parts of the world. England, the exploiter, the modern Carthage, was now slipping into wealthy decadence. Let the Reich assert its power and the German Eagle would prevail. One of the most convincing, urbane and learned critics of British imperialism was Gerhart von Schulze-Gaevernitz, a German university professor. Schulze-Gaevernitz made ample use of Hobson and of the writings of other British radicals and socialists. He argued that British industry was losing its lead. Industrial exports played a diminishing role in the British economy, compared to the island's home market. Britain was approaching the state of capitalist decadence. Having ceased to be the world's workshop and having become the world's banker instead, England had come to depend more and more on tribute from colonial and foreign borrowers. Modern British luxury styles and ease of living, even the art of William Morris with its insistence on quality goods, were but the fruits of this fundamental change.[1]

The concept of a decadent Carthaginian oligarchy that exploited the tropical treasures of the world profoundly affected right-wing as well as left-wing critics of British imperialism in Germany and elsewhere in Continental Europe. German scholarship created an equally powerful ideological tool in the concept of the 'proletarian people'. German nationalists were the first to claim this status for their own country. As Max Ferdinand Scheler, a German philosopher, put the matter in a

[1] See *Britischer Imperialismus und englischer Freihandel zu Beginn des zwanzigsten Jahrhunderts* (Leipzig, 1906).

wartime publication, 'the German worker nation, in a certain sense, is the same among the great nations as the proletariat is within each nation'.[1]

Theoreticians within the Marxist camp formulated their assumptions in similar terms. In 1910 Rudolf Hilferding, an 'Austro-Marxist' and later a German cabinet minister, thus produced a brilliant pioneer study of finance capital which analysed the cartelization of industry and the dominant role of the banks (a marked feature of the German though not so much of the British economy of his day). He agreed with Hobson that modern imperialism was the product of capital exports. He shared also Hobson's reformist view that the rich had a choice in the matter, that imperialism was not an absolute necessity for the continued existence of capitalism.[2] Hilferding's theory of imperialism was, in other words, a vehicle for publicizing the doctrines of reformist socialism, just as Hobson's interpretation accepted a consumptionist prescription for Britain's social ills.

Lenin later made extensive use of works published by scholars such as Hobson and Hilferding, but at the same time gave a revolutionary twist to their findings. Lenin's thesis is so well known that it requires but a brief and summary recapitulation. According to Lenin, technological and organizational developments inexorably transform competitive capitalism into monopoly capitalism. Production becomes concentrated in cartels and trusts. The banks steadily increase their influence over industry and form great financial combines which in turn control the governments. The capitalists pay their workers less than the workmen's labour is worth. The capitalists find that profits diminish at home and are therefore forced to invest their financial surplus abroad; for Lenin assumed, like all the other right- and left-wing advocates of the tropical treasure house theory, that lenders would secure greater returns in exotic countries in Africa and Asia than at home. Loans might be placed in 'semi-colonies' such as Egypt. But capitalists would normally make their greatest gains in territories subject to their direct political control. The need to export capital, to secure more raw materials and larger protected markets necessarily led to the 'new imperialism', of which the scramble for Africa formed but a part.

[1] *Die Ursachen des Deutschenhasses: eine national-pädagogische Erörterung* (Leipzig, 1917), p. 61.

[2] *Das Finanzkapital: eine Studie über die jüngste Entwicklung des Kapitalismus* (Vienna, 1910).

The system, however, could not last. Capitalism developed in an uneven fashion. The capitalist have-nots were bound to challenge the capitalist haves. Imperialist competition inevitably led to world wars; world wars in turn would lead to a revolutionary overthrow of the system. Lenin—unlike Hobson or Hilferding—believed that capitalism could not be reformed, that the capitalists had no choice in formulating their imperial policies, and that only the revolutionary class struggle could break the grim cycle of exploitation, empire and war.

Lenin's doctrine marked a major departure in the development of Marxist doctrine. Marx, with his nineteenth-century optimism and his Eurocentric orientation, had still believed that Western capitalists were as yet performing a progressive function in backward countries with feudal or tribal systems of government. He had looked with approval, therefore, upon the work of, say, British railway builders in India. Lenin now denied that capitalists could do any good in the colonies. Even railway building in the colonies had simply become an instrument of oppression; Lenin thereby cut Marx's doctrine of economic progress from its economic moorings. To Lenin the achievements of capitalist railway companies in providing employment, facilitating trade, relieving slave porters of their backbreaking burdens, had become irrelevant. He maintained at the same time that the system of bourgeois capitalism formed a cohesive whole that was ready for overthrow. Rebels in backward capitalist states need not therefore wait until the proletariat of the advanced countries had mounted the barricades. They should start sawing through the weakest link of the capitalist chain. Even in a peripheral empire such as Russia, a great revolutionary success might set off a series of explosions that would blow the world capitalist system sky-high. What mattered was the existence of a revolutionary situation and the ability of a disciplined communist party to mobilize and lead the masses. Lenin's doctrine thus led to a Copernican revaluation of Marxist thought; Western Europe no longer dominated the revolutionary state; the underdeveloped countries were allotted a crucial role.

Lenin's doctrine purported to explain also why the Western workers had not revolted earlier, and why they were fighting for their imperialist masters in the Great War. Imperialism, with its super profits, had enabled the capitalists to bribe some of their wage slaves and thereby split the workers' ranks. Some countries were distinctly more bourgeois than others. Lenin's views in this respect, therefore, bore some resemblance to Germanic concepts of bourgeois and proletarian nations, adding a vertical as well as a horizontal division to the international framework of revolution.

Lenin's famous *Imperialism; the highest stage of capitalism* (1917) was not a scholarly treatise but a tract for the times, designed to rouse the masses to action. Had the author failed to seize power, his book would probably be forgotten today. But he lived to become the greatest revolutionary leader of the twentieth century. His work on imperialism thus acquired a prestige that no academic monograph could match. His arguments came to dominate the debate on colonialism, whereas the contributions of other socialists such as Helphand, Rosa Luxemburg, Bukharin, Kautsky and others now gather dust in the back of political science library stacks. Yet applied to the scramble for Africa, Lenin's theses make but little sense. Economic pressure groups—as we shall see—did play an important part in the partition of Africa. But in the latter half of the nineteenth century Europe was not bursting at the seams with surplus funds seeking outlets in the Dark Continent. As many other writers have pointed out, the bulk of British exports before the First World War went to the Americas and to other regions of white settlement outside Africa. Britain's greatest individual borrower was the United States. German colonization in the Bismarckian era took place at a time when the Reich had relatively little capital to spare for overseas loans. The large-scale cartelization of German industry and the decisive role therein of big banking—which Lenin heavily emphasized—dates only from the beginning of the present century. German lenders who risked their money abroad preferred the Americas or adjacent countries in central and eastern Europe. French financiers were not particularly interested in their colonies; tropical Africa especially remained the neglected stepchild of the Paris Bourse. Leopold II of Belgium was a 'projector' of the eighteenth-century variety and had no banking capital behind him when he started his Congo project. Applied to Italian or Portuguese imperialism, the financial interpretation makes even less sense. Italy was chronically short of capital, whereas Portugal was a poverty-stricken country, and her imperialism was strictly of the uneconomic kind.

The Hobson–Lenin thesis moreover does not explain the exact *modus operandi* employed by the Stock Exchange lords in shaping the partition of Africa. Economic pressure groups did influence national policy. But statesmen also had many other lobbies to consider. The financial bourgeoisie was itself riddled by internal dissensions, and never acted with the cohesion of well-drilled party cadres. Imperialist-minded politicians were in fact more likely to manipulate the bankers than to be manipulated by them. Salisbury was not subservient to the firm of Rothschild. Bismarck did not act just to please the house of Bleichröder.

Lenin assumed also as a self-evident fact that direct political domination would enable the capitalists to maximize their profits. There is little historical evidence, however, for this assumption. The British South Africa Company exerted full administrative control over the two Rhodesias. But even Rhodes's concern, the most successful of the numerous chartered companies formed during the scramble, found the cost of administration an intolerable burden. The company's commercial representatives in Rhodesia became convinced that company rule, far from promoting the company's economic interests, in fact made their work more difficult, with the result that the chartered company soon became anxious to lay down the burden of government, provided it could secure an adequate return on the capital already invested.

The Hobson–Lenin doctrine, moreover, is obliged to postulate a caesura in the story of Europe's expansion in Africa. From about 1870 onwards, the 'imperialism of free trade' (as it has been subsequently styled in a somewhat loose fashion), supposedly gave way to a 'New Imperialism', annexationist and war-minded in character. The realities of African history lack this dramatic touch; there was no sudden break. The number and extent of Europe's colonial acquisitions made in Africa during the earlier nineteenth century alone, during the so-called pre-imperial era, make up an impressive list. They range afield as far as Natal and Algeria, and their configuration had considerable influence on the course of the scramble. It is easy, therefore, to exaggerate both the financial factor and the element of novelty in the new imperialism.

The concept of colonial super-profits clothed the tropical treasure house theory in new dress. Some ventures, such as the diamond and gold industries of South Africa, did in fact yield enormous gains. The South African 'Rand Lord', with his soaring bank balance and his sumptuous mansion in Park Lane, became, for many British radicals, the very prototype of the bloated, war-mongering exploiter with a cigar and a top-hat. But even on the Witwatersrand, large dividends in some mines were balanced by low profits or losses in others. According to S. H. Frankel, Professor of Colonial Economic Affairs at Oxford, the mean annual yield of capital in the Rand mines during the first forty-five years of their effective exploitation amounted to no more than 4·1 per cent. Most British investors preferred smaller risks, even though these entailed smaller profits. The gold-speculator willing to put up risk capital took second place to the *rentier* anxious to secure a modest but safe income. In 1911, Sir George Paish, a British expert, thus calculated that over 60 per cent of Britain's foreign investments had gone into the construction of railways. Most of this money had been placed outside Africa and yielded only modest dividends. Much in fact was lost.

Victorian company promoters and their socialist critics were indeed often united in a common error of judgement. They stressed the profits made in Africa. They never spoke of the lenders and entrepreneurs who lost their money in Africa. All too often they forgot that well-paying investments in Africa required extensive social and economic overheads —schools, hospitals, power plants, harbours, roads and railways. In most parts of Africa this infrastructure had to be created from scratch. Hence many early investors failed to make money during the scramble. In this connexion, we should mention also the great financial *demi-monde* of imperialism, the shady share-pushers who, far from exploiting Africans, robbed none but their own shareholders. In Rhodesia, for instance, this was done with such effect that by the late 1890s Rhodesian gold shares were said to 'stink in the investors' noses'!

The classical theories of socialism moreover were just as 'Euro-centric' as those of the most rabid imperialists. Socialist historians, like their bourgeois Victorian and Edwardian counterparts, saw the coloni-zation of Africa almost entirely in metropolitan terms. Local factors— the Boer trekkers' search for land, the Arab slave-traders' search for labour, the remorseless movement inland of the 'gunpowder frontier', the internecine struggles between indigenous communities in Africa— are largely left out of the picture. There is no mention of local African powers such as Zanzibar, Egypt, Ethiopia or Liberia, all of which extended their domain during the partition period. Black people rarely take their place on the stage of history, except as exploited labourers under the white man's lash, as romantic warriors fighting for a lost cause, or as drunken chiefs signing away their people's birthright for a keg of rum or gin.[1]

---

[1] The traditional Eurocentric outlook still dominates the works of many prominent contemporary communist historians such as Endre Sík, *The history of black Africa*, trans. by Sándor Simon (Budapest, Akadémiai Kiadó, 1966–), 2 vols.

Lenin, too, like many conservatively-minded imperialists of the pessimistic school, failed to allow for the recuperative capacity of the capitalist system. The communists believed, like many advocates of colonial expansion, that the capitalist countries had more or less reached the limit of their economic expansion; hence empire was the only way out of their predicament. In Lenin's view, the contradictions of capitalism had become unmanageable; future progress could only come under a new socialist dispensation that would smash the existing shackles on production. In fact, however, the major capitalist states, Germany, Britain, France, Italy and the U.S.A., not to speak of minor countries such as Sweden, or capitalist colonies and 'semi-colonies', all continued vastly to expand their gross national product. The growth rates of the various capitalist countries bore little relationship to the extent of their colonial possessions. The history of European investment abroad, moreover, revealed no *necessary* relationship between capital investment and political influence. During the nineteenth century Prussia and, to a much greater extent still, the U.S.A., absorbed vast quantities of British capital. Yet British lenders were never able to pull the strings at Berlin or Washington, though they might bully small and weak powers such as Egypt.

Lenin was equally mistaken when he argued that working-class reformism was nothing but the bastard offspring of imperialism. In fact European working-class militancy never actually mirrored the size of empire. Norway, Sweden, Switzerland and Denmark all lacked colonies. Yet the workers of these countries were no more inclined to mount the barricades than were their British comrades. Both Portugal and France had cut off large slices of the imperial cake. As German imperialists never tired of pointing out, the French and Portuguese colonies were considerably larger in relation to the size of the mother-land than were Germany's. Yet French and Portuguese proletarians were, on the whole, much more militant than were those of northern Europe.

We may therefore turn aside from Lenin to consider some rival interpretations of imperialism. Their number is legion; in fact a casual reader might easily gain the impression that more people wrote on imperialism than ever fought on its behalf. The present survey can mention only a few authors; but one of the most outstanding was Karl Kautsky, a moderate German socialist, now mainly remembered for Lenin's polemics against him as a renegade. Kautsky stood for a reformist course at home and a pacific, Anglophile and anti-annexationist policy abroad. During the Great War he bitterly opposed German chauvinism and, like Lenin, sought to buttress his programme by a new interpretation of imperialism. In 1915 he published a small, now forgotten, monograph that deserves to be remembered as a classic on the subject of imperialism.[1] Kautsky's treatise first analysed pre-capitalist modes of imperialist expansion and tried to show that most modern forms of imperialism were still influenced by archaic motivations. The ancient forms of empire had rested on military power, on exploitation through tribute or forced labour, or through levies on trade. (This analysis—one might add—was also perfectly applicable to many indigenous forms of African imperialism of the kind typified by the ancient states of Ghana and Mali.) A subsequent form of European expansion was linked to mercantile monopolies and to the search for luxury goods such as furs, ivory and spices. British, French and Russian frontiersmen occupied vast areas; i.e., the British in North America, the French in Canada, and the Russians in Siberia. The rush for ivory and rubber helped to open up Africa. But colonization based on such simple robber economies could not last long; the treasures of nature were quickly exhausted, while modern technology and advanced methods of agriculture provided adequate substitutes.

Mercantilist economies, based on trade monopolies, necessarily displayed a warlike character. In Kautsky's opinion, however, industrial economies tended towards pacific expansion. Factory owners gained no advantage from wars that would only disrupt world trade and impoverish their customers. 'There are those who pretended that this was a war intrigued and organised and dictated by financiers...' wrote Lloyd George about the First World War.

I was Chancellor of the Exchequer and, as such, I saw Money before the war; I saw it immediately after the outbreak of war; I lived with it for days, and did my best to steady its nerve...; and I say that money was a frightened and trembling thing: money shivered at the prospect [of war]...Big business everywhere wanted to keep out of it...Here were no eager men praying for the hour to arrive when they could strike down a great commercial rival.[2]

Military and naval power was almost irrelevant in such considerations. The merchant fleets of Norway considerably exceeded in size those of

[1] *Nationalstaat, imperialistischer Staat und Staatenbund* (Nürnberg, 1915).
[2] *War memoirs of David Lloyd George* (London, 1933), I, 74.

much bigger powers like France and Italy. Yet Norway needed neither a large navy nor a colonial empire. Kautsky at the same time denied that the export of capital must inevitably lead to imperial domination. The British example seemed to prove the opposite. The most important British imperial territories, from the point of view of investment and trade, were the white settlement colonies. Indeed, the relative importance of Canada and Australia as borrowers of British capital had been going up in recent years, while the value of India and other colonies had diminished, as shown in the following tabulation:[1]

	1908–1910	1911–1913	Increase or decrease
	(£ millions)		(%)
Canada	91·5	132·3	+ 40·8
Australia	28·9	35·4	+ 7·5
South Africa	20·9	14·5	− 6·4
India	46·4	12·7	− 33·7
Other colonies	38·0	18·8	− 19·2

These white settlement territories were not, however, acquired as the result of modern finance capitalism. Neither were they colonies in the true sense of the word. The white dominions were now self-governing democracies of an advanced kind, tied to the motherland through a loose association. Leagues of states (run on what we would now call commonwealth lines) corresponded in Kautsky's views to the highest state of capitalism: 'an association of states, not a nationally mixed state like the Austrian Empire, is that form of empire which capitalism requires to attain its last and highest form, before the proletariat will take over'.[2]

Kautsky's interpretation of the scramble for Africa was equally interesting. He opposed the view put forward by so many of his fellow-socialists, that colonial empire building was occasioned primarily by the export of capital, and by the fusion of industrial and agrarian protectionism. Britain, the most highly developed capitalist state at the time of the partition, did not in fact take the initiative in the race for African colonies. According to Kautsky, the joint interests of British working-class consumers and shipowners, both more powerful in the island kingdom than anywhere else, prevented the country from adopting protective tariffs, and forced its industrial capitalists to find

[1] The figures are quoted by Kautsky, *Nationalstaat*, p. 38.
[2] Kautsky, *Nationalstaat*, p. 75.

new markets with free trade methods. The bulk of the British possessions in Africa had been acquired primarily to safeguard the route to India, with British strategy hinging on the Cape and the Suez Canal. (Kautsky's interpretation thus basically agrees with the thesis put forward in *Africa and the Victorians*, concerning imperialism in the Dark Continent (New York, 1961) by Ronald Robinson and John Gallagher, two modern British scholars who arrived at similar conclusions on the basis of a vast amount of documentary material not available to Kautsky.)

It was France, not Britain, which set off the scramble. The root cause of French imperialism was not, however, financial. France ruled no colonies in the then accepted sense of the word. French colonialism, Kautsky argued, was originally archaic in character, resembling more closely the Russian variety. The French empire, by increasing the number of salaried posts, served the interests of the army and the bureaucracy, and of those classes from which the military and civil service drew its recruits—that is to say, the intellectuals, the petty bourgeoisie and agrarian groups. It was only subsequently that French imperialism became a tool of industrial and finance capitalism. Germany too, after a period of initial reluctance, acquired considerable possessions in Africa; but German hopes for vast wealth to be drawn from the Dark Continent were doomed to disappointment. In relation to the total trade of the imperialist powers, her African commerce was quite insignificant. Kautsky showed, for instance, that in 1912 France exported goods to the value of 6,234 million francs. Of these, 108 million francs were exported to French Africa. The French export to Belgium alone was ten times as large, amounting to 1,024 million francs in 1911. Germany's total exports in 1913 amounted to 10,773 million marks; of these exports, goods worth only 54 million marks went to her African colonies.[1]

According to Kautsky, the relative insignificance of the African trade explained the fact that, despite recurrent crises like the Fashoda and Morocco conflicts, African problems never led to war between the great powers. Imperial disputes between the great powers had in fact all been settled before the war broke out, for the risks inherent in war were out of proportion to the stakes involved. The only territories which, at the time Kautsky wrote, were really valuable for the purposes of European capitalism were South Africa, Egypt and Algeria. South Africa, however, had already attained political independence; Egypt

[1] Kautsky, *Nationalstaat*, pp. 53, 70–1.

was approaching that status, and Algeria would in time follow suit. Once these countries had become masters in their own house, they would maintain home rule against all comers. German wartime dreams of a new, profitable African empire, Kautsky implied, were therefore quite unrealistic.

Kautsky's theory has many merits. Lenin's portrait of imperialism is drawn in monochrome: the monopoly capitalists are fundamentally all alike; their exploited native victims similarly form an undifferentiated mass. Kautsky's picture, by contrast, is multi-coloured, at least as far as the European scene is concerned; he places stress on the multitude of pressure groups that had an interest in imperial expansion.

It is indeed tempting to describe imperialism, especially the French, German, Italian and Portuguese variety, as 'the highest stage of nationalism'. The nationalist metal, of course, was never unalloyed with economic components. The advocates of colonial expansion often had something of the outlook of real estate speculators gambling on a rise. Africa, as we have seen, was considered a vast potential treasure house. Using a different metaphor, we might say that it was looked upon in some sense as a vast unappropriated estate whose indigenous rulers had no true legitimacy. It therefore behoved the white patriot to stake out as large a territorial claim as he could, lest foreigners should step in and exclude their competitors by prohibitive tariffs or indirect forms of economic favouritism.

Kautsky did not take much account of what might be called the municipal colonialism displayed by certain merchant cities such as Bordeaux and Bremen. In addition, specific economic interests generally played a part in peculiar instances of annexation. Traders such as J. C. Goodefroy and Adolf Woermann had a share in winning over Bismarck to a policy of colonial expansion; French businessmen like Victor Régis with an interest in the West African peanut trade strongly favoured a forward French policy in the Senegal. But even so, within the total framework of Western capitalism, men like Goodefroy, Woermann or Régis were small fry who controlled but an insignificant portion of their country's wealth, and did not represent bourgeois interests as a whole. It is indeed dangerous to identify sectional interests within a class with the general interests of a class. These usually diverge, especially when there is no central decision-making unit to coordinate the demands of a class as a whole.

Neither France, Germany nor Italy had much need of African

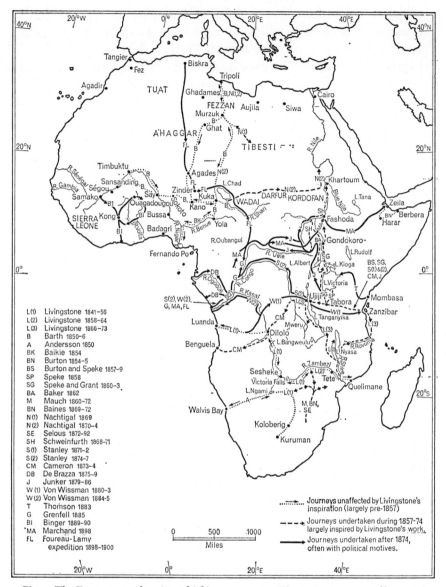

L(1) Livingstone 1841–56
L(2) Livingstone 1858–64
L(3) Livingstone 1866–73
B   Barth 1850–6
A   Andersson 1850
BK   Baikie 1854
BN   Burton 1854–5
BS   Burton and Speke 1857–9
SP   Speke 1858
SG   Speke and Grant 1860–3
BA   Baker 1862
M   Mauch 1860–72
BN   Baines 1869–72
N(1) Nachtigal 1869
N(2) Nachtigal 1870–4
SE   Selous 1872–92
SH   Schweinfurth 1868–71
S(1) Stanley 1871–2
S(2) Stanley 1874–7
CM   Cameron 1873–4
DB   De Brazza 1875–9
J   Junker 1879–86
W(1) Von Wissman 1880–3
W(2) Von Wissman 1884–5
T   Thomson 1883
G   Grenfell 1885
BI   Binger 1889–90
MA   Marchand 1898
FL   Foureau-Lamy
      expedition 1898–1900

................▶ Journeys unaffected by Livingstone's
                inspiration (largely pre-1857)

– – – – –▶ Journeys undertaken during 1857–74
            largely inspired by Livingstone's work.

━━━━━▶ Journeys undertaken after 1874,
         often with political motives.

0   500   1000
          Miles

Fig. 5. The European exploration of Africa, 1850–1900. The major journeys of historical importance are listed. Many others took place but could not be shown on a small map.

colonies; colonialism was a form of 'conspicuous consumption'[1] closely interlocked with policies at home but not required to satisfy the need for massive investments abroad. The French economy remained largely self-sufficient. The great majority of French businessmen had little enthusiasm for colonies. French farmers inclined toward protection and feared colonial (above all Algerian) competition as much as competition from foreign countries. As Henri Brunschwig shows in Chapter 4, the rising colonial movement in France found its principal supporters among journalists, bureaucrats, geographers and other academicians who preached imperialism as a means of restoring national greatness and of winning back the glory lost at Metz and Sedan. The typical agents of French imperialism were military and naval officers, technicians and teachers, 'the exportable surplus of its standing army and efficient education, not those of its economy'.[2] Algeria was a military march protected by the bureaucracy from political interference. In 1881 this particular form of French imperial enterprise was extended to neighbouring Tunisia. Frenchmen later employed the same technique to conquer yet another military fief in the western Sudan. Military and naval imperialism of course usually blended with economic motives. Paris would listen to the appeals on the part of expansionist-minded young officers for the creation of new fortified posts in West Africa, only when such calls responded or at any rate appeared to respond to the economic interests of well-placed Marseille or Bordeaux merchants. Colonization, however, was expensive. The bourgeoisie as a whole was taxed to pay for annexations that were of direct benefit to only a small section of the French middle classes. Hence special mercantile lobbies could never sway French policy on their own; they required the support of a wider military, bureaucratic and opinion-making constituency to enforce annexationist policies on the French bourgeoisie at large.

The German experience was similar. Germany too had small economic pressure groups with a stake in a forward African policy. But German colonialism, like Pan-Germanism, found most of its supporters among nationalist professors, school-teachers, civil servants and soldiers more than among bankers. Throughout the formative

[1] Richard J. Hammond, 'Economic imperialism: sidelights on a stereotype', in *Journal of Economic History*, Dec. 1961, 21, no. 4. pp. 582–9.
[2] Quoted from the introduction by Ronald E. Robinson to Henri Brunschwig, *French colonialism, 1871–1914: myths and realities*, revised ed. trans. by William Granville Brown (London, 1966), p. 1.

years of a colony such as German East Africa, the characteristic agent of German imperialism was the *Schutztruppenoffizier* rather than the banker, merchant or farmer. It was only from the turn of the present century, some twenty years after the original annexation, that German planters began to achieve some success in the commercial cultivation of sisal and coffee, and that administrative power was 'civilianized'.

Portuguese colonialism throughout this period was even more a matter of prestige than of profits. Portugal's colonies in Africa had their origins in a mercantilist empire based on the commerce in gold, spices and slaves. This empire subsequently crumbled, but the Portuguese held on to a few remnants in a spirit of national inertia. They did not move to expand their possessions on a large scale until foreigners began to challenge Portugal's title-deeds and thereby provoked an intense nationalist reaction, especially among students, military officers, journalists and academic men.

Many modern historians have accordingly tried to explain the scramble and its aftermath in terms of irrational factors, as a movement born of 'international hysteria', an interpretation that goes well with a post-colonial mood of imperial abnegation in the West. Many late nineteenth-century imperialists indeed suffered from a form of national anxiety neurosis, and looked to dominion abroad as a cure for their country's social and economic ills at home (ills that were often already on the road to being cured). Rhodes, like many empire builders of his vintage, was more 'future directed', and in a way more pessimistic than, say, David Livingstone with his serene mid-Victorian confidence in England's future. Rhodes wished to forestall foreigners in the grab for African territory, lest Britain should go empty-handed and her empire should decay. Friedrich Fabri, a German advocate of colonization, was equally fearful of the consequences of a policy of colonial abstention. Fabri thus deplored the departure of so many Germans to foreign shores, where their skill and money would build up Germany's rivals, and where their persons would be lost to *Deutschtum*. He anticipated that urbanization would prevent the Reich from supplying its future citizens with sufficient food, while German factories would no longer command adequate markets abroad. Fabri also held that colonization would counteract the threat of social revolution by providing the country with a safety valve, thus foreshadowing Lenin's theory of the use of colonial profits to bribe the workers of the West. His speculations, however, bore little relationship to contemporary realities. When Bismarck founded the German empire, the stream of German emigration was already drying up, as German countryfolk went to seek their fortunes in the growing industrial cities of the Fatherland. Advances in agricultural science, agro-chemistry and farming techniques were adding substantially to Germany's crop yields. Her industrial products had become vastly improved in quality, and were finding ready customers, especially in other industrialized countries such as Great Britain. Similarly, the era of great internal risings was already over, and Bismarck's fears of great social insurrections had already become as unrealistic as the sanguine hopes of Marx.

Some writers, however, went a good deal further. In 1919, for instance, Joseph Schumpeter, an Austrian scholar of pacific leanings, published a brilliant little work, *Imperialism and social class*, which described imperialism as a form of social atavism. Schumpeter to some extent agreed with Marx. He argued that the system of production prevalent in any given society would produce a certain ideological superstructure. In Schumpeter's view, however, the roof did not necessarily cave in when the foundation had decayed. Certain attitudes might survive in an 'objectless' manner long after the original conditions justifying their existence had passed away. Imperialism, according to Schumpeter, stemmed from pre-capitalist, war-oriented forces; empire was a social atavism, and—under modern conditions—an essentially irrational phenomenon. Schumpeter clearly went too far with his stress on irrational or archaic forces. Nineteenth-century Britain, for instance, was not run by a professional warrior class; yet the British did add vastly to their imperial possessions during the past century, and some British capitalists certainly had a financial stake in imperialism. Schumpeter moreover overlooked the realities of imperial diplomacy. Imperialist statesmen, according to Schumpeter's interpretation, seem to embark on specific policies without sound reasons. Yet men like Rosebery, Salisbury and Bismarck argued quite rationally for or against the acquisition of specific territories. Many of Rhodes's financial supporters may have failed to make the profits they anticipated; but their calculations were not irrational. Schumpeter ignored also the philanthropic and the missionary element in imperialism: the campaign against the slave-trade which played a considerable part in West African colonization, for instance, and the steady lobbying on the part of humanitarian pressure groups anxious to force the British government into apparently unprofitable regions at great expense to the British taxpayer for the assumed benefit of indigenous tribesmen. Finally, Schumpeter had nothing at all to say of the idealism of missionaries and colonial officials who sometimes played an important part in the politics of the scramble.

Many theoreticians, of course, have interpreted missionary endeavour simply as part of the ideological superstructure of capitalism. The image of the British missionary with his Bible in one hand and his cotton bale in the other forms part of pan-German as well as of Marxist folklore! But the realities of mission enterprise were much more complicated. The financial supporters of the African Lakes Company in late nineteenth-century Nyasaland, for example, did not seek for higher returns in Central African trade than were available to them in Scotland; instead they were prepared to shoulder financial losses in order to support the Christian missions by Lake Nyasa and to help in the extirpation of the slave-trade. If anything, the African Lake Company was the economic superstructure of an ideological base.

Admittedly, policies of missionary expansion, like those of territorial expansion, were closely intertwined with political, social and economic problems at home; but the relationship was not simply one of profit and loss. The British missionary movement, for instance, was to some extent a spill-over of domestic reformism in the eighteenth and nineteenth centuries into the foreign field. From converting working-class infidels and giving succour to the poor in England, it was but a short step to converting and uplifting the heathen abroad. Missionary enthusiasm in turn seeped back into the domestic field, setting up a complex relationship between religious and social reform in England and the colonies. In the United States, to give another example, the Afro-American missionary impulse was part of a wider movement for improving the Negro masses in North America. There was a similar kind of interaction between mission movements in continental Europe and European reformism, whether of the liberal or the conservative kind. In Germany, for instance, Friedrich von Bodelschwingh (1831–1910), an aristocratic farmer turned clergyman, founded Bethel, the greatest charitable institution of the German *Innere Mission*, as well as workmen's homes. At the same time Bodelschwingh took a leading part in German missionary enterprise in East Africa, which in turn owed a considerable debt to the German domestic example.

In countries as far afield as Uganda and Barotseland, missionary enterprise influenced the direction and strategy of imperial expansion.

The majority of missionaries looked to the secular sword of Europe to crush the slave-trade, to extirpate internecine African warfare and to end blood-stained customs such as the poison ordeal, the execution of alleged witches, the killing of twins, or the practice of ritual cannibalism. The missionaries, like the traders, wanted to remove traditional obstacles to the movement of persons and property. They looked to a free labour market, to a free exchange of ideas, to freedom from traditional caste restraints such as the sumptuary legislation that existed in some of the more highly stratified African societies. Missionaries occasionally became king-makers in Africa; sometimes they even set up small theocracies of their own. But by and large they lacked armed force, and they commonly turned to European administration for direct or indirect help in the task of evangelizing Africa. In many instances pioneer missionaries were first on the African scene, and European administrators only followed in the evangelists' footsteps.

Once European supremacy had been established, white clergymen often acted as a brake on abuses committed by local white administrators and settlers. The missionaries thus wittingly or unwittingly made imperial rule more acceptable to the indigenous people; and in some cases their intervention prevented insurrections, thus rendering imperial conquest less costly and more humane. Missionary concepts moreover influenced many secular officials who frequently shared the clergymen's predilection for moderate and non-revolutionary reforms at home and abroad. Indeed a surprisingly large number of empire builders had clerical connexions of some sort. Rhodes and Lugard both were parsons' sons. Lyautey, as a student at Saint-Cyr, had founded a group for social action and had taken part in the activities of Workers' Circles started by Albert de Mun, a Catholic, a royalist and himself a former cavalry officer.

No scholar has as yet undertaken an exhaustive comparative investigation into the social background of all the senior administrators employed in Africa by the various European nations. An inquiry would probably show that once the rough-riding period of early occupation was over, once the big-game hunters, the mercenaries, the tough labour recruiters and traders turned officials had given way to professional civil servants, a large percentage of the colonial administrators came to be drawn from what might be called the reformist but non-industrial portion of the bourgeoisie. The colonial services did not so much—in the words of the well-known radical *bon mot*—provide outdoor relief for sons of the upper classes. Rather they gave employment to the children of regular officers, civil servants, professional men, and landowners. Colonial administration, like the mission societies, also attracted people animated by the ideal of service. Whether a religious believer or not, the colonial ruler believed himself to be serving both his country and its colonies. He felt that money-making alone could never be a sufficient excuse for empire. The conqueror had a mission too; to rule was also to serve. Most administrators felt ashamed of individual outrages that white men might commit against black men. But their consciences were clear concerning colonial rule as a whole. Empire represented progress; progress was sacred; progress lay with Europe. Throughout the earlier history of African imperialism, the ideological initiative lay with the white man; and the intangible factor of morale, strengthened enormously by religious, philosophical or political convictions, favoured the ruler against the ruled.

Space permits only the briefest reference to the interaction between the missionary and the administrative frontiers. Missionaries helped to provide Africans with pioneer social services such as education and medical attention. The civil servants in turn often tried to influence missionary policy; they frequently furnished financial subsidies for missionary schools, hospitals and agricultural institutes. In addition, the missionaries commonly acted as the eyes and ears of imperialism, gathering intelligence about the indigenous people of Africa, and shaping public opinion in the metropolitan countries concerning African questions.

The missionary impact upon Africa was uneven in its effects. The evangelization of Africa was part of a long-drawn-out process whose results are as yet uncertain, while the military and administrative occupation of Africa was a more straightforward and more easily definable process. Nevertheless, there were some similarities between the two areas. The pioneer clergymen had to build a network of mission stations, stores, schools and sub-stations. The pioneer administrators had to create a far-flung network of administrative, police and military posts. The governmental occupation of Africa was just as uneven in its effects as the clerical variety; many parts of Africa were but lightly held, while others experienced occupation of a much more thorough kind. Similarly, effective administrative occupation did not come all at once; one or even several decades might pass until the vast territories of Africa, painted over on the map by European cartographers in British red or German blue, had come under effective European governance.

We may therefore speak of missionary, military and even civil service frontiers in Africa, using American and Australian concepts of the kind first applied to Africa by Sir Keith Hancock. Like most generalizations, the term 'frontier' of course invites criticism. In F. J. Turner's usage, for instance, the word lacks precision. Turner used the term to indicate both empty or near-empty land on the farthest edge of American settlement, and also to designate a social process entailing colonization and institutional readaptation. Nevertheless, the term frontier, with its emphasis on geographical movement and social change, is a useful one. The frontier thesis emphasizes local responses to local problems; it stresses the dynamism of the frontier in terms of local factors; and is therefore a useful corrective to a purely Eurocentric interpretation of colonial history in Africa.

The hunters' frontier, for instance, was of a multi-racial kind. In the nineteenth century, Africa was the world's largest supplier of elephant tusks. The expanding luxury industries of Europe required a great deal of ivory for piano keys, billiard balls, fans and ornaments. Indians bought enormous quantities of rings, left over from the turning of billiard balls, which were sold in bazaars as women's bangles. Afrikaners and English-men, East Coast Arabs, Portuguese half-castes, Mbundu and Yao all tried to cash in on the expanding demand for ivory, and steadily to expand their sphere of operations as the great beasts were 'shot out' in the more accessible regions. The trade in ivory was often associated with the traffic in slaves (who were used as porters in areas where animal disease prevented the use of ox-drawn or horse-drawn wagons); the ivory trade was closely tied in, too, with the commerce in rifles, blunderbusses and ammunition.

Historians might accordingly speak also of the 'gun powder frontier' which swept into the interior of Africa as white men, Arabs and others sold blunderbusses and rifles in exchange for local African products. The new fire-arms affected the balance of power within the African communities touched by the trade. Chiefs and war-lords who managed to benefit from their connexion with a world-wide exchange economy furnished their followers with more effective weapons than those available to their ordinary subjects. In addition they acquired significant military advantages over adjacent communities who still relied on bows, spears and javelins. Other tribes in turn acquired the new arms, lest they succumb to foreign raiders. The use of fire-arms accordingly spread farther inland, introducing profound changes in many indigenous tribal structures long before the first white district commissioner had made his appearance on the local scene.

The trader's frontier is an equally valuable concept. It assumed multifarious forms in the modern history of Africa. It was associated first of all with the commerce in slaves, rubber and ivory, and subsequently with the traffic in tropical goods such as palm-oil and peanuts. Men of many different nationalities—Englishmen, Frenchmen and Portuguese, Sierra Leonian creoles and Bantu entrepreneurs such as the Bisa of south-east Central Africa or the Nyamwezi of what is now Tanzania—all played their part in the commercial penetration of nineteenth-century Africa.

Africa also experienced many different kinds of agricultural frontiers. Cattlemen as diverse as the Afrikaners and the Somali looked for new pastures; planters of many different nationalities sought land to produce cocoa, coffee, tea and tobacco and other commodities for an expanding world market. Equally important was the miner's frontier. Europeans, with their superior technology, necessarily assumed a leading role in Africa's modern mining industry. To some extent their enterprise was associated with the export of capital from Europe, and therefore fits more or less into the Leninist categories. The miner's frontier, like other economic frontiers, however, also had a self-financing element. A considerable part of the wealth accumulated by South African firms in the Kimberley diamond industry was later used in the development of the Witwatersrand gold mines. Profits from the Rand in turn helped to finance mining enterprise in Rhodesia and the Copper Belt of what is now Zambia.

No frontier, of course, operated in a vacuum. Planters and prospectors, miners and missionaries all had to contend with a multiplicity of local African communities, ranging in size from powerful monarchies such as the Ashanti to stateless societies such as the Tonga. Some academic writers may indeed have over-compensated to some extent for the Eurocentric failings of their Victorian forebears, and may have seen the partition and the subsequent patterns of imperial rule too much in terms of African responses. African statesmen, of course, did play an important part in shaping the outlines of empire. Lewanika, the calculating sovereign of the Barotse in Northern Rhodesia, for instance, had excellent internal and external reasons for seeking British rather than

Portuguese protection. His intervention in the politics of the scramble was a matter of considerable local importance and indirectly helped to determine the frontiers of modern Zambia. But even the strongest of tribal kingdoms generally wielded but limited power. The initiative generally lay with the invaders from overseas with their superior technology, their arts, their science, their superior economic and organizational resources and their superior military potential.

The partition provides only a few instances of major military miscalculations made by the imperial powers. The French failed to allow for the stubborn resistance of Algeria's Muslim people and had to fight much harder for the country than they had anticipated. The British gravely underestimated the fighting potential of the Boers, the white Africans in the southern portion of the continent, and unsuspectingly slithered into what was in terms of manpower and *matériel* the greatest overseas military adventure hitherto undertaken by a great power. The Basuto in South Africa acquired ponies and fire-arms that gave them considerable powers of resistance. The Italians made an even more disastrous mistake about the military capacity of the Amhara in Abyssinia. By and large, however, the men from Europe came to hold the whip hand. Local administrators might not have many troops at their command at any given time, but the white men's *potential* military power was usually irresistible. The partition was made possible by the profound weakness of most indigenous African political systems, and by their inability to cope with the economic, military and political problems arising from direct contact with the Western world. The clash of cultures produced not one but many European imperialisms; it also created many different economic frontiers, all of them inextricably interwoven with local African, metropolitan and international threads.

A more detailed discussion of the general causes of imperialism would take us even farther afield. We might emphasize, for instance, technological factors such as developments in shipbuilding, railway engineering, or the impact made by the construction of the Suez Canal. We should have to stress the enormous cultural as well as military discrepancy between late nineteenth-century Europe and indigenous Africa. For, it must be remembered, the scramble involved African as well as European empire-builders. The Ethiopians, above all, greatly expanded their possessions, first of all in response to internal pressures within their own country, later in part as a reaction to the threat posed by European imperialists. The Ethiopians, like the French, had their

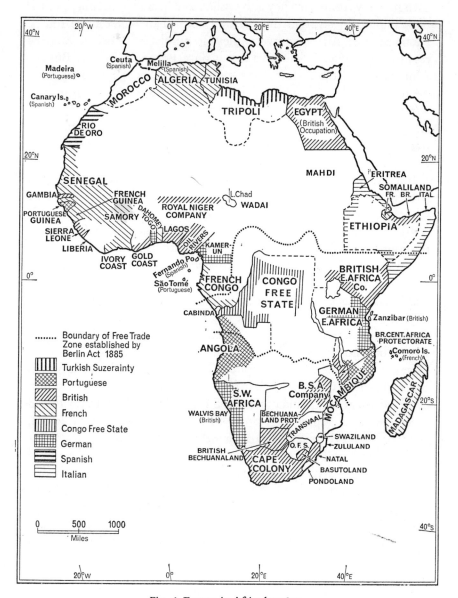

Fig. 6. Europe in Africa by 1891.

own military frontiers. They also wished to expand the number of their tax-paying subjects; and they desired control of wider trade routes. Alone among African powers, they accumulated sufficient military resources to inflict a definitive defeat on a European power. But the Amhara lacked the men and the means that enabled European competitors to make such substantial contributions to mining, agronomy, Western education, medical services and other specialized fields. The Abyssinian empire therefore generally tended to conform to more traditional military patterns, even though it also acted to some extent as an instrument of cultural transfusion.

But having taken all these factors into consideration, we should still have to explain why the scramble took place just when it did. One school of historians makes a great deal of the part played by strategic considerations, by 'the obsession with security, a fixation on safeguarding the routes to the East'.[1] Strategic considerations impelled the British to seize the Cape. Even more important, from the standpoint of strategy, was Egypt. The British, having sent troops to carry out what was intended as a temporary occupation, found compelling reasons to stay. By the early 1880s, British naval planners no longer regarded Constantinople as the key to the Eastern Mediterranean and the Middle East. They now looked to Alexandria, and they regarded the Suez Canal as the spinal cord of empire. The British moved into Egypt in order to protect the seaways to India. But intervention in Egypt in turn involved them in Uganda and the Sudan. British action also forced other countries, especially France, to seek compensations in Africa, and thereby played the major part in determining the time and manner of the scramble. The Egyptocentric case, which also links the rise of empire in Africa with the decline of the Ottoman empire, has been ably argued with a wealth of detail by Robinson and Gallagher. The strategic thesis is, however, too all-embracing in character. It overstresses the role of Egypt, fundamentally a Middle Eastern country, in the history of sub-Saharan Africa. It does not devote sufficient attention to the motives of Great Britain's foreign competitors, especially to their insatiable search for prestige. Nor does it always give sufficient weight to other factors, such as the changing local balance of power within the framework of so many African polities in other parts of the continent.

A second school believes that the partition was set off by the appear-

[1] Ronald E. Robinson and John Gallagher, with Alice Denny, *Africa and the Victorians: the official mind of imperialism* (London and New York, 1961), p. 470.

ance on the African scene of two new competitors—Belgium and Germany. To quote from Roland Oliver and John Fage's excellent *Short history of Africa*, 'it was this that upset the pre-existing balance of power and influence, and precipitated a start of international hysteria in which all powers rushed in to stake claims'.[1] But the Belgo-German' interpretation explains too much by too little. Belgium did indeed play its part, but recent research has emphasized, for example, the major role played by earlier French colonization in the Congo before King Leopold of Belgium had begun to seek sovereignty in order to keep his stake in the Congo.[2]

All things considered, a pluralistic explanation appears to make more sense. One must take into account a multiplicity of local factors, including the politics of the African communities. No history of the scramble can be complete, moreover, that fails to take account of the white men on the spot, the people who acted as the middlemen of Western civilization. There were—as we have said—the frontiers of the mariner, of the missionary merchant and of the miner. There were the farmers and the cattlemen, the soldiers and the administrators. There were the pressures of the turbulent frontier which, in regions as far afield as the Cape and Senegal, sucked the white invaders inland in their attempts to pacify the border areas. There was also competition between the local representatives of rival European powers, who might react to foreign conquests by expanding their own spheres of influence. Many problems arose from commercial contacts between Europe and Africa. Finally no historian of Africa will ever complete his account of the scramble and partition without ploughing his way through tomes with such delightfully Victorian titles as *The Ivory Coast in the Earlies; The Narrative of a Boy Trader's Adventures in the Seventies, through which Runs the Strange Thread, that is the History—Meagre, but All that is Available—of a Young English Gentlewoman* ! In fact, there were not one, but many European imperialisms, all of them interwoven with missionary, military or mercantile strands, with metropolitan, local and international threads. All these strands combined to produce the pattern of white expansion. European empire-building in Africa, which had begun as a slow and almost imperceptible process, began to pick up momentum; and by the early 1880s a convergence of many forces resulted in the rapid partition

[1] *A short history of Africa* (Harmondsworth, Middlesex and Baltimore, 1962), p. 182.
[2] Jean Stengers, 'L'impérialisme colonial de la fin du XIXe siècle: mythe ou réalité?' *Journal of African History*, 1962, **3**, no. 3, pp. 469–91.

of Africa. Each of these forces had multiple causes. Each one in turn requires a pluralistic explanation. Each one of them contained an element of the fortuitous. As a modern Soviet historian has put it in a different context:

Every historical event is the result of a convergence of many contributing conditions. A different convergence might result in a different event which, influenced by all the remaining factors, would in turn lead to consequences different from those that in fact occurred and, thus, there would begin an entire chain of events and phenomena—a different variant of development... [1]

The history of European imperialism can therefore be written only in a polycentric fashion. Whether we deal with white expansion in Africa, or with any other great instance of cultural diffusion on a continental scale, no unitary theory will ever untangle for us the richness and variety of the historical skein.

BIBLIOGRAPHY

Brunschwig, Henri. *French colonialism, 1871–1914: myths and realities.* Revised ed. Trans. by William Granville Brown; introd. by Ronald E. Robinson. London, 1966.

Curtin, Philip D. *The image of Africa: British ideas and action, 1780–1850.* Madison, University of Wisconsin Press, 1964.

Feis, Herbert. *Europe, the world's banker, 1870–1914: an account of European foreign investment and the connection of world finance with diplomacy before the war.* New Haven, Yale University Press, 1930.

Fieldhouse, D. K. '"Imperialism": an historiographical revision', *Economic History Review*, 1961, ser. 2, **14**, no. 2.

The theory of capitalist imperialism. London, 1967.

Frankel, Sally Herbert. *Capital investment in Africa: its course and effects.* London, Oxford University Press, 1938.

Gann, Lewis H. *A history of Southern Rhodesia: early days to 1934.* London, 1965.

Gann, Lewis H., and Peter Duignan. *Burden of empire: an appraisal of Western colonialism in Africa south of the Sahara.* New York, 1967.

Gillessen, Günther. *Lord Palmerston und die Einigung Deutschlands: die englische Politik von der Paulskirche bis zur Dresdener Konferenzen (1848–1851).* Lübeck, 1961.

[1] A. Ya. Gurevich in *Voprosy istorii*, 1965, no. 8, translated and quoted by Arthur P. Mendel, 'Current Soviet theory of history: new trends or old?' in *American Historical Review*, Oct. 1966, **72**, no. 1, p. 55.

Hammond, Richard J. 'Economic imperialism: sidelights on a stereotype', *Journal of Economic History*, Dec. 1961, **21**, no. 4.

Portugal and Africa, 1815–1910: a study in uneconomic imperialism. Stanford University Press, 1966.

Hilferding, Rudolf. *Das Finanzkapital: eine Studie über die jüngste Entwicklung des Kapitalismus.* Vienna, 1910.

Hobson, John Atkinson. *Imperialism: a study.* London, 1902.

Kautsky, Karl. *Nationalstaat, imperialistischer Staat und Staatenbund.* Nürnberg, 1915.

Landes, David S. 'Some thoughts on the nature of economic imperialism', *Journal of Economic History*, Dec. 1961, **21**, no. 4.

Lenin, V. I. *Imperialism, the highest stage of capitalism: a popular outline.* New, revised trans. New York, 1939.

Leroy-Beaulieu, Paul. *De la colonisation chez les peuples modernes.* 6th ed. 2 vols. Paris, 1908.

Lloyd George, David. *War memoirs of David Lloyd George.* 6 vols. London, 1933–6.

Luxemburg, Rosa. *Die Akkumulation des Kapitals: ein Beitrag zur ökonomischen Erklärung des Imperialismus.* 2 vols. in 1. Leipzig, 1921.

Mendel, Arthur P. 'Current Soviet theory of history: new trends or old?' *American Historical Review*, Oct. 1911, **72**, no. 1.

Nussbaum, Manfred. *Vom 'Kolonialenthusiasmus' zur Kolonialpolitik der Monopole: zur deutschen Kolonialpolitik unter Bismarck, Caprivi, Hohenlohe.* [East] Berlin, Akademie-Verlag, 1962.

Oliver, Roland, and John D. Fage. *A short history of Africa.* Harmondsworth, Middlesex and Baltimore, 1962.

'Parvus' (pseud. of Alexander Helphand). *Die Kolonialpolitik und der Zusammenbruch.* Leipzig, 1907.

Marineforderungen, Kolonialpolitik und Arbeiterinteressen. Dresden, 1898.

Robinson, Ronald E., and John Gallagher, with Alice Denny. *Africa and the Victorians: the official mind of imperialism.* London and New York, 1961.

Scheler, Max Ferdinand. *Die Ursachen des Deutschenhasses: eine national-pädagogische Erörterung.* Leipzig, 1917.

Schulze-Gaevernitz, Gerhart von. *Britischer Imperialismus und englischer Freihandel zu Beginn des zwanzigsten Jahrhunderts.* Leipzig, 1906.

Sík, Endre. *The history of black Africa.* Trans. by Sándor Simon. 2 vols. Budapest, Akadémiai Kiadó, 1966– .

Stengers, Jean. 'L'impérialisme colonial de la fin du XIXe siècle: mythe ou réalité?' *Journal of African History*, 1962, **3**, no. 3.

Zeman, Z. A. B., and W. B. Scharlau. *The merchant of revolution: the life of Alexander Israel Helphand (Parvus), 1867–1924.* London, Oxford University Press, 1965.

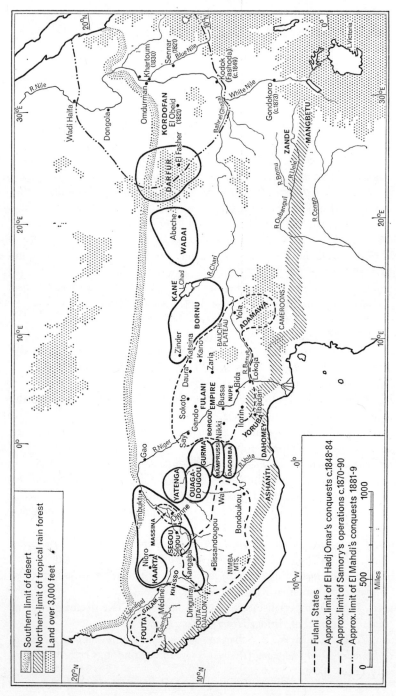

Fig. 7. States of the Sudan in the nineteenth century.

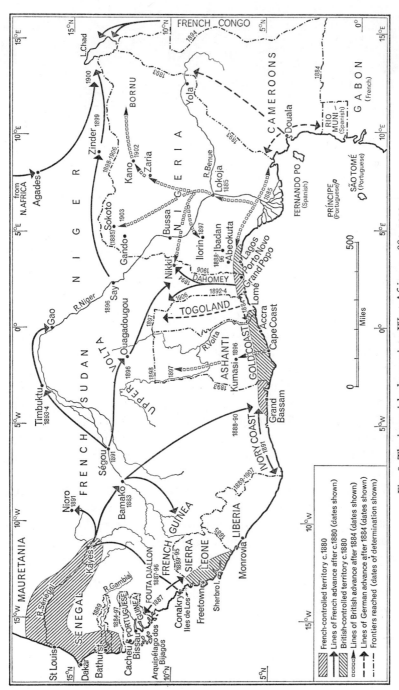

Fig. 8. The imperial advance into West Africa, c. 1880–1900.

CHAPTER 4

FRENCH EXPLORATION AND CONQUEST IN TROPICAL AFRICA FROM 1865 TO 1898

by HENRI BRUNSCHWIG

During the nineteenth century France did not have the same impelling reasons as Great Britain for interesting herself in Black Africa. In the first place, French commerce with the Dark Continent was limited. Moreover, the French had not become greatly aroused about the suppression of the slave-trade, even though they had agreed in principle to its prohibition at the Treaty of Vienna and though French laws had prohibited the traffic from 1821 onwards. If France was nevertheless active in the tropics, even outside Senegal, her oldest settlement, it was because of her relations with Great Britain. The long-standing sense of rivalry between the two navies was strengthened after 1815 by the unwillingness of British administrators to return to France the stations held in 1792. In fact the British did not give them all back. The Treaty of Vienna excepted from the *status quo ante* Mauritius, which contained the only good harbour in the Indian Ocean. French sailors regarded this as an insufferable affront; and once the navy had been reconstituted, they attempted to compensate for their loss by occupying the Bay of Diego-Suarez in Madagascar and, earlier, the Islands of Nossi Be (1841) and Mayotte (1843).

When one considers the small amount of French trade with Africa or with India, it is evident that French intervention was mainly a question of prestige. Indeed, French action arose from the same proud defiance of the British that had led the French to found, in 1844, the three forts of Grand Bassam, Assinie and Gabon. It is true that traders to the Senegal coast had asked for an investigation of the commerce on the shores of Guinea, and that one of the ships engaged in the suppression of the slave-traffic had been entrusted with this task. But the result of the first voyage made by the *Malouine* (1838–9) had not been encouraging, and the treaties of protection concluded between 1839 and 1842 by Edouard Bouët, its commander, were never ratified. It was only when a British Parliamentary Select Committee issued a report recommending treaties with the black chiefs and the re-occupation of forts previously abandoned by the British to replace the infamous commerce in slaves by legal trade that the French government decided urgently upon setting up the three forts.

In the meantime the nationalist enthusiasm of the sailors could not make itself felt except with the consent of the Ministry of Foreign Affairs. But right up to the end of the century the ministry subordinated the activity of the navy in tropical Africa to the ministry's general policy of avoiding any conflict with Britain. Thus Guizot, who was Minister of Foreign Affairs in 1844, had the treaties of protection revised and assured London that the sovereignty acquired by France would be an 'external sovereignty'. This 'did not imply any idea of interfering with the internal affairs of the country'; it would respect unlimited freedom of commerce and would suppress the slave-trade.[1]

At the same time there was little curiosity about Africans, little desire to establish trading posts and to develop them into colonies, and little commercial expansion. Budgetary deficits were ever-present; and in 1871 the French abandoned Grand Bassam and Assinie, though reserving their rights of sovereignty over these areas. South of Gabon two naval officers explored the coast between the estuary and the mouth of the Ogooué (Ogowe). In 1862 Souriau, a naval lieutenant, and in 1868 Serval, a captain of engineers, signed treaties similar to those concluded in Gabon with the chiefs of Cape Lopez and Fernan Vaz. The officers were welcomed with open arms by the local Africans, whom the abolition of the slave-trade had deprived of commerce with Europe but who had become dependent on European products. Here also France, in practice, limited herself to an 'external sovereignty' and did not trouble to explore the interior.

But Senegal was the only exception. There Louis L. C. Faidherbe's campaigns created a colony around the *comptoirs* that had been traditionally devoted to trade in gum, gold and ivory. Whites settled alongside blacks and mulattoes at St Louis, and the South Atlantic fleet was based at Gorée. The mulattoes, born in the country, familiar with the local dialects, and yet culturally assimilated to the whites, played an essential role. They organized the convoys up the river to Bakel and the country of Galam; they made up the militia for the campaigns against the Moors or against El Hadj Omar (Al Hajj 'Umar); they bore witness

[1] Henri Brunschwig, *L'avènement de l'Afrique noire du XIXe siècle à nos jours* (Paris, 1963), pp. 60–1.

to the value of a liberal policy of assimilation. In 1837 they comprised 7,653 out of 12,101 inhabitants at St Louis; and, after the emancipation of the slaves in 1848, French citizenship was conferred on all citizens of the old *comptoirs*. They elected deputies to the National Assembly (1848–53), and thereafter to the Chamber of the Third Republic (from 1879 on). The laws of 1872 and 1880 gave municipal status to Gorée, to St Louis, and thereafter to Rufisque and to Dakar (founded in 1857); other mixed communities, directed by an administrator assisted by a partly elected council, were created in 1852. An elected General Council was set up in 1879 similar to those that had been reorganized in the French Departments by the law of 1871.

It was also the mulattoes who supported Faidherbe's policy of conquest in order to free themselves from the Moors, whose exactions from the river-traffic and frequent incursions in the south hindered trade. The mulattoes undoubtedly persuaded Faidherbe that the colony had a brilliant future. Their voyages had acquainted them with the importance of the trade with the Sudan and thence across the Sahara. They had the best of reasons to believe current stories about Sudanese gold, for they had exchanged salt and cloth for the gold dust of Bouré. Faidherbe had effected a partition between Senegal under Christian administration and the kingdom of El Hadj Omar, whose advance had been halted at the gates of Medina in 1857. The mulattoes considered that, as a natural consequence of Faidherbe's achievement, Senegal should become the chief outlet of the commerce carried on by the numerous caravans operating at that time between the great curve of the Niger and the Guinean coast. This design should be accomplished by the creation of a trade-route guarded by fortified posts all the way from Medina to Bamako.

Shortly before his term of office ended, Faidherbe entrusted E. Mage, a naval lieutenant, with a mission to the Niger. Mage set out in November 1863 with Quintin, a ship's doctor, and reached Ségou in February 1865. Ahmadou (Amadu), El Hadj Omar's son, welcomed them, without telling them that the king had been killed during a campaign against the rebels of the Macina. He extended hospitality to them until 1866, when he agreed to sign a commercial treaty, whose terms, however, were extremely vague and which produced no concrete results.

Another outlet for the trade with the Sudan was in the so-called Rivières du Sud ('Southern Rivers')—Nunez, Pongo (Pongas), and Mellacorée—which from the beginning of the century had been sought out from time to time by the traders of St Louis. The caravans would bring down the gold, ivory and hides from the Upper Niger and from the Fouta Djallon to the European 'factories'. Those belonging to the French were the most important, especially those in Mellacorée (Gaspard Devès).

The development of the ground-nut trade after 1860, the interest taken both by the Senegalese and by the trading firms of Marseille and Bordeaux in the cultivation of ground-nuts and coffee at Rio Nunez caused Faidherbe to envisage annexing to Senegal all the streams enclosing Portuguese Guinea, from the Casamance, controlled since 1838 by the fortified post of Sedhiou, down to the northern boundary of Sierra Leone. In 1860 Faidherbe sent Lieutenant Lambert to explore the Fouta Djallon: 'It is through its defiles', Lambert reported, 'that the European trade from the coast will find the most direct and sure route to reach the markets of the Upper Niger and of the Sudan, towards which, after nearly a century, it is beginning to find its way.'[1]

Pinet-Laprade, who was governor of Senegal from 1865 to 1869, made treaties of protectorate with the chiefs of the three rivers and founded the military posts of Boké (Nunez), Boffa (Pongo), Benty (Mellacorée). However, local disorders, rivalry between tribes and wars made this dominion precarious. The British government did not share the anxiety of the Sierra Leone traders, who were rivals of the French on all sides, in Mellacorée, in the Scarcies, and in Forecariah. Hence Faidherbe's dearest wish was to obtain little Gambia, a British enclave in Senegal, in exchange for the French possessions of Assinie and Grand Bassam. In 1866 France agreed to add her fortified posts in the Rivières du Sud to the list of dependencies to be handed over to the British. Discussions broke down, but were resumed in 1870, and France agreed to cede Gabon instead of the Rivières du Sud. An understanding had almost been reached when Britain, after a new interruption, demanded Gabon, the Ivory Coast and the Rivières du Sud as well as a monetary compensation; and in 1876 the talks were finally broken off.

At the time of the founding of the Third Republic, French Tropical Africa consisted of a compact colony in course of formation, with a policy of assimilation and a programme of expansion which a historian (Bernard Schnapper) has described as 'Senegalese imperialism'. The French had also three small protectorates in the Gulf of Guinea claiming 'external sovereignty' which had neither great economic nor great

[1] M. Lambert, 'Voyage dans le Fouta-Djalon', *Le Tour du Monde*, 1861, **3**, no. 1.

strategic importance. The whole was administered by the Directorate of Colonies in the Ministry of Marine. It was this ministry that appointed the officials who maintained French sovereignty on the spot and who, except in Senegal, did not concern themselves with exploration. The navy had other fields of action—Indo-China, the Antilles, even Réunion. It participated also in the more distant ventures of the Second Empire— in Syria, China and Mexico—where more laurels could be won. In the eyes of the navy, as well as of the Quai d'Orsay, Black Africa was of little importance. As for public opinion, it had long since become dubious of far-off expeditions because of the Mexican fiasco, and mistrusted colonial enterprises on account of the recurrent and endless difficulties in Algeria since 1830. French public opinion was concerned only with internal politics; and was much more interested in the transformation, effected at long last after the plebiscite of 1869, from a liberal to a parliamentary empire, than in the rivalries between sailors and traders in far-off regions whose very names were often difficult to find on maps.

The crisis of 1871 and the formation of an imperialist public opinion

Three factors contributed significantly toward awakening in French public opinion a sustained interest in colonization: the outstanding technical achievements in the world at large; the discovery of diamonds and then of gold; and finally, the strong nationalistic spirit engendered in the French people by the defeat of 1871.

First of all, the year 1869 saw some remarkable technical achievements in the world at large. In that year the Union Pacific rail line, which was to link New York with San Francisco, was begun. It thenceforth became a model for the trans-Asiatic and trans-African railroads to come. In the same year the representatives of all the great powers opened the Suez Canal, on which work had begun ten years before. Its promoter, Ferdinand de Lesseps, was neither an engineer nor a banker. His career in the consular service had been modest, but his energy and diplomatic ability had won for him the title of 'the great Frenchman'. He was the most decorated man in Europe, the capitalist whose peaceful activities on an international scale appeared more effective and more glorious than military success. This great civilian was the inspiration of young explorers who dreamed of becoming rich and famous. Almost all those who travelled across Africa between 1875 and 1890 followed his example. All the great technical projects that fired the public imagination—the trans-Saharan and trans-African railroads, the canal from the Gulf of Syrtes to the Tunisian *schotts*, or from Lake Aoussa to Tadjoura Bay—drew inspiration from him. 'The true conquests of the present epoch', wrote Paul Soleillet in the preface, dated 1879, of his *Voyage à Ségou*, 'are not military, but industrial and commercial accomplishments. Lesseps has done as much for his country's glory as Turenne and Bonaparte. All nations have sung his praise, for all can profit from his work.'[1]

One of the many unsuccessful promoters of colonial public works was Alphonse Beau de Rochas, an engineer who had ruined himself with concession projects at Obock and with railroads in Central Africa. At the age of seventy-two, Beau de Rochas was directing what he called 'the French task of penetrating the African continent by railroads, conceived essentially as a work of peaceful penetration'. In 1886 he offered De Brazza plans for a narrow-gauge railway (2/3 metre) from Sétif to Didjeli in Algeria. He concluded his offer by saying: 'All this is important, very useful, very much in the public interest and, moreover, very simple and very easy to carry out, if only some one had the will to do it. It goes far beyond Suez and Panama, but I am not Monsieur de Lesseps although you are Monsieur de Brazza...'[2]

Numerous explorers also elaborated projects for canals and railroads. Aimé Olivier, an engineer, followed up in Guinea the exploration of Lambert (1860). Olivier considered that the Sudan might be reached by means of a railroad from the coast to Timbo, Dinguiraye, and thence to the confluence of the Tinkisso and the Niger, a much easier and less costly route than that from Senegal to Bamako. These pioneers were often highly imaginative. The Suez project was simple. That of E. Roudaire, who wanted to create an inland sea in the Tunisian *Sahel* and speculated about changes in climate and the fertilization of the desert that would result from it, was less so; while Denis de Rivoyre observed 'that it would be easy to change the course of the Nile so as to turn Egypt into a desert in case England attempted to take it'![3]

The same ingenuity was displayed by another engineer, Amédée

---

[1] *Voyage à Ségou, 1878–1879, rédigé d'après les notes et journaux de voyage de Soleillet par Gabriel Gravier* (Paris, 1887), p. xvi.

[2] S.O.M. Brazza (Paris, Archives Nationales), 3rd Mission, VII.

[3] Minister of War to Minister of Foreign Affairs, 24 Nov. 1881, *Mémoires et documents, Afrique* (Paris, Archives Affaires Etrangères), vol. 64.

Sébillot. Sébillot thought up a new scheme after the destruction of an expedition led by Colonel Paul F. X. Flatters to the Hoggar in 1881, and after the abandonment of the well-studied project by A. Duponchel, an engineer, for a trans-Saharan railroad. In 1893 Sébillot proposed the construction of a trans-African railroad with a gauge of 2 metres. The route would run from Algiers to Agades. There it would divide—one branch going to Obock, the other to Ouidah (Whydah). At this point it would branch out a second time, for the Chad and Johannesburg, respectively. The express trains that would run on these lines at 100 km an hour would cut the journey from Bombay, by Obock, to London from twenty-four days to eleven; the trip from the Cape to London would take twenty days instead of thirty-five, and that from Rio de Janeiro via Ouidah to London, fourteen days instead of eighteen. 'Mobile forts', i.e., armoured trains, would ensure the security and the wealth of the African continent; and the ability of its 200 million people to travel would guarantee the profitability of the enterprise.

As late as 1914, still another project was promoted by Commandant Roumens, who urged the construction of two trans-African railroads, one from Algiers to the Cape by Katanga, the other from Bizerta to Conakry by Timbuktu. And all these projects were welcomed by the public, now showing a sympathy for colonial matters that had not existed in France before 1870.

A second major cause for the arousing of French colonial sentiment was the discovery of diamonds (1867–72) and then of gold (1886) in South Africa. The rush of immigrants to the Transvaal, the prodigious gains of a Barnato or a Rhodes, laid hold of men's spirits and caused the legend of the Sudanese gold to be revived. Dr Paul Colin hoped to exploit this in 1888:

In a few days from now [he wrote], I shall have a treaty signed with Kassama, the chief of Diebedougou at Famale that will concede to me the rights of commercial and mineral exploitation. With this treaty and the samples of gold ore and of gold-bearing earth that I shall bring back, I hope to be able to constitute a powerful company in France for the exploitation of the area.[1]

The first colonists of Obock were much taken up with mining concessions, for they believed that rich gold deposits would be found in the region. One of them, Godineau de la Bretonnerie, an associate of Beau de Rochas in 1872, vainly tried to obtain from the government

[1] G, 108, 2nd dossier, item 29 (Dakar Archives).

a concession in the Isle of Dissé in Adulis Bay, which did not belong to France. In August 1873 he wrote to the President of the Republic:

If France should renounce this gift of property, the chiefs of Sinafé have conceded to me lands along the coast from Zoula Bay to Amphila Bay, with the purpose of building a 'factory' that I shall call Vendôme, in comemoration of my native town where my father was *maire* for thirty years. The coal mines that I shall establish will soon attract all the ships that pass these ports of call; this traffic will soon bring life to the *comptoir* of Vendôme, to the Red Sea and to Ethiopia, a country peopled by 15 million Christians and very little known to the rest of the civilized world.[1]

Lastly, the defeat of 1871 and the loss of Alsace-Lorraine evoked in all classes of the population a nationalist outburst that was peculiarly French in character and that was of capital importance. What had been hitherto a trait confined to sailors or soldiers, for whom national prestige was associated with professional success, now became national in character. To prove to the world that conquered France remained a great nation, that she was still capable of expansion, that she too had a civilizing mission, became a necessity in the eyes of all. Needless to say, Frenchmen sought to justify these conquests by economic arguments. The doctrines expounded from 1874 onwards by Paul Leroy-Beaulieu contrasted the traditional settlement colonies with colonies based on capital investment and occupation. The latter variety was regarded as modern, liberal and beneficial to colonized and colonizers alike. In his often-quoted speech of July 1885, and in his book *Le Tonkin et la mère Patrie*, Jules Ferry repeated the economic arguments that learned societies, colonial associations and the press had previously disseminated. He took great pains to synthetize the three fundamental themes of imperialist nationalism—the humanitarian argument, the argument of political prestige and the argument of economic need. Nevertheless, these works have sometimes been misinterpreted by historians. Scholars have inferred from them that the cause of expansion was above all economic. But the date of Ferry's syntheses—after the Berlin conference, which took place during 1884 and 1885—suggests that they were designed to appeal to financial circles which hitherto had watched colonial expansion without participating in the process.

The most striking characteristic of this period was the nationalist feeling that expressed, as if by reflex action, the common desire to compensate for the loss of Alsace-Lorraine. As Gambetta wrote on the

[1] *Mémoires et documents, Afrique* (Paris, Archives Affaires Etrangères), vol. 63, p. 427.

morrow of the establishment of the protectorate over Tunis, 'The pessimists must recognize the facts. France is once again taking up her place among the great powers.'

Enough has already been said about the prominence of this argument in the deliberations of the learned societies and in the press, but we shall also find it almost always manifest in the mind of the solitary explorer departing on his expedition. Questioned about the reasons which motivated his great mission, Capt. L. G. Binger said: 'I was an Alsatian, France welcomed me, and to show my gratitude I tried to gain for her by persuasion a nice piece of Africa.'[1] When Dr Colin sent to the officer commanding in Upper Senegal the treaties concluded on his own initiative with the chiefs of Tambura and of Diebedougou, in Bambuka, in 1883, Commandant Boilève was upset and wrote to the governor: 'I don't know if Dr Colin takes what he has done seriously, but I know that he has said to one of my officers that like any other explorer he intended to return to France with treaties.'[2]

'Any other explorer' might have included De Brazza, making treaties in 1880 with the chief of the Bateke, Makoko; or Soleillet, taking possession in 1882, 'in the name of the French people', of the Suba Islands in the Strait of Bab el Mandeb and (a few months later) of the port of Sagallo on Tadjoura Bay; or Aimé Olivier in Guinea.

This lust for territory, that equally distinguished the Germans and Leopold II, stood out as one of the characteristics of the new imperialism. Among the French it was not occasioned only by the desire for personal enrichment or glory; it had also a moral justification. It responded to a special need; it expressed the desire to recover the national dignity impaired on the battlefields of 1871. In the preface of his oft-reprinted book on *Les colonies françaises* (1880), Professor Paul Gaffarel declared:

The ancient soil of Gaul cannot be extended: too many jealous neighbours watch our every movement. While they expand, we remain stationary. Russia annexes little by little the immense territories of Central Asia. Germany rounds herself off at the expense of her neighbours. England and the United States seize everything that seems to them good to take or to keep. Austria, Greece, and even Italy have found and will find means of territorial expansion at the expense of the Ottoman Empire. It is absolutely necessary that France in her turn augment her domain and she cannot do it except by acquiring new colonies.[3]

[1] *Une vie d'explorateur: souvenirs extraits des carnets de route...* (Paris, 1938), preface.
[2] I, G, 65 (Dakar Archives).   [3] *Les colonies françaises*, 6th ed. (Paris, 1899), pp. i–ii.

These quotations might be multiplied indefinitely. They characterize a new, empire-oriented generation of Frenchmen. Intoxicated by the immense possibilities of the new technology, envious of the riches concealed in unexploited mines, galvanized by the defeat of 1871, explorers rose up from the ruins created by the war, confident in their star, enthusiastic, inexperienced, with their heads full of projects and their hands empty.

Outside the restricted groups of activists who were fired with enthusiasm over colonization, this imperialism was, however, no more than a consequence of nationalism at home. The masses, on patriotic grounds, ceased to oppose colonial expansion; they accepted it for the prestige it gave to the weakened mother country. But the French people as a whole were not interested in colonization for its own sake but only in relation to everyone's major preoccupation—the German menace.

France and African exploration

Before 1870 France had not distinguished herself in the exploration of Africa. Until that time, exploration had been mainly the concern of soldiers or sailors charged with missions of reconnaissance or—more rarely—of commercial inquiry, in the course of their official business and at the expense of their departments. France could boast of René Caillé, of Duveyrier, of a number of travellers who were members of the Institut like the brothers d'Abbadie, or a number of admirals. But what were these people compared with Mungo Park, Barth, Livingstone, or even contemporaries like V. L. Cameron, H. M. Stanley, G. Nachtigal and G. F. Rohlfs? In the field of exploration France was backward, just as the Geographical Society of Paris, founded in 1821, was far behind the Royal Geographical Society of London.

It was only after 1871 that the exploration movement began to develop, and that geography, 'the philosophy of the earth', became the first among the humanities. After that year special credits were granted to scientific missions, of which the explorers might make use.

A commission for scientific and literary voyages and missions was created in 1874 in the Ministry of Public Instruction. It received a grant of 200,000 francs per annum, of which only a trifle was devoted to exploration. In 1883 the Ministry of Marine and Colonies set up a special commission for colonial missions. Its initial annual appropriation was 100,000 francs. In 1895 this increased to 250,000 francs, but fell to

130,000 in 1903, to 61,000 from 1907 to 1910, and to 45,000 from 1911 to 1914. The grants were divided among too many applicants—11 in 1895, 42 in 1903, from 35 to 25 between 1907 and 1910, and from 35 to 11 between 1911 and 1914. The subventions were accordingly never sufficient for their purpose. The commission could never allot more than partial subsidies and never had any real control over the organization and management of expeditions.[1] Hence would-be explorers applied also to other ministries: to Public Instruction, to Foreign Affairs and to Public Works; and also to the Admiralty, which granted free passage and encouraged the colonial authorities to co-operate.

To these public funds explorers might add grants from learned societies. The first in point of time, apart from the Geographical Society, was the Society of Colonial and Maritime Studies, founded in 1876. In 1885 it had 673 members, each paying 20 francs in subscription per annum. It included all the official élite. It sponsored Soleillet and the trans-Saharan railroad, and it pursued its propagandist activity after the creation of the French African Committee in 1890 and the French Colonial Union in 1893. These organizations opened public subscriptions and distributed funds without ever controlling entirely any one expedition. Hence it is impossible to set up a balance sheet of French exploration, for it was not planned, as was so much of Great Britain's.

The most reputable explorers sacrificed part of their private fortune to their life work. De Brazza, for instance, in the course of his first mission, undertaken with a subsidy of 26,000 francs, actually spent 42,000. Aimé Olivier bore the whole cost of his journeys in Guinea. Less scrupulous men like Paul Soleillet 'fed at more than one trough' and made a good thing out of their profession of 'African traveller'.[2] Between these two extremes one may find in varying proportions all the ingredients: disinterested patriotism, economic prudence, and careerist ambition.

But almost always—up to the time of the great colonials whose missions were not merely exploratory, notably that of Marchand and the mission toward Lake Chad, after 1895—French exploration had, so to speak, an amateur character. The travellers scraped up funds as best they could, bought their equipment in specialized Parisian stores, went forth alone or in tiny groups, without serious preparations, without experience and without sufficient means. They trusted their star; and

[1] S.O.M. Missions 100 (Paris, Archives Nationales).
[2] S.O.M. Missions 2 (Paris, Archives Nationales).

whether they were adventurers, traders, scholars, or even old soldiers, they generally finished by falling foul of those who sought to monopolize the control of exploration and of policy, of those whose business and privilege it was to enlarge the national territory, namely, the soldiers and sailors. These latter were the people who controlled West Africa and who after long effort ended by controlling the formation of Equatorial Africa.

When in 1874 the Minister of Marine, Admiral Montaignac, entrusted a mission to Ogooué to Pierre Savorgnan de Brazza, a young officer of Italian origin who had only recently been naturalized, the bureaucrats in the Admiralty did not look upon the decision with favour. They would still have liked at that time to exchange the French possessions in the Gulf of Guinea for Gambia. Gabon was of no interest whatever, and there was thought of abandoning it along with Assinie and the Grand Bassam. What was the point of incurring the expense of a journey when, just recently, neither the Marquis de Compiègne and the naturalist Marche, nor the German explorer Lenz had been able to get beyond Lambarené on the lower Ogooué? Only the personal friendship of the minister with De Brazza, whom he had met in Rome, could justify such an enterprise, that otherwise ought to have been entrusted to an older and more tried officer. The young man set out with a doctor of the same age, Noël Ballay, and an adjutant, Hamon. And no more was heard of him until his return at the end of 1878.

At any rate, De Brazza succeeded in getting up past the Ogooué and the Passa to the Bateké plateau. He reached the Alima tributary of the Congo at the same time as Stanley, who had followed the Congo, reached the mouth. De Brazza thus discovered a means of access to the enormous navigable network of streams between Stanley Falls and Stanley Pool that avoided the impassable rapids between the Pool and the estuary. It was an important discovery; but the acclaim it achieved is inexplicable except in the context of the shift in public opinion since 1871. De Brazza's performance would place France in the first rank in a field where she had not hitherto attained international status. Now beside a Stanley, a Baker, a Rohlfs, Frenchmen could boast of the merits of a compatriot. And what merits! He was young, he was good-looking, he was aristocratic. He had chosen to be a Frenchman. He had made his journey without firing a shot, he had liberated slaves, had enriched the collections of the Museum of Natural History, and had made a number of geographical observations. He was perfect. He became famous overnight. Like a modern film star or popular singer, honours were showered upon him. France had her explorer at last.

This first mission was significant because De Brazza set a fashion. His emulators—even, indeed above all, those who were jealous of him and criticized him—conformed to it and followed the same *cursus honorum*: an inconspicuous departure, a long silence broken by alarming rumours concerning the probable death of the courageous pioneer, an unexpected return; then the gold medal of the Geographical Society, a solemn lecture at the Sorbonne, a reception by the City Council of Paris, the Legion of Honour, the publication of large illustrated books with gilt-edged pages given to the best pupils at prize-givings. Such, after De Brazza had shown the way, was the fortune of Binger, of Monteil, of all who succeeded in the great career of explorer.

The peculiar characteristics of French exploration thus become apparent. On the one side we have a traditional military procedure: missions entrusted by the high command, under the aegis of the minister concerned, to officers who were given precise instructions and provided with the necessary means. The purpose of such missions, which were dominated constantly by suspicion of the British or of colonists who were more interested in their material interests than in national prestige, was essentially political.

On the other side there were the 'profiteers', half-adventurers, half-idealists, who were averse to the use of force, since they had none at their command. They were always impecunious and seemed undisciplined by nature. They were actually obliged to solicit the support of the administrators and the soldiers on the spot. Although they could put pressure on local men through metropolitan protectors such as the learned societies, through friends at court and in the press, they did not, however, get very far. Their names will be found in the archives, not in the public memory. But their attitude of mind, reflecting that of public opinion, their essentially personal and adventurous method, gradually found its way into the establishment and ended by winning over the soldiers and the sailors. And the man who made all this possible was De Brazza.

The Senegalese thrust

While De Brazza, amid general public ignorance and indifference, was carrying out his first mission to the Ogooué (1875–9), Colonel Louis Brière de l'Isle, a native of the Antilles who was governor of Senegal (1876–81), involved France in an imperialist policy by attempting to extend the boundaries of Senegal toward the Rivières du Sud and the Niger.

On the Guinea coast he came up against the governor of Sierra Leone, Sir Samuel Rowe (1876–81), who sought to establish British control over the coast between the Pongos and Freetown. The French, however, had a firm hold over Benty, and their trade dominated Mellacorée and the Scarcies. Brière sent his political director, Captain C. Boilève, to renew and multiply treaties with the native chiefs, who often tried to play off one European rival against the other. The local conflict lasted until 1881, and reached its climax when Boilève, on 14 March 1877, occupied by force the isle of Matacong (north of Benty), where Rowe was getting ready to set up an English customs post.

However, W. H. Waddington and Lord Salisbury, the two foreign ministers concerned, were anxious to maintain good relations between Britain and France. The two countries had co-operated at the Berlin Congress of 1878, where France had obtained a promise of benevolent neutrality should she intervene in Tunisia. The two powers had co-operated also in Egypt, where the Franco-British financial condominium was organized in 1879. The ministers refused to go to war about a coast that had no economic importance. Waddington ordered that Matacong be evacuated, pending the result of negotiations. Brière de l'Isle complied with bad grace (2 June 1879), and afterwards asked authority to establish a customs barrier at the mouth of the Mellacorée 'so as to show the natives that we intend to maintain ourselves on that river and not to leave it, as the English have been saying for thirteen years that we would, much to the detriment of our interests'.[1] He returned to the charge on several occasions, demanding as late as October 1880 that treaties be made with the local chiefs so as to 'affirm our sovereignty over the coast which extends from the Rio Pongo to Forrécarieh'.[2]

[1] *Mémoires et documents, Afrique* (Paris, Archives Affaires Etrangères), vol. 50, p. 48.
[2] Brière de l'Isle to Jauréguiberry, 20 Oct. 1880, *Mémoires et documents, Afrique* (Paris, Archives Affaires Etrangères), vol. 50, p. 246.

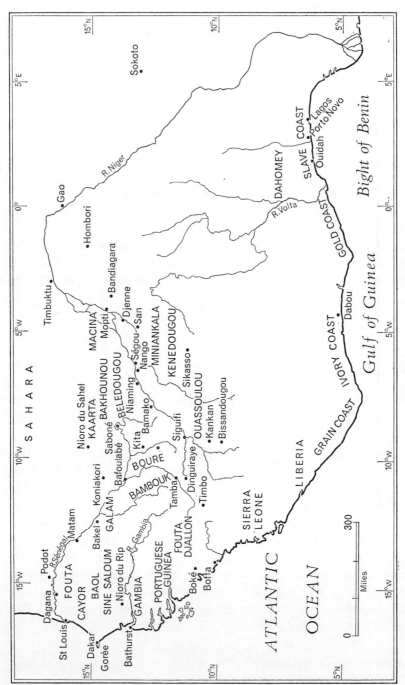

Fig. 9. West Africa in the late nineteenth century.

Nothing was done. The two governments appointed a mixed de-limitation commission which met in May 1881 and fixed the frontier, leaving the Scarcies to Sierra Leone; the Mellacorée with the coast north to the Rio Nunez, including Matacong Island and the Iles de Los, to France.

The project of extending the Senegal colony to the Niger was like-wise discouraged. It had begun when Brière de l'Isle received a visit from Paul Soleillet, who had made his name in France with a project for building a railroad between Algeria, Timbuktu and Senegal. This adventurer was supported by learned societies; and, in spite of his want of culture and his incompetence, he had succeeded in getting himself accepted as a great explorer. With funds obtained from the General Council, as well as with the support of the governor, he set off for Ségou. He was welcomed there on 1 October 1878 by Ahmadou, but he could not go on to Timbuktu on account of the troubles in Macina, and returned to St Louis on 21 March 1879.

Brière had given him 8,000 francs, so that he might recuperate in France. He promised him a further 12,000 francs thereafter if he would attempt to reach Timbuktu directly by way of Mauritania. Soleillet thereupon craftily induced the Ministry of Public Works to put him on the 'Commission for the Trans-Saharan Railroad', formed to study the much more serious project of Duponchel, an engineer. Soleillet also wangled a ministerial promise of 30,000 francs for a new expedition. When Brière learned of this, he withdrew the proffered subsidy, despite protests from Soleillet, who in the meantime had also obtained the offer of a grant from the Ministry of Public Instruction. Soleillet's second mission, however, rapidly turned into a fiasco. He left on 16 February 1880, but was robbed before he could reach Adrar and returned to St Louis on 12 April.

The Ministry of Public Works thereupon awarded him a further 20,000 francs to start again, this time from the upper river. But before taking off he published articles hostile to the military and to their policy of conquest which so alienated Brière that he brought the mission to an end. Soleillet was informed of this at Medina, from which he was repatriated in December 1880. He obtained an indemnity of 10,000 francs from the Ministry of Public Works, however, and started an action against the Governor of Senegal for having seized his baggage. The sums spent in a single year by this adventurer, who pursued his career to Obock and in Abyssinia, total more than 80,000 francs.[1]

[1] S.O.M. Missions 2 (Paris, Archives Nationales).

Despite all this, however, Brière de l'Isle sent his political director Captain J. S. Gallieni, who had succeeded Boilève, to pioneer the way toward the Niger and to re-establish contact with Ahmadou. Very little was known at that time about the Tukulor (Tokolor, Toucouleur) state, a Fula empire founded by El Hadj Omar (c. 1797–1864) in the first half of the nineteenth century. Omar was the son of a marabout, that is to say, a travelling Islamic preacher. He was educated in the teachings of the Tijaniyya, a Puritanical Muslim brotherhood with egalitarian leanings that wished to restore Islam to its pristine purity. Like other Muslim state-builders of this period, Omar obtained a good deal of support from the more mobile elements in Sudanic society, from traders and from the Muslim intelligentsia as against the more traditional leaders. He proved an able soldier, and his cavalry, well supplied with fire-arms, subdued a large area. Omar established control over the smaller Bambara and Mandingo communities in the upper Niger and upper Senegal valleys. Later he successfully warred against the larger Bambara states of Kaarta and Ségou; finally he established his capital in Ségou.

Omar tried to promote trade with the Atlantic region and to spread Islam among his subjects; but his fiscal exactions proved unpopular. Many of the conquered pagan peoples tried to reassert their traditional beliefs and ethnic identity against their overlords. There were dissensions within the ruling strata themselves, and the very size of the empire militated against its territorial cohesion. When Omar died in 1864, his son Ahmadou had to face numerous revolts. The Quadiri Fula of Machina were up in arms; so were the Bambara. Ahmadou's brother Aguibou, who ruled in Dinguiraye, was menaced by two rivals, Mahmadou Lamine, a Sarakole who in 1884 carved out a kingdom for himself between Faleme and the upper Gambia, and Samory, a Mandingo warrior and state-builder. Samory established himself at Kankan in 1879 and proved a formidable soldier. Samory, though far from being a Muslim fanatic or even a scholar, honoured the marabouts, professed to fight a jihad or holy war against the unbelievers and built mosques in the lands he conquered. His state, like Omar's, depended on the successful deployment of warriors wielding fire-arms, on the collection of tribute from the conquered and on foreign trade, including the traffic in slaves which continued to ravage parts of the area.

Gallieni hesitated about what line to take towards the Tukulor empire, menaced as it was by so many enemies. Was Ahmadou still sufficiently powerful to warrant the support of France, which could progressively extend her hegemony over the Sudan in alliance with Ahmadou? Or should the French precipitate his fall by encouraging uprisings on the part of the Mandingo and the Bambara, who were anxious to free themselves? Gallieni began by defeating a group of Tukulor at Sabouciré in 1878; and the following year he set up a fortified post at Bafoulabé, in spite of the protests of Ahmadou, who invoked the Mage treaty of 1886.

Gallieni then set off as envoy with 150 men and with presents for Ahmadou, at the same time representing himself to the Bambara as their protector against the Tukulor. But the Tukulor became suspicious when they saw that Gallieni was holding back his best presents. Thus, when, having passed Kita, he pursued his journey towards Ségou, he was attacked at Dio on 11 May 1880. He lost twenty men killed; twenty others were wounded, the baggage was lost, and the delegation reached Bamako in a sorry state. Ahmadou would not let him go on to Ségou and kept him in semi-captivity at Nango until Lieutenant Colonel G. Borgnis-Desbordes appeared with a relief column at Kita and set up a fort there (February 1881).

Negotiations begun at Nango led to a treaty of alliance by which, according to its Arab text, France promised to furnish arms to Ahmadou and to construct no forts on his territory. She received in exchange the exclusive right of establishing *comptoirs* and of opening trade routes between Senegal and the Niger. This policy of friendship would have sustained Ahmadou and would have extended the influence of France up to Timbuktu and the western limits of the Fouta Djallon, which were being guarded by Aguibou, brother of the Sultan of Ségou. But the Minister of Marine did not seek ratification of the treaty, for he did not wish to abandon those Mandingo and Bambara who had become allies of France or to destroy the forts of Bafoulabé and Kita. Nevertheless relations between France and the Tukulor empire remained officially cordial. France was thus enabled to turn her attention towards the Fouta Djallon, which she believed was coveted by the British, while the Tukulor became more and more preoccupied with the progress of Samory.

Borgnis-Desbordes, head of the Haut Fleuve district from 1880 to 1883, was a soldier to whom the new ideas about colonization were of no interest. To him Gallieni's political speculations were so much hot air. What really mattered was to reach Bamako and to win some victories in which the country might take pride. In 1882 the Minister of Marine, Admiral J. B. Jauréguiberry, gave him instructions to advance to Bamako. Later on he was to set up a post at Niagassola, between Kita and Bamako, thereby surrounding 'the Tokolor citadel of Mourgoula', which would ultimately fall by itself. Emir Abdallah, who ruled at Mourgoula, was a friend of France. He had maintained good relations with Valière, Bayol and Gallieni; he had not protested against the setting up of Kita, which had deprived him of various tributes from the Bambara. His city depended above all on caravan trade and was prosperous. In spite of all this, Borgnis disregarded his instructions and acted on his own initiative. In January 1882 he began by making a thrust towards the south in order to vanquish Samory, who had set out from Kankan and had begun to lay siege to Kéniéran. Encouraged by this success, Borgnis suddenly appeared in December before Mourgoula, summoned the Emir, and reproached him both for his tyrannical administration and for his relations with Samory. Abdallah and the notables of Mourgoula were taken completely off-guard by this show of force on the part of the French, whom they had considered to be allies. Unable to offer resistance, Abdallah and his leading dignitaries were forced to withdraw to Nioro, and were conducted there by Dr Bayol. Mountaga of Nioro received them with bad grace and protested violently against these abuses. But Mountaga was no more able to meet force with force than had been Abdallah. The letter by which he broke off relations with the French reached Borgnis at Bamako on 1 February 1883. Ahmadou, on whom both Mourgoula and Nioro were dependent, did not budge because Fabou, Samory's brother, was threatening Bamako. Titi, the Bambara chief of that city, thus welcomed the French with relief; and when Fabou had crossed the Niger he was beaten by the French on 12 April. But for Borgnis, Fabou would have taken Bamako. The most pressing danger for Ahmadou was Samory. Thus he allowed Borgnis to build a fort while Bayol and Lieutenant Quiquandon were concluding numerous treaties of protection in the Bélédougou area, between the Niger and the Baoulé. Here the French, under Commandants G. Boilève and A. Combes, who succeeded Borgnis, continued to make scattered gains between 1884 and 1885.

A new threat gave additional impetus to this piecemeal progress. A Sarakole marabout by the name of Mahmadou Lamine (Mamadu Lamina) resisted Samory's advance, seized Senoudébou and even ventured forth up to the very walls of Bakel. This imbroglio of inter-African disputes afforded the French an opportunity to play the role of arbiter. In 1885 Commandant H. Frey, trying once again to link politics with war, established French authority. He fought Samory near the small French fort of Niagassola on the Bakhoy, and threw back Mahmadou Lamine towards the upper Gambia, where Gallieni continued to pursue him until Mahmadou's death on 12 December 1887. At the same time Frey was carrying on negotiations with Ahmadou, who was being threatened by both. He thereby prepared the way for Gallieni, who returned in 1886 with the rank of lieutenant-colonel and the title of *Commandant supérieur du Soudan français*.

The three years of Gallieni's rule (1886–9) inaugurated a period of pacification during which Gallieni sketched out the system used in Tonkin and Madagascar that was later to bring him fame. His objectives were to make a show of strength in order not to have to use it, to give priority to politics over war, to encourage economic and cultural penetration by peaceful means, to keep alive the suspicions between black rivals, and to see to it that the British did not advance from Sierra Leone towards the Sudan via the Fouta Djallon. He succeeded in concluding successively treaties of peace, protection and commerce with the important chiefs who controlled the main caravan routes.

In March 1887 at Bissandougou Samory agreed to accept as boundaries with France the Tinkisso and the Niger. The region of Ouassalou south of the Niger was, however, treated as an exception and placed under a French protectorate. In May 1887 at Gouri, Ahmadou likewise accepted a rather vague French protectorate, without a resident, over the whole of his possessions. In March 1886 at Dinguiraye, Aguibou received a mission led by Captain Oberdorf, who promised him French protection without, however, getting him involved with Ahmadou, on whom he depended and with whom the French were negotiating at the time.

Politically speaking, all this remained rather vague. The French and Arab texts of the treaties did not always agree. The equilibrium remained unstable and required constant watching. The French, however, could hope for a stabilization that would permit gradual economic and cultural penetration. This would require time, continuity and active collaboration among the representatives of the civil administration who were advocating the new colonization. Unfortunately the financiers did not keep in step with the political theorists. Gallieni did not find any merchants who were willing to make the required investments to develop the Sudan. One of the few colonials who did help Gallieni was Dr Paul Colin, who stood out as a fine example of those Frenchmen who had more imagination than cash.

The conquest of the Sudan and of French West Africa was essentially the achievement of the military. The civilians who had sought adventure in the country had never succeeded in conquering it. The most curious attempt was undoubtedly that of Colin, who was active during the frustrating period between 1883 and 1888. These were the years when the French and Tukulor were eying one another while the spotlight of history was being turned upon the new figure of Samory, of whom it could not yet be said whether he was a friend or an adversary of the French. After the Conference of Berlin in 1885 the scramble for the coast took up most of the attention of the powers, while private explorers again ventured forth to the borderlands between the upper Senegal and the Ségou empire.

Colin had been an assistant surgeon in the navy, at posts at Bakel, at Medina and at Kita. He had seen the gold-dust brought by the caravans from Bouré. He knew about the trade routes used by these caravans to the upper Senegal or to the Rivières du Sud. He had heard the complaints of the traders of Medina against soldiers who were forever promoting military operations that shed glory upon themselves but that diverted caravans and hindered commerce. Like all explorers, Colin had a lively imagination with which he combined a deep patriotism and legitimate ambition. When the Commission for Exploration was set up in the French Admiralty, Colin offered to explore the Bouré. The Ministry gave him the 20,000 francs in grants that were at the disposal of Senegal. It also authorized him in vague terms to establish relations with the chiefs of the Bouré, 'the richest gold-bearing country of the West Sudan', to 'conclude treaties that would grant us the right to exploit the gold reefs, or at any rate authorize our nationals or people travelling under our flag to do business in the country, and would guarantee our security'.[1] With the help of the local authorities, he succeeded in reaching not Bouré, but Bambouk. But the military became alarmed when he went so far as to negotiate with Samory and sketched a grand design for encircling the Tukulor by means of a coalition comprising Samory, the rebels of Macina and the sheik of Timbuktu (August 1883). The Governor of Senegal reminded him that political matters were the

[1] S.O.M. Missions 2 (Paris, Archives Nationales); I, G, 65 and I, G, 108 (Dakar Archives).

province of the commandant of the Upper River and were not his concern. Be that as it may, Samory did not respond to his advances. Colin could do no more than sign treaties of protection with the chiefs of Tambura and of Diebedougou (November 1883); and he returned to France on bad terms with the military authorities.

Despite his good relations with the chiefs of Bouré and assumed support from the ministry, Colin vainly sought for capital to colonize the region he had explored. He wanted, at one and the same time, to set up a plantation, to install a *comptoir* at Kassama, the capital of Diebe- dougou, and to control gold production there. When Gallieni became commandant of the Upper River, he undertook to help Colin, to whom the cotton industry of Normandy had lent cloth with which to start his *comptoir*. Gallieni granted him a subsidy of 10,000 francs and promised him help in various forms—transport, food supplies, and troops—on condition that Colin would complete before 1 June 1888 a mission of exploration and of route-marking in the south of Bambuka, between Faleme and Bafing. However, made mistrustful by Colin's earlier activities, Gallieni gave him very precise instructions. These stipulated that the political initiative lay with the commandants of the posts of Bakel, Kayes, Medina and Bafoulabé, 'in that which concerns their relations with the chiefs of Bambouk', that he was not an 'official personage'. Once Colin's mission had been accomplished, he was not to count on any subsidy to assist the commercial operations that he was privately undertaking with the aim 'of halting (at Kassama) the caravans of the region that were bound for Gambia or Sierra Leone...to take away from English traders the export of the products of Bambuka and particularly of the gold that is abundant there'.[1]

Colin had more imagination than common sense. He chose his personnel badly. He suffered numerous vexations that for lack of space we cannot enumerate here. He committed the gross error of publishing in the home country articles hostile to military conquest and to Gallieni and styled himself an official 'representative of France'. He signed a treaty that gave him personally 'the rights of mining and commercial exploitation' of Diebedougou (January 1888), which France did not recognize. The mill-owners who, under the name of 'Société Flers exportation', had entrusted him with linens, calicoes and 'guineas' (a type of cloth), refused him the capital that would be

[1] S.O.M. Missions 2 (Paris, Archives Nationales); I, G, 65 and I, G, 108 (Dakar Archives).

required for the creation of depots and of a regular trading network. His topographical mission was limited to discovering 'the division of the Upper Faleme, which had been believed until this time to extend in a direct line towards Labé'.[1]

Colin returned home a ruined and disillusioned man. Colonel Archinard, Gallieni's successor, as a result of his dealings with Colin, had become decidedly hostile to any interference in the Sudan by traders. The Sudan thenceforth became the private hunting-ground of the military, whose troops were to pursue Samory for the next ten years.

The Congolese thrust

The exploration of the Congo basin coincided with military expansion in the Sudan. The initiative, however, did not lie with the government. Jauréguiberry, the Minister of Marine in 1880, was annoyed by the fuss that had been made over De Brazza and gave no thought to sending him back to Gabon. However, Leopold II, the King of the Belgians, who had founded the International African Association in 1876 and the Comité d'Etudes du Haut Congo in 1878, succeeded in securing for the latter the assistance of Stanley. He sent him secret instructions through Colonel Strauch, the secretary-general of the Association and president of the Comité. Stanley and Colonel Strauch met at Gibraltar in September 1879 when Stanley was on his way back from recruiting African troops and porters at Zanzibar for his new mission to the Congo. His orders instructed him to lay out a trail between the estuary and the Pool and to obtain rights of sovereignty from the black chiefs. In this way, free states would be created that could be joined in a federation, whose head would be named by the Committee.

De Brazza, much disturbed by the thought that the collaborators of Leopold might establish themselves on the Pool, approached the French Committee of the I.A.A. and the Geographical Society for funds to permit his return to Africa. Lesseps, the president of the Committee, proposed that De Brazza should choose the sites of one or two medical and scientific stations that the I.A.A. wished to found in West Africa. The Committee was not well endowed, and De Brazza did not have time to wait for the government to increase the subsidies he had been promised. He set off in haste, with 20,000 francs and with promises, but without written instructions, and, worse still, without any

[1] S.O.M. Missions 2 (Paris, Archives Nationales); I, G, 65 and I, G, 108 (Dakar Archives).

official assignment. Jauréguiberry did not dare, however, to refuse the Committee material help from the Gabon Colony in the form of troops, arms and scientific instruments. The explorer went up the Ogooué again and in June 1880 founded Franceville on the Passa; thence he wrote to the Committee asking that they send out at once Ensign Mizon, who had requested leave from the navy in order to join the Committee's service. After that, De Brazza reached the Lefini and once more met the Bateke chief, Makoko. On 10 September 1880 De Brazza, in the name of the French government, concluded a treaty with Makoko that gave France sovereignty over 'the country situated between the source and the mouth from Lefini to Ncouna' (on the Stanley Pool). Three weeks afterwards, on the Pool, he took over by a second treaty the concession where he wanted to establish a French post, leaving Sergeant Malamine and two native soldiers to guard the flag. Of all this he reported not a word to Stanley, whom he met subsequently at Vivi, nor to the Commandant of Gabon, where he arrived at the end of December. As Mizon had not yet come, he returned to await him at Franceville where he found letters from the Committee telling him that government support was not forthcoming.

Although the government was officially left in ignorance of De Brazza's activities, he sent several reports to the Committee, some of whose members were at the same time members of the Geographical Society or members of Parliament. Savants, deputies and admirals were thus aware of his activities, and it was doubtless at their instigation that the long, moving letter he wrote from Franceville in April 1881, expressing disappointment at receiving no support, was duplicated and distributed. The campaign in favour of the ratification of the treaties that he had not been empowered to sign was already well under way when he returned to France in June 1882.

During his isolation at Franceville, the explorer had occupied himself by opening up a passage between the Passa and the Alima, on which he wished to put the steam-launch that Dr Ballay, sent out by the Ministry of Public Instruction, was to bring him. Connexion would thus be ensured between Gabon via the Ogooué, Franceville, the Alima, the new passage and the post at Stanley Pool. Gabon would therefore become the outlet for the trade of all the central Congo basin. At length Mizon arrived; and, without authorization from the new commandant of Franceville, De Brazza left for the coast, revictualling Malamine en route. He discovered the route of Niari-Kouilou (Kwili), shorter even than that of the Ogooué, and returned to France completely exhausted.

De Brazza's lengthy reports of August 1882 pleaded for ratification of the treaties. Jauréguiberry, disgruntled at being confronted by a subordinate officer with a *fait accompli*, refused to allow his hand to be forced. The government had not charged De Brazza with acquiring territories in Central Africa, and it was aware that such acquisitions held forth no promise of appreciable economic advantage.

Between the months of July and November 1882, however, the political picture changed. In Egypt a nationalist party had been formed, and organized opposition to Franco-British financial control. Riots had broken out, and on 11 June a hundred Europeans were massacred at Alexandria. The British proposed to the French that a joint demonstration be made. Freycinet, the Prime Minister, could not obtain the necessary funds from the Chamber, since the need for haste prevented him from presenting himself as the representative of all the creditor powers. The British therefore intervened unilaterally, occupying Alexandria in July, and subsequently, after their victory of Tel-el-Kébir, Cairo and the Suez Canal (13 September). The Freycinet ministry was overturned in August and replaced by a ministry under Duclerc that lasted six months.

Public opinion strongly resented the expulsion of France from Egypt. Colonial circles deplored the evacuation of Matacong and the refusal of the government to occupy the territory of Obock. This region, though acquired in 1862, had not been developed despite frequent demands for concessions there by traders or adventurers attracted by the supposed resources of Abyssinia. In May, the Rivière expedition to Tonkin had met with disaster. Despite the success of the Tunisian affair, it seemed that France was retiring on all fronts.

Just at this moment, the Makoko treaty supervened. No great power was interested in the Congo at this point. The Quai d'Orsay, in ratifying the treaty, was not breaking with its traditional policy of *entente cordiale* with Britain. At the same time, nationalist sentiment acquired a new, immense colony to feed on. Then, instead of ratification by simple decree, as had been the custom for African protectorates, a great show was made. The Chamber was in raptures. Leopold II unwisely tried to block ratification. But he merely helped thereby to give wide circulation to the Epinal prints that popularized the heroes of the affair. In one scene De Brazza was portrayed coming forward in a chivalrous manner to shake the hand of Stanley, who had just delivered a lecture in Paris in English which made offensive and ironic remarks at De Brazza's expense. In another picture Malamine was shown in rags, under the tricolour, his arms crossed, barring passage to Stanley's well-equipped force. And a third scene portrayed the Bateke chiefs at Brazzaville receiving French flags from De Brazza's hands.

In spite of Leopold's effort to block 'the policy of penetration in Africa', the treaties were ratified (21 November 1882). Captain Cordier was sent out to sign treaties with the chiefs of Loango and Pointe Noire so that France would be assured control also of the route via Niari-Kouilou (March–June 1883). From that time on, rivalry persisted between Stanley and De Brazza, who had been sent back to Africa with the title of Government Commissioner in West Africa. A veritable steeplechase began between the two groups, each of the respective commanders sending out explorers to make treaties and to establish military posts. De Brazza began by concentrating his effort on the triangle bounded by the Ogooué, the Likouala and the Congo. Jacques de Brazza explored the valley of Likouala (1885–6). Dolisie disputed with the Belgians over the valleys of Niari-Kouilou, of the Sangha and of the Oubangui.

After the boundary on the Oubangui had been agreed upon in principle at the Conference of Berlin, De Brazza, in his capacity as General Commissioner of the government in the French Congo, together with Dr Ballay as Lieutenant-Governor of Gabon, concentrated his effort on the north. P. Crampel went up the Sangha, Fourneau up the Como to the Rio Muni in Spanish Guinea, and Dolisie up the Oubangui. Madame Coquery has just completed a critical history describing this huge movement of conquering exploration from 1883 to 1885. In a few years French and Belgian historians will have thrown a closer light on what lay behind the scenes of this conflict between eager protagonists.

The Congolese and Senegalese thrusts then began to merge. After 1890, projectors interested in the trans-Saharan and trans-African railroads distinguished between the Nigerian and the 'Chadian' Sudan, which they described as the French or the Black Indies. The Franco-British treaty, which drew a straight line on the map between Say on the Niger and Barroua on Lake Chad, had the effect of turning exploration activities towards Chad, the centre, so to speak, of a French bloc in tropical Africa that, in the words of Commandant Roumens, would set the boundary of 'Greater France at Dunkirk and Brazzaville'.

During his great journey of exploration between 1890 and 1892, Lieutenant Monteil prepared the way for the conquest. Starting out from St Louis, he reached Ségou, cut across the bend of the Niger by the Mossi country (Ouagadougou), then reached Lake Chad via Sokoto and the Bornu. Thence he struck directly northward to Tripoli by the caravan route. Crampel, for his part, attempting to reach Chad from the Congo, was massacred by the emissaries of the black Sultan Rabah (1891). It was a slow and painful process to reconnoitre the upper Sangha (De Brazza 1892 and Clozel 1894) and the country between Oubangui and Adamawa (Maistre 1892–3). Emile Gentil succeeded at length (1895–7) in joining the Oubangui to Chari and to Chad. It now became possible to mount the three great expeditions, which started respectively from southern Algeria (Foureau-Lamy), from the Niger (Joalland-Meynier) and from the Chari (Gentil); they then joined at Chad and defeated Rabah, who was killed on 22 April 1900 at Kôussari.

The advance along the coast

Though no great power protested against the French occupation of the Congo, the Portuguese were disturbed. They had historical claims to this coast, which they had discovered in the sixteenth century, and they had occupied Angola farther south. Their requests for information on the activities of Stanley were side-tracked by the Belgian government, which was not officially concerned in the projects of the I.A.A. On the other hand, Portugal had been negotiating since 1879 with Great Britain about the boundaries of Transvaal and Moçambique. She became more conciliatory when she found that she could count on British support on the Congo. An Anglo-Portuguese treaty, signed on 26 February 1884, recognized the sovereignty of Portugal over the coast between the parallels of latitude 5° 12' south and 8° south. The territory thus defined comprised the whole of the estuary and the lower Congo up to Nokki. As a jurist of the period said: 'King Leopold's domain has been put in a bottle and England has sealed it with a Portuguese cork.'

The Belgians in Leopold's entourage were not the only ones to protest. In England the shipowners, who were friendly to Leopold, and the Protestant missionaries were disturbed to see Catholic Portugal take control of their activities. The government did not persist with the treaty and did not ask Parliament to ratify it. But Bismarck, who was seeking a *rapprochement* with France, took advantage of the opportunity. Germany and France jointly invited the powers to an international conference with the aim of ensuring freedom of navigation on the Niger and the Congo, freedom of commerce in the Congo Basin, and of defining the formalities to be observed before fresh occupations on the African coast should be considered effective. The conference met from November 1884 to March 1885; behind the scenes the diplomats pursued the negotiations which led to the formation of the Congo Free State, laid down the principles of notification (of protectorate) and of effective occupation, and consequently impelled the interested parties to dispute the last unoccupied areas on the African coast.

It was obvious that matters would not rest there, and that the nations concerned would seek to gain control over the hinterlands which would make the coast worth having. To the French, dominated as they were by the idea of a solid mass of African territory that would link all their possessions between the Niger and the Congo, a joining of the coast settlements and the 'black Indies' was imperative. The treaty of August 1890, negotiated by the Quai d'Orsay behind the back of the under-Secretary of the Colonies, would halt French expeditions coming from the north on the line from Say to Barroua. But the colonies on the coast could serve as point of departure for the penetration from the south towards the rich countries of the Niger bend. The push inland from the coast between 1885 and the end of the century completed the French empire in tropical Africa.

First of all there was the brilliant mission of Gustave Binger, an officer who had served in Senegal and had become the collaborator of Faidherbe in Paris. In order not to arouse the attention of the British, he left Bamako in July 1887 in the direction of the Ivory Coast, where the French forts had been evacuated in 1871 and where France was represented by Marcel Treich-Laplène, the agent of the trading-firm of Verdier. Travelling alone, Binger reached Kong, where he failed to find the mountains alleged to exist by geographers. Treich-Laplène, who had in the meantime slipped out of Grand Bassam, joined him at Kong in January 1889. The two explorers returned to the coast with treaties of protectorate that allowed them to set up in 1893 the colony of the Ivory Coast, of which Binger was the first governor.[1]

[1] Paul Atger, *La France en Côte d'Ivoire de 1843 à 1893: cinquante ans d'hésitations politiques et commerciales* (University of Dakar, 1962), pp. 117–36; S.O.M. Missions 12 (Paris, Archives Nationales).

In the same year, Dr Bayol, who had explored Guinea from the coast to Timbo, became Governor of French Guinea and began the construction of the railway dreamed of by Olivier de Sanderval.

De Sanderval is certainly the most remarkable example of an engineer-explorer who worked on his own and whose failure was due more to want of official support than to the excesses of his imagination. He was born Aimé Olivier, studied at the Ecole Centrale and married the daughter of one of the Pastré brothers of Marseille, whose firm ran *comptoirs* on the coast of Portuguese Guinea. Drawing inspiration from the journey of Lambert to Timbo in 1860, he set out in 1879 at his own expense, and in June 1880 obtained from the Almamy Ibrahim Saury of Timbo, and in July 1881 from his successor, Ahmadou, a concession for a railroad into the Sudan. On his return, the Portuguese conferred on him the title of Comte de Sanderval.

The French government then ordered Dr Bayol to negotiate for a protectorate. But Bayol was forestalled by an English mission sent from Gambia to Sierra Leone under the direction of the administrator, W. S. Gouldsbury. The Almamy signed treaties of commerce and friendship with both (March 1881); but these agreements appeared of doubtful value to the experts of the Foreign Office and the Quai d'Orsay. Olivier afterwards made several voyages and obtained in 1888, in full sovereignty, a small territory of 200 square kilometres upon the plateau of Kahel. He proclaimed himself king and sought vainly for capital to construct his railroad. He had not succeeded in getting his rights recognized when Bayol, who was now Governor of Guinea at Conakry (1893), reached Timbo and set up a French protectorate there. Construction of the railroad began in 1897 with public funds.

In Dahomey, which offered the readiest means of penetrating through the jungle to the bend of the Niger, the French did not hesitate to declare war on Behanzin, the King of Abomey. Colonel Alfred Dodds directed these operations in 1892, starting from the 'Etablissements du Golfe de Bénin', which had been constituted in 1890 around Porto Novo and Cotonou, over which Behanzin had recognized French sovereignty. In 1893 the 'Etablissements du Golfe de Bénin' stretched as far as Abomey. Subsequent expeditions rapidly pushed towards the north, thereby extending the colony of Dahomey, formed in 1911, as far as the Niger. Lastly, Mauritania was explored and pacified by Coppolani between 1899 and 1904.

At the monent when this triple thrust had accomplished the formation of the African empire, there occurred the only serious crisis that obliged France to withdraw in the face of a foreign menace. The confrontation of Fashoda resulted rather from the want of coherence between the views of the Ministers of Foreign Affairs and of the Colonies, and from the unforeseen circumstances that delayed the progress of Marchand's column between 1895 and 1898, than from the espousal by government and public opinion of a project linking the French Sudan and Djibouti across the Egyptian Sudan. When A. A. G. Hanotaux at the Quai d'Orsay approved the mission to Djibouti in 1896, he saw it mainly as a means of reopening the Egyptian question. The British were not then in occupation of the Egyptian Sudan, which was in the hands of the Mahdists, who had revolted against the Khedive in 1883. The British, however, sent out Kitchener to crush the Mahdists, and subsequently he met Marchand at Fashoda in September 1898. The detailed history of the affair is now known. Despite the clash of chauvinistic sentiment, neither Hanotaux, and certainly not his successor T. Delcassé, ever seriously considered war with Britain. The agreement of 21 March 1899, which may be linked with that of 14 June 1898 on the northern boundary of Dahomey, was a prelude to the *Entente cordiale* of 1904. France had succeeded in penetrating into the Niger bend beyond the Say-Barroua line of the treaty of 1890. She had renounced any intention of intervening in the Egyptian Sudan, and had saved face.

The year 1898, which put an end to the great projects of expansion, is important in the history of French Africa. It may be considered also as the beginning of the intervention of large-scale capitalism in these colonies. The law authorizing chartered companies to be set up in the Congo appeared at long last to justify the views of Leroy-Beaulieu and of Jules Ferry on the necessity of colonization to the metropolitan economy.

Lastly, it was during this period that the great federations of French West Africa (1895) and French Equatorial Africa (1910) were organized. The problems of economic exploitation and of administration now came to the forefront. At the same time, the completion of the conquest, juridically described as 'pacification', imposed French domination on any Africans who might still resist.

Considered as a whole, this huge movement of expansion and conquest that took place between 1865 and the end of the century impresses us at first glance by a certain incoherence. Strictly speaking, during this period there was no such thing as colonial policy, much less an African policy. There was no general plan, only a series of projects often contradictory and by no means all the result of government initiative. Without the intervention of De Brazza, acting in an unofficial capacity, there would have been no French Equatorial Africa. The rivalries and the devious actions of the Minister of Marine or of the Colonies were often pursued behind the back of the Council of Ministers. If in the last analysis the Ministry of Foreign Affairs always had the final word and did not always ratify the *faits accomplis* with which it was presented, this does not efface the impression of disorder and of improvisation that the historian finds in the records of the archives.

Behind this incoherence, however, one finds a public opinion where apparent ebbs and flows are illusory. Actually public opinion was strongly united. In its deepest and most unconscious reflexes, it was the most profoundly patriotic public opinion that contemporary France had known. There was room for discussion on whether this or that conquest was opportune, on the methods of this or that pacification, on the abuses committed by this or that individual. But there was general accord on the need for France to take her place in the world, on the palpable superiority of Western civilization over the culture of primitive peoples, on the new greatness that the conquest of Africa brought to the nation and on the benefit that the blacks would derive from French rule.

If the adventurers, the traders large and small, the industrialists had hoped for profits, and indeed had sometimes realized their expectations, they generally did so only after much delay and at the expense of the official budget. During this first period of exploration and conquest there is no evidence of economic interests bringing pressure to bear on the government, certainly not to the extent that a historian may attribute an overriding initiative to such lobbies. The conquest of French tropical Africa was a political rather than an economic achievement. It resulted from a policy pursued without interruption by reason of its appeal to all Frenchmen, however sharply the French might have been divided by political questions at home.

BIBLIOGRAPHY

Atger, Paul. *La France en Côte d'Ivoire de 1843 à 1893: cinquante ans d'hésitations politiques et commerciales.* University of Dakar, 1962.

Berge, François. 'Le sous-secrétariat et les sous-secrétaires d'état aux colonies: histoire de l'émancipation de l'administration coloniale', *Revue Française d'Histoire d'Outre-Mer*, Paris, 1960, nos. 168–9.

Binger, L. G. *Du Niger au Golfe de Guinée par le pays de Kong et le Mossi, 1887–1889.* 2 vols. Paris, 1892.

Une vie d'explorateur: souvenirs extraits des carnets de route. Paris, 1938.

Brunschwig, Henri. *L'avènement de l'Afrique noire du XIXe siècle à nos jours.* Paris, 1963.

'Les cahiers de Brazza, 1880–1882', *Cahiers d'Etudes Africaines*, 1966, **6**, no. 22.

Mythes et réalités de l'impérialisme colonial français, 1871–1914. Paris, 1960.

'La négociation du traité Makoko', *Cahiers d'Etudes Africaines*, 1965, **5**.

Deschamps, Hubert. *Les méthodes et les doctrines coloniales de la France du XVIe siècle à nos jours.* Paris, 1953.

Désiré-Vuillemin, Geneviève. *Contribution à l'histoire de la Mauritanie de 1900 à 1934.* Dakar, 1962.

Gaffarel, Paul. *Les colonies françaises.* 6th ed. 2 vols. Paris, 1899.

Hargreaves, John D. *Prelude to the partition of West Africa.* London, 1963.

West Africa: the former French states. Englewood Cliffs, N.J., 1967.

Lambert, M. 'Voyage dans le Fouta-Djalon, exécuté d'après les ordres du Colonel Faidherbe, Gouverneur du Sénégal', *Le Tour du Monde*, 1861, **3**, no. 1.

Leroy-Beaulieu, Paul. *Le Sahara, le Soudan et les chemins de fer transsahariens.* Paris, 1904.

Mage, A. E. *Voyage dans le Soudan occidental (Sénégambie, Niger), 1863–1866.* Paris, 1868.

Méniaud, Jacques. *Les pionniers du Soudan, avant, avec, après Archinard, 1879–1894.* 2 vols. Paris, 1931.

Monteil, Parfait-Louis. *De Saint-Louis à Tripoli par le Tchad: voyage au travers du Soudan et du Sahara, accompli pendant les années 1890–91–92.* Paris, 1895.

Murphy, Agnes. *The ideology of French imperialism, 1871–1881.* Washington, D.C., The Catholic University of America Press, 1948.

Rivoyre, Denis de. *Mer Rouge et Abyssinie.* Paris, 1880.

Roumens, Etienne C. V. *L'impérialisme français et les chemins de fer transafricains.* Paris, 1914.

Saint-Martin, Yves. *L'empire toucouleur et la France: un demi siècle de relations diplomatiques (1846–1893).* Dakar, Faculté des Lettres et des Sciences Humaines, 1967.

Sanderson, G. N. *England, Europe and the upper Nile, 1882–1896.* Edinburgh University Press, 1965.

Sanderval, Aimé Olivier, vicomte de. *De l'Atlantique au Niger par le Foutah-Djallon: carnets de voyage.* 2nd ed. Paris, 1883.

Conquête du Foutah-Djallon. Paris, 1899.

Soudan français: Kahel, carnet de voyage. Paris, 1893.

Schnapper, Bernard. *La politique et le commerce français dans le Golfe de Guinée de 1838 à 1871.* Paris, Ecole Pratique des Hautes Etudes, 1961.

Sebillot, Amédée. *Le transafricain: les grandes lignes commerciales de la Méditerranée au Golfe de Guinée et à l'océan Indien.* Paris, 1893.

Soleillet, Paul. *Voyage à Ségou, 1878–1879, rédigé d'après les notes et journaux de voyage de Soleillet par Gabriel Gravier.* Paris, 1887.

CHAPTER 5

FRENCH COLONIZATION IN AFRICA TO 1920: ADMINISTRATION AND ECONOMIC DEVELOPMENT

by CATHERINE COQUERY-VIDROVITCH

On the eve of the partition of Africa, about the year 1880, tropical Africa was almost entirely independent. Thirty-five years later, the two federations of French West Africa and French Equatorial Africa were well constituted colonies, administered by an organized cadre of colonial officials. Great trading societies covered the country with a network of stations the general lines of which would not thereafter be modified. Subsequent policies or reforms were often no more than the application of previous decisions or simple changes of detail. The basic structure of the colonial edifice was firmly established from that time on; and it remained either to profit from the achievements or to pay for the mistakes of a system whose genesis belonged entirely to the first period of colonialism, 1880–1920.

Apart from an active minority of convinced expansionists, metropolitan public opinion, although favourable to a policy of African grandeur, had not adopted the colonial idea without reservations. Statesmen who for many years had supported the device of protectorates disliked the cost of a forward policy, while businessmen feared excessive control from the metropolis. Thus the country, taken unawares by the rapidity of its conquests, lacked the required policy-making and executive cadres.

The Ministry of Marine was of course the traditional protector of the colonial *comptoirs*, but its organization, entirely military, was demonstrably outmoded and its officials were overwhelmed with work. Within a few years, the authorities had to improvise a specialized staff belonging to an independent ministry. Being forced to innovate, the first pacifiers (Brazza in the Congo, Binger in the Ivory Coast, Ballot in Dahomey) were led to replace naval officers by civilians, who, in that time of extreme nationalism, were no less attached to the honour of the flag than the sailors, but were freer of routine and more attentive to economic problems. At the same time the advocates of capitalist colonization, whether defenders of the liberalism dear to the Senegalese colonists or supporters of the great colonial companies of the Congo, asked Paris to create a colonial organization of a new type more suited to their purposes. The struggle for power between the civilians and military, between businessmen and the armed forces, dominated the period during which colonial rule was set up. The civilians prevailed; but their doctrine had yet to be worked out. It was only after much groping and many contradictory experiences that the French established, from the administrator in the bush to the man at the top of the federal hierarchy, that uniformity of cadre and that organization of the territories which symbolized their famous assimilative centralism.

West Africa, gradually organized around the old prosperous Senegalese *comptoir*, became a model colony, where the firmness of administration justly tempered the dynamism of a trading economy. Equatorial Africa, on the other hand, a wretched field for unfortunate improvisations, was left without effective control to businessmen who were more often than not ill-informed and short of capital, and whose activities would soon show the failings of an excessively harsh and coercive system.

THE BEGINNINGS OF THE ADMINISTRATION: THE MINISTRY OF COLONIES AND ITS STAFF. In 1880 the conquest of the Senegalese hinterland had barely begun. On the frontier of Samory's territory, power remained in the hands of the military. Samory was a Diula ruler who founded a great empire around Ségou in the Sudan between the Kong and the Niger; he was not captured until 1898. Along the Bight of Benin, the 'French establishments on the Gold Coast and along Gabon', supervised by the head of the naval division of the West African coast, counted for little. They comprised a mere handful of traders and a few more or less neglected fortified posts. Direct administration by the admiralty was considered a guarantee of honesty and security.

At the very beginning of the imperialist era, however, the first effort was made to free the direction of the colonies from admiralty control. In 1881, at the moment when Francis Garnier reached Hanoi, when Jules Ferry occupied Tunisia, and when Brazza carried out his second mission to the Congo, Gambetta set up the Ministry of Trade and Colonies. The Under-Secretary of State for the Colonies, Félix

Faure, a businessman and a leading member of Le Havre Chamber of Commerce, represented the interests of this seaport in the same way as his minister, M. Rouvier (later an influential member of the Colonial Party), represented those of Marseille. Crude and premature as it was, his effort had no future. It did not diminish the antagonism that existed between the businessmen, who were pacifist through self-interest, and the naval officers, who by reason of their calling professed a haughty nationalism. The vested interests were determined not to be displaced. The suggestion of a link with the Ministry of Commerce was not renewed before 1889; and twelve years were to pass before the French authorities (by the law of 14 March 1894) created the Ministry of Colonies.

Nevertheless, the death knell of Ministry of Marine supremacy was sounded with the second Jules Ferry ministry (1883–5). In the new cabinet Félix Faure now addressed himself to ensuring the autonomy of the new civilian form of government and entrusted the study of projected reforms to the Conseil Supérieur des Colonies. This was a consultative body that since 1893 had included the senators and deputies from overseas, elected delegates from other colonies, as well as higher officials and leading men of affairs. The Minister of Marine could thus no longer control the activity of a subordinate whose authority had extended in ten years over numerous governors, enormous territories and a variety of peoples; and in the end the minister refused to bear the sole constitutional responsibility.

The decisive change resulted from the conquest and organization of Indochina, which allowed Eugène Etienne, at that time Under-Secretary of State for the Colonies, to establish, in 1887, the framework of the new ministry. But it was in Black Africa that a new type of colonial civil servant first appeared on the scene. In Senegal, established traders like the directors of the Société Maurel and Prom or of the Compagnie Française d'Afrique Occidentale (C.F.A.O.) actively supported the business-deputies who, in Paris, stood for the primacy of economic and social considerations over political or military imperatives.

In 1883 the crisis broke out over the Congo. Then, and for the first time, the conflict was resolved in favour of the civilians. The government was well aware that public opinion, rendered restive by the costly pacification campaign of 1881 in Tunisia, was still hostile to colonial conquest. The authorities were determined to avoid in the Congo the difficulties that had been made inevitable by the military in Tonkin.

Hence a civilian mission was entrusted with the task of maintaining the French presence in Equatorial Africa. The 'West African Mission', directed by Brazza, a naval officer detached from the service for the occasion, was to set up a score of stations that 'would spread out in all directions and would make known in a short time the country, its products, its needs, its means of communication; would train inter-preters and would establish the best relations with the local population, etc...'[1] These economic and scientific objectives were made a pretext for placing the mission under the exclusive control of the Ministry of Public Instruction.

The defeated navy viewed the triumphant role played by Brazza with disfavour. The Commander of Gabon declared bluntly that 'the presence of the Mission...on the territory of the colony [was] contrary to the general good of the service'[2] and refused to collaborate. In 1884 these shabby quarrels all but brought about the failure of the expedition. Three ministries (Public Instruction, Marine and Foreign Affairs) all became involved. An urgent choice became necessary between two contradictory conceptions: traditional occupation resting on scattered fortified posts, or effective occupation requiring the governance of native tribes, who hitherto had been ignored. Brazza succeeded in getting the second solution adopted, but he could not prevent the new colony from being placed under the Ministry of Marine.[3]

Thereafter, a civil administration had to be improvised. The new post of Commissaire, afterwards Commissaire-Général of the Government, was created for Brazza. This title, which the authorities had also intended to confer on a proposed governor for Obock,[4] revealed the transitory character of the organization. The administrative personnel was of the most miscellaneous kind. In a short space of time Brazza had to recruit sufficient staff to occupy territories as large as France; and in the absence of an existing service he was forced to rely on his connexions with the geographical societies and on the advertisement columns in the newspapers. Attracted by the explorer's reputation,

[1] J. L. Dutreuil de Rhins, text of his lectures to the Sociétés de Géographie, *Fonds Brazza*, 3rd mission, II, Archives Nationales, Section Outre-Mer.

[2] Commandant Cornut-Gentille to Minister of Marine, 7 Aug, 1884. *Gabon–Congo*, III, 6(b), Archives Nationales, S.O.M.

[3] He tried in vain to have West Africa put under the Quai d'Orsay. *Fonds Brazza*, 3rd mission, III.

[4] Freycinet, Minister of Foreign Affairs, to Jauréguiberry, Minister of Marine, 5 April 1882, *Mémoires et Documents, Afrique*, LXIV, 234, Archives des Affaires Etran-gères.

by a taste for adventure, or by a more trivial desire for gain, all manner of men—journalists, students, lawyers, engineers, people of the most diverse backgrounds—sent in their applications.[1] Many of these recruits had to be dropped. Thieves, drunkards or incompetents were sent back to France. When Brazza left the colony in 1885, he was forced to keep officials on the job beyond their agreed eighteen-month period of employment. He could only achieve his aim by appealing to the loyalty of civil servants who were now better selected but physically exhausted.[2]

The authorities could not go on indefinitely in this haphazard fashion. The presence of civilians overseas compelled the government to define their status and to regulate their recruitment. The projects that Félix Faure had not had time to complete included one for a school of administration serving Indochina. When in 1888 Faure once again became Under-Secretary of State, he was at first content to rename the former Cambodian mission (now reserved to colonial students) 'Ecole Coloniale'. This became the future *section indigène* of the institution that P. Dislère, by means of the *décret organique* of 22 November 1890, turned into a great school of administration to serve the entire empire. Between 1893 and 1894, Guinea, the Ivory Coast, the French Sudan and Dahomey, the new colonies of Black Africa, all began to draw on the Ecole Coloniale for officials.

For a long time, however, graduates from the school remained in a minority among French colonial administrators. The first high officials obtained their training on the spot, including Brazza and his companion Noël Ballay, a navy medical officer, V. Ballot, a former minor official, and others. In 1907, out of 489 officials in French Black Africa, there were 200 men with university degrees or their equivalent; of these only 70 came from the Ecole Coloniale.[3] Symbol of imperial unity, the Ecole trained the senior officers. Herein lay both its glory and its weakness. The French had aimed at creating at one stroke a unique institution, a school devoted to the training of officials who should be interchangeable and versatile, capable of exercising the most diverse functions (administrative, judiciary, etc.) throughout the empire. The immensity of this empire and its diverse character—with a

[1] *Fonds Brazza*, 3rd mission, v.
[2] The French system of commissioners makes a very interesting parallel with the commissioners under the British Foreign Office in both West and East Africa at this time.
[3] Note 2, Association Professionnelle des Administrateurs des Colonies, *Bulletin*, 13 July 1907.

black or Moslem world in Africa and an Asian world in Indochina—made this enterprise a gamble. It had 'the enormous inconvenience of being a perpetual incitement to join, to assimilate, what ought to have been kept separate or conceived as different'.[1] Hence, teaching at the Ecole was concerned almost exclusively with general culture, initially to the detriment of the study of those civilizations in the midst of which the future official would have to serve.

The French approach thus differed fundamentally from that of the British, who had no Ecole Coloniale and who, from the very beginning, had distinguished between areas that were geographically and ethnographically distinct. The members of the Indian Civil Service were drawn from the great British universities. Eclecticism was the rule in the choice of British administrators in Black Africa. The Colonial Office first considered the background, the experience, and the recognized qualifications of the candidate. Then it evaluated reports on the candidate from former employers, and it judged on the impression made by the applicant at interviews. Though British pragmatism did not exclude a certain amount of favouritism, it had the great advantage of encouraging the colonial civil servant to make his career on the spot, and thus went contrary to that passion for centralization and administration ('no promotion without a transfer') that dominated the French colonial administration for many years.

THE 'BROUSSARD', THE HEAD TAX AND NATIVE POLICY. Colonial government depended on that jack-of-all-trades, the *broussard*, or district officer. Set at the head of a huge *circonscription* (the 'circle' introduced by Faidherbe), the *broussard* held all powers of administration, justice and police over several thousand people, for whom he was the sole link with higher authority. This combination of executive and judicial power was of course nothing new to Africans, whose chiefs were at once leaders and guarantors of public order. In African eyes, however, the *commandant* seemed in practice to have only one objective —the collection of taxes. This was an ungrateful task to which the administration attached much importance. In the first place, the colonies were poor. But according to contemporary doctrine, they were supposed to be self-sufficient. Once conquered, a country was thus promptly subjected to a head tax. This impost, together with the customs duties, was the sole form of local revenue. Taxation, moreover, was for a long

[1] Emile Gaston Boutmy, *Le recrutement des administrateurs coloniaux* (Paris, 1895), p. 115.

time the only means of economic development used by the metropolitan country in its overseas dependency. Initially the French imagined that if they would only create new needs for the Africans, the indigenous people would go out to work. When this did not happen, the French introduced taxes so as to make Africans earn wages.

Between 1900 and 1910 the head tax was introduced everywhere. In Haute-Sangha in the French Congo the first levy was made in 1898 (producing 37,000 francs and a ton of rubber). In the Ivory Coast, an order dated 4 May 1901 assessed 'the contribution due from each native inhabitant, man, woman and child aged ten or over' at 2.50 francs per year. The authorities imposed taxes in money so as to encourage the introduction of a modern cash economy; but at first rubber, ivory, gold or any other product was accepted at market price. The district officer assumed the complex and formidable task not only of making a census of the taxable population, but also of collecting the taxes and of selling the revenue paid in kind through commercial channels.

In Equatorial Africa, the need to make good the alarming financial deficit of the colony caused Commissaire-Général Gentil to address to his staff the notorious circular of 19 March 1903: 'I shall not hide from you that my opinion of your performance will rest chiefly on the results that you obtain with respect to the native tax [3 francs a head], which should be the object of your constant attention.'[1] This opened the door to all the abuses already practised in the Congo Free State, where the district officer was also responsible for the production of rubber. Ordered to find money, officials found it by force. Villages were terrorized through searches conducted by Senegalese troops; recalcitrant natives were beaten with rawhide whips; forced labour was used to transport the produce. When to this was added, as in Chari, the obligation of provisioning the Chad troops, to the tune of 3,000 loads per month of 25 to 30 kilograms a head, the moral pressure experienced by district officers caused some of them to employ illegal means, such as summary executions or the taking of hostages.

The result was flight from, or revolt against the *commandant*, who had become an object of fear. As late as 1911 the Gouro refused to pay taxes, to supply carriers, or to execute *corvées*. Large-scale pacification campaigns alarmed the people affected to such an extent that they

---

[1] *L'Humanité*, 27 Sept. 1905. The rate of the tax was fixed at 3 francs by the circular issued by Gentil on 19 July 1904, which forecast its being raised to 5 francs on 1 Jan. 1905; but this measure was not applied until 1908 (circular of 3 Sept. 1907).

scattered into the jungle and were not disarmed until 1914. In Equatorial Africa, from the time of the passage of the Marchand expedition and the Gentil troops (1897) to 1920, more or less widespread uprisings were continual. Insurrections broke out in the Sangha in 1904, in the Lobaye between 1904 and 1907, in the Oubangi between 1906 and 1907, in the Woleu-Ntem, the Upper Ngounié and the Lobaye between 1908 and 1910, in Mayombe between 1909 and 1911, in Ivindo and the Middle Ogooué. 'Although the French conquest of Equatorial Africa was essentially peaceful, this did not preclude a long and arduous work of pacification.'[1]

Under these conditions, it was difficult for the district officer to win over the population by a coherent native policy; yet he was the only one in a position to do so. One of the major concerns of the colonial administration was to harmonize French law with local institutions. Such a policy presupposed a knowledge of local conditions on the part of the only man who was in continual contact with the Africans. This the first explorers had generally possessed. Enthusiasts for the discovery of a new world, they described it with a degree of precision and care in ethnographic matters that was remarkable for the time (for instance, the reports of the members of Brazza's West African expedition).[2] There were worthy successors among the next generation of officials. The most eminent were Georges Bruel and above all Governor Maurice Delafosse, whose work on the Upper Senegal–Niger region for a long time stood unsurpassed, and whose translations of Arab texts were among the leading contributions to African studies, then in their infancy. Some reports that have remained unpublished were no less remarkable; they were the fruit of numerous tours of duty, often long and arduous but always fruitful when they had not the purpose of levying taxes.[3] But these studies, which generally were not undertaken before World War I, derived their value entirely from the personal qualifications of the administrator. The general assumption was that the native was an overgrown child, idle and turbulent, who needed above all to be subdued and disciplined. The special qualities of African civilizations were either unknown or they were described in terms of cruel or stupid superstitions that should be wiped out. This

[1] H. Ziegle, *L'Afrique équatoriale française* (Paris, 1952), p. 100.
[2] *Fonds Brazza*, 3rd mission, VII.
[3] 'Tours undertaken solely for the purpose of making a visit and getting better acquainted with conditions', recommended by Governor-General of French Equatorial Africa Merlin, circular of 1 Aug. 1909, J.O., p. 259.

misunderstanding led the men on the spot to favour Islam, for the conquest of Algeria had already accustomed the French mind, with its devotion to order and logic, to a civilization whose apparent uniformity was more attractive than 'the mysterious rumbling of the religions derived from the soil'.[1]

In any case, the goodwill of the colonial officials was powerless in face of the French passion for direct administration. Native policy consisted most often in eliminating traditional authorities, which were mistrusted. Administrative chieftainships were instead given to docile leaders, who were shunted aside in their turn as time went on. At first the rapidity of conquest had obliged the French to use existing local governments. But from 1900 onwards the authorities began to favour the elimination of the great chiefs, who were gradually replaced by French officials. The authority of the chiefs was fragmented 'to the point where the village became the administrative entity'.[2] In 1900 the kingdom of Abomey was suppressed and King Agoliagbo was deposed, though he had been appointed by the French. King Makoko, whose prestige was undiminished in the eyes of the Bateke, was forgotten once he had ceded his territory and the French had no further need of him. It is true that the authorities continued to make use of solidly organized kingdoms such as the Mossi, the Abron and the Agni. Where such polities existed, the *chefs de canton* were usually chosen from the great hereditary families. But since the administration lacked personnel, it had to rely on the *chefs de village* for maintaining contact with the people. These lowly dignitaries, poor devils, were carefully selected and held responsible for the family heads. They became ill-paid, petty functionaries, miserable despots, charged with imposing taxes, forced porterage and *corvées*. Deprived of their former prestige, they had no authority of their own, for 'there are not two authorities in the circumscription, the French authority and the native authority; there is only one. The district officer alone commands and alone is responsible. The native chief is simply a tool or an auxiliary.'[3]

[1] P. Alexandre, 'L'Islam en Afrique noire', *Marchés Tropicaux du Monde*, 12 Oct. 1957, no. 622, p. 2385.
[2] Rapport d'ensemble de la Guinée française en 1906, Conakry, 1907, as quoted by Jean Suret-Canale, *Afrique noire, occidentale et centrale*, vol. II: *L'ère coloniale, 1900–1945* (Paris, 1964), p. 96.
[3] Circular of 15 Aug. 1917, in *Une âme de chef, le Gouverneur général J. Van Vollenhoven: à la mémoire du capitaine J. Van Vollenhoven, Gouverneur général des colonies, tué à l'ennemi* (Paris, 1920), p. 207.

Because of transport difficulties and delays in communication, the greatest possible political initiative was left to the district officer. Having been invested with absolute power, subject only to the tardy control of the governor, he tended to turn his circumscription into a personal fief, with 'his' natives, 'his' guards, 'his' agricultural officer. The system inherently generated abuses. It was imprudent to leave the task of directing so vast a territory to men who, though often enthusiastic and capable, did not always have sufficient education or the qualities of mind required to exercise an authority founded on coercion. In 1905 scandals going back to 1903 came to light in the Congo: three administrators of Fort-Crampel, the starting-point of the portage to Chad, were implicated. One, Proche, had caused two Africans who had fled on the arrival of the guard to be shot without trial. A second, G. Toqué, had allowed a black man guilty of stealing a few cartridges to be drowned. The third, Gaud, was accused of having, with Toqué's complicity, made a 'boy' drink a soup made from a skull and of having blown up a prisoner with dynamite, as a way of celebrating Bastille Day.[1] The trial caused a great stir. It occasioned a mission of inspection by Brazza and a virulent press campaign in France; but the affair, which was connected with the problem of concessionary companies, was suppressed when the Chamber of Deputies refused to publish the report of the mission. This was not an isolated example; André Gide in *Voyage au Congo* bore witness to the same sort of thing as late as in 1927.

However that may be, the doctrine was henceforth established: the power of the *commandant* symbolized the triumph of direct administration. From the local chief to the governor-general, by way of the administrator of the subdivision, the administrator of the circumscription, and the governor of the colony, French authority was organized in a strictly hierarchical pyramid; the African seldom played any part in it except at village level.

THE FEDERATIONS. After the federations of French West Africa and French Equatorial Africa had been set up, French Africa was unified in its higher administration as well as in its personnel. From 1895 onwards in West Africa, and from 1908 in Equatorial Africa, the governors of individual colonies were subordinated to a governor-general. This

[1] *Le Temps*, 23 Sept. 1905, as quoted in Jules F. Saintoyant, *L'affaire du Congo, 1905* (Paris, 1960).

policy was adopted partly on account of the influence of the Indo-chinese Union, but mainly because of successive local experiences. The origins of French West Africa, which developed from a number of distinct colonies towards a more unified association, differed essentially from those of French Equatorial Africa. Right to the end, French Equatorial Africa oscillated between the most complete union of its territories and the most liberal autonomy for each of them.

From its very beginning, French West Africa experienced a tenacious rivalry between the civilians of Senegal and the military of the barely-pacified zones of the upper river. The federal constitution of 1895 is revealing in this respect. The new governor-general, Chaudié, who was still also governor of Senegal, was given authority only over the military powers of the lieutenant-governors of the colonies and of the Sudan. He lacked financial means and was assisted only by a Conseil de Gouvernement, composed of administrators and officers from Senegal, without any representatives from the other territories. Chaudié therefore had no powers to handle the political or military differences between the colonies. But on 17 October 1899 a new decree divided the Sudan territory between the neighbouring colonies in order to end the 'very human tendency which leads combat officers to seize the occasion to distinguish themselves by actions which are always glorious but frequently useless'.[1] This was 'the beginning of the era reserved to traders and engineers'.[2] Henceforth, successive governors-general, free from responsibility for Senegal itself, succeeded in whittling away the power of their subordinates and began to turn the over-loose and lax Federation into a more and more solid and coherent whole. The governorship-general was at last set on solid financial bases by the decrees of 1902 and of 18 October 1904, which assured to it the revenue from all indirect taxation—including the consumption tax (in fact a covert import duty). The governors-general were now in a position to promote a true economic federation capable of planning and financing public works such as railroads and ports. This was the principal advantage of French West Africa. The chief weakness of this arrangement was that it ignored the most elementary demographic and ethnic requirements. It aimed to impose peace and French civilization on a

[1] Final report of the federal commission to the Minister of Colonies, Sept. 1899, as quoted in Colin W. Newbury, 'The formation of the government general of French West Africa', *Journal of African History*, 1960, I, no. I, pp. 111–28.
[2] Report by Destenave, Commandant of the Eastern Macina, to the Minister of Colonies, Paris, 1899, as quoted in Newbury, 'French West Africa', p. 119.

territory nine times as big as the metropolis and peopled by about twelve million inhabitants, unevenly scattered from the dense forests to the fringes of the desert. It was only between the two world wars that the vanity of this ideal began to be apparent.

The same preoccupation with uniformity led somewhat later and more hesitantly to the creation of French Equatorial Africa. There the task appeared even more complex. From the Congolese jungle to the Sahel of Chad, vast climatic and cultural disparities and almost insurmountable difficulties of travel rendered anomalous the peripheral position of the successive capitals (Libreville, and after 1903 Brazzaville). In face of the country's poverty, the want of organization among its people, and the inexperience of the great companies charged with its development, the only resource of the State was administrative reform, a policy which it pursued vigorously. From 1883 to 1910 there were some eight reorganizations. In contrast to French West Africa, organized around Senegal, French Equatorial Africa, already handicapped by a deplorable economic system, suffered from the lack of an appropriate administrative structure. The authorities were content to imitate either their Congolese neighbour, whose success after 1895 aroused the envy of all, or, after the régime of concessionary companies had broken down, the model of West Africa.

In 1881, there was as yet no question of making Gabon into an independent colony. The *comptoir* of Gabon was economically negligible. It barely managed to subsist on a metropolitan grant in aid of its meagre import duties, totalling altogether less than 300,000 francs annually. The establishment of the new colony of 'West Africa' finally led to the suppression of the military régime in Gabon. In 1886 the colony was put under a lieutenant-governor, subject to the commissary general. But the powers of the lieutenant-governor were ill-defined. Brazza was a bold explorer, but a reckless, domineering man and a poor administrator. His collaborator therefore could not cope with muddle and lack of discipline. In 1897 the authorities therefore embarked on a policy of complete unification. However, the adoption of a common budget, which was also inadequate for its purpose, proved disastrous. The revenues were all spent on the occupation of new territories (Chari and Chad). The French experienced similar difficulties in Senegal and the Sudan; and the commissary of Chad, invested with exceptional military powers, enjoyed too much freedom of action. The reform of 5 July 1902 restricted his powers by decreeing that the autonomous budget of Chad should be submitted for the approval of the commissary general.

Under the influence of the example of French West Africa, the authorities in 1903 began looking for a federal solution to the problem. The commissary-general was placed at the head of the colony of Middle Congo, but was relieved of the direct administration of the other territories (Gabon colony, Oubangui-Chari, and Chad). The profound shock of the Gaud and Toqué scandal once more produced a sharp reversal of policy. The existing system perforce left too much freedom to the local administrator. Hence reform was sought by strengthening the hand of the commissary-general, who in 1908 became Governor-general of French Equatorial Africa. French Equatorial Africa thus always followed in the wake of French West Africa. In the beginning of the century, Equatorial Africa had imitated West Africa's policy of decentralization. When French West Africa adopted a new course, Equatorial Africa again followed the leader. The French therefore at last managed to ensure the unity of an empire that aimed at an identical system of government, no matter whether in Indochina or in Africa.

Economic development in French West Africa

Dissimilarities in natural conditions and in methods of economic development made the two federations fundamentally different. French West Africa formed an unequal whole, but conditions were relatively favourable both from the climatic and economic points of view. To the products gathered by Africans (rubber, palm-kernels) were soon added export crops, especially ground-nuts, which were to make the fortune of the colony. French traders who had long been established on the coast (Maurel and Prom in the Senegal, Verdier on the Ivory Coast, V. Régis—afterwards Mantes and Borelli—in Dahomey) remained faithful to the economic liberalism that had made their fortunes. They knew how to make use of the 'French peace', and in their hands the federation became a remarkable instrument of economic advance.

In French West Africa the administration was all-powerful. In French Equatorial Africa, on the other hand, the authority of officials remained uncertain and limited until a relatively late date. At least until 1910, power lay in the hands of enormous but disreputable monopolistic companies organized on the model of the Belgian Congo: The policy of scuttle adopted by the government completely paralysed the economy.

THE TRADING HOUSES. The establishment of colonies facilitated the development of West Africa, but economic life retained the spirit inherited from the age of the *comptoir* and of the coast trade. The merchants had dealt first in slaves, then in ivory, gold or gum. Later they had turned to palm produce, peanuts and cocoa. Anxious only to get the maximum immediate advantage by all possible means, the trader had no interest in the organization of production, which was left in the hands of the Africans. Installed in his 'factory', at once office, trading-post, and wholesale and retail outlet, the merchant paid out as little money as possible and recovered most of it promptly at his shop, stocked with imported goods.

For a long time the most celebrated trading house in Senegal was that of Maurel and Prom, who in the nineteenth century had started to deal in ground-nuts. In the same way the firm of Régis promoted on the Slave Coast the commerce in palm-oil. The firm of Maurel kept pace with the extension of French control over the country, set up agencies or traders, developed the traffic in rubber in Sudan, and carried its activities as far as the Niger (gums, peanuts, and later cotton). In 1923 the company had 150 *comptoirs* in West Africa, together with 60 ships; and its wharves were found wherever coastal or river navigation was practicable.

It was mainly at the very end of the nineteenth century that economic imperialism began to flourish. In 1887 the Compagnie Française d'Afrique Occidentale, with a capital of 30 million francs, replaced the Company of Senegal and the West African Coast, founded in 1881 by a businessman from Marseille. In 1906, the S.C.O.A. (Société Commerciale de l'Ouest Africain) with a capital of 3 million francs, took over the house of Ryff, Roth and Company, which had managed several 'factories' since 1899, and gradually covered the whole of French West Africa with a closely-knit network of establishments. The French Company of the Niger, whose powerful resources—its capital was largely British —would make it one of the three 'greats' of Black Africa, was founded in 1913. Commercial expansion stimulated banking: from 1901 onwards the B.A.O. (Banque d'Afrique Occidentale), with E. Maurel as chairman of the board of directors, extended the hitherto modest operations of the former Bank of Senegal. In this period firms of a modern type accordingly made their appearance. They soon dominated the colonial economy by purchasing the export crops, by distributing imported merchandise such as cloth, spirits, ironmongery and canned goods, and by controlling their prices through mutual agreement. These enterprises rested on a 'singularly primitive and sluggish trading economy'.[1] Between 1900 and 1914 eleven trading societies were founded in French Tropical Africa, compared with only three plantations, two forestry, two mining and four transport companies. They nevertheless represented a considerable investment: the total capital involved was estimated in 1916 at 1,112,000 francs, of which 403,000 francs was placed in trading companies and 257,000 in the timber trade.

PUBLIC WORKS. At the close of the century the private companies, whose rising power was to weigh more and more heavily on the colonial administration, were operating only on the coast or along the rivers. The expansion of these enterprises depended on means of communication: the Senegal river was navigable for only two to three and a half months out of twelve, and the other colonies were without any great waterways. The growth of the rubber trade and the extension of cultivated areas in the Sudan opened up possibilities for additional business, once the system of human porterage was replaced by more effective and less costly means of transport. Mercantile interests therefore played a major role in the policy of great railroad works undertaken after 1890.

Up to the end of the century, the state had put its faith in private capital, and it did not intend to modify this policy. Railway entrepreneurs, more often than not, had taken their chance 'at their own risk and peril'. Even after the beginning of the imperialist era, public opinion objected to sinking money in Africa, and until the First World War successive Chambers had cut down colonial budgets to the minimum. Trading companies applied a similar doctrine: their policy was mercantilist; their objective, immediate profits. However, while during the previous century France had imported more from the colonies than she had exported to them, the trend was suddenly reversed: West Africa absorbed more products than she sent out, and could only pay with money furnished by the metropolitan country,

[1] Jean Dresch, 'Sur une géographie des investissements de capitaux: l'exemple de l'Afrique noire', *Bulletin de l'Association des Géographes Français*, Jan.–Feb. 1946, nos. 177–8.

which 'employed in judicious investments would bring in ultimate returns'.[1] But once the assumption had been accepted that colonization by capital was necessary, it remained to be seen who would provide the funds.

The state would have liked to see the traders pursue the development of virgin soils, the expense of which public authority did not wish to incur itself; such was the object of the policy of forming great concessionary companies that had been adopted in 1898 in the Congo Free State. In French West Africa, T. Delcassé, then Under-secretary of State for Colonies, had made a tentative beginning in 1893 by granting to the firm of Verdier a concession over an enormous territory (5·5 million hectares); but protests from the other Ivory Coast houses obliged him to annul this grant three years later. The Committee on Colonial Concessions returned to the question in 1900. It examined evidence furnished by various informed persons on the question of whether or not territorial concessions should be granted in the West African colonies other than the Congo.[2] The project failed on account of the fierce opposition of the colonists. They feared that the appearance of monopolies, even if limited to the Sudan, would damage their trading network. They were certain, moreover, that no private company would risk its capital in undertaking those great public works which the colonists considered essential. Their pressure was the more effective because since 1893 the *Union coloniale*, 'an association of the principal French houses having interest in our colonies',[3] supported their representations in France. They ultimately succeeded in bringing about a more positive policy toward colonial loans: three loans, of 65 million francs in 1903, of 100 million francs in 1907, and of 167 million in 1913, were guaranteed by the metropolitan country. Out of this total, 179 million was devoted to public works, including 125 million for railways.

The line from Dakar to St Louis was completed in 1885, and aroused the hopes of businessmen by turning the Cayor plain, hitherto barren and unsubdued, into a leading exporter of ground-nuts. But except for this venture, the railway programme had hardly got under way at the beginning of the twentieth century. The main railway development in French West Africa took place between 1902 and 1910. It included the Senegal–Niger link (completed in 1905), the line following the river from

[1] Henri Brunschwig, 'Colonisation—décolonisation: essai sur le vocabulaire usuel de la politique coloniale', *Cahiers d'Etudes Africaines*, 1960, I, no. 1, pp. 44–54.
[2] Ministère des Colonies, Commission des Concessions Coloniales, *Procès-verbaux des séances*, April and May 1900.
[3] Comité de l'Afrique Française, *Bulletin*, Aug. 1893.

Kayes to the junction at Thiès (only finished in 1924), and the railroads of Guinea, of the Ivory Coast and of Dahomey, as shown in Fig. 11.

The government had tried at first to entrust the construction and management of the lines, in one form or another, to private enterprise. It was forced, however, to admit failure and, whenever possible, to cancel the concessions and undertake the work itself. Such difficult construction projects not only required substantial outlays of capital (each kilometre of track cost on the average some 80,000 gold francs), but also entailed a considerable lapse of time before the investment paid off. In addition to this, only the state or federation was capable of drawing up a comprehensive plan. Although the designs for a trans-Saharan line, much canvassed in the 1880s, had been abandoned, experts still entertained the hope, on the eve of World War I, of unifying the existing stretches into an ambitious trans-Sudanian railroad that would penetrate the interior. The high cost of such works and the appearance of the first motor trucks doubtless explain why the rail network in French West Africa was never expanded.

The railways, even though cheaply built and of limited extent, none the less, as they became arteries of trade and of transit, required maritime outlets. Along with railways, therefore, the Federation favoured large-scale harbour works. The most important of these were undertaken at the neglected port of Dakar. The authorities decided in 1898 to turn Dakar into a naval station, whereupon the merchants succeeded in securing a revision of the initial scheme that would ensure the future of the commercial harbour. This was made possible by the allocation of 10 million francs from the loan of 1903. The works were completed in 1910.

GROWTH OF AGRICULTURAL PRODUCTION. The result of these efforts was not slow to appear; between 1900 and 1920 production expanded enormously.[1]

	Imports	Exports
	(in millions of francs)	
1895	47·8	38·9
1909	118	109
1920	654	589

While exports of rubber inexorably declined after 1910, exports of palm products from Dahomey and above all exports of ground-nuts

[1] Agence Générale des Colonies, *Renseignements généraux sur le commerce des colonies françaises et la navigation en 1921* (Paris, 1923); and G. Hervet, *Le commerce extérieur de l'Afrique occidentale française* (Paris, 1911).

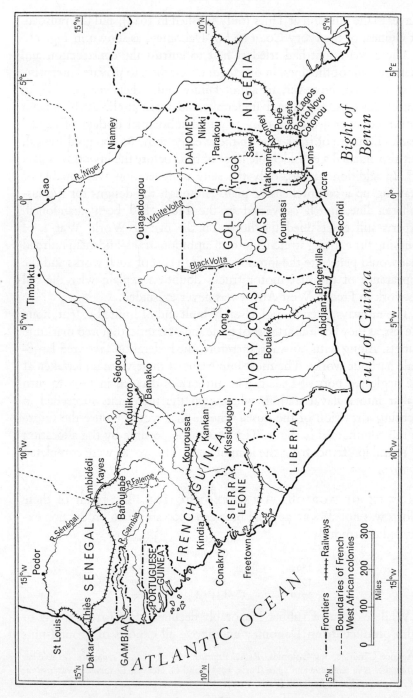

Fig. 10. West African railways after the First World War.

from Senegal continued to rise sharply. However, the hardwoods of the Ivory Coast, like the cotton plantations of Sudan and the tropical fruits of Guinea, represented as yet no more than an economic aspiration.

The hopes placed in the latexes of the Guinea area and also in the rubber vines of the Sudan proved to be ill-founded. From 1890, when 830 tons were exported, wild rubber had constituted the principal means by which the African paid for his taxes and for imported goods. Rising rubber prices had occasioned feverish activity. Rubber was sought farther and farther inland as the railroads were extended. In 1910 the product brought between 13 and 20 francs a kilogram on the European market and accounted for 60 per cent of exports by value. Production reached a peak in 1906 and yet another peak in 1909–10 (4,000 metric tons). But the plantation rubber of Asia, which in 1910 had accounted for only 12 per cent of world consumption, supplied about 50 per cent three years later. Simultaneously, the production of wild rubber in French West Africa fell to 2,500 metric tons and the price crashed to 7 francs per kilogram. A far-reaching social crisis resulted, for people had neglected less remunerative crops. In Guinea they were obliged to return to rice, sesame, ground kernels and copal. In Fouta farmers concentrated on millet and stock-raising. Elsewhere, for instance in the Sudan and the Ivory Coast, the want of any substitute made wild rubber, even at 3 or 4 francs per kilogram, the principal cash crop. However, in 1920 French West Africa exported only 770 tons, worth 3·8 million francs.

By contrast, the growth of ground-nut cultivation was prodigious. The increased production kept pace with the extension of the railroad from Senegal to Niger, and rose from 50,000 metric tons in 1897 to 240,000 in 1913. From then on, however, the output was restricted by soil depletion and by unprogressive methods of cultivation. In 1920 it had reached only 300,000 metric tons.

Palm products, the staple crop of the coast of the Gulf of Benin, reached record figures in 1911–12 (12,000 metric tons of oil and 30,000 of ground kernels at Dahomey, nearly 7,000 metric tons of each product in the Ivory Coast). The increase in exports in 1920 was due to the acquisition of Togo, representing 4,000 tons of oil and 10,000 tons of palm-kernels. The palm forest of Dahomey, densely populated and situated only a short distance from the coast, had been left to itself since the time of King Ghezo. The oil, pressed out by hand, was mediocre in quality and its yield was very low. Although the area of gathering or of native cultivation had increased by 1914, production methods had not changed since the middle of the nineteenth century. The few ventures undertaken by European planters in growing bananas or cotton met with failure, as did attempts to train African agricultural workers in improved methods.

THE UNHAPPY LOT OF THE PRODUCER. Because the colonies contained enormous areas of uncultivated land, a policy of immediate exploitation was undertaken, without regard to the infertility of the soil, the conditions under which crops were grown, or the sparseness of the population. The native producer was neglected, since he was considered lazy, blind to progress, and incapable of understanding where his true interests lay.

The government made up for lack of funds by using coercion. In 1910, a typical year, the Government General allotted to the Bureau of Agriculture no more than 24,000 gold francs out of a budget of 18·6 millions, or 1·3 per cent, sufficient only to support a few plantations and three or four European experts. In these circumstances the district officer would call together the chiefs, preach to them the advantages of this or that crop and order them to grow it. The *broussard* would distribute seed and order his guards to supervise the carrying out of his instructions. Officials changed frequently and with them the cropping programme. Each year the 'commandant's fields' accounted for thousands of hectares and constituted a heavy burden on the Africans, all the more so since they only received a miserable price for their efforts. In 1900 the Association Cotonnière du Soudan bought 'obligatory cotton' at 15 centimes per kilogram although the local market price was 30 or 40 centimes. Only 20 to 30 centimes was paid per kilogram for kapok fibres delivered to administrative centres situated as much as two or three days' walk from the place of production.

The system reached its apogee in World War I, when the French were determined to increase crop production to the maximum in order to feed the metropolitan country. The government, moreover, raided the reserve granaries, with the result that during a subsequent famine only 4,000 tons of cereals was available to relieve distress, and that only because the Sudan had had neither the time nor the means to send these stores to France. The economy accordingly remained fragile.

The desire for gain seized both the trading houses and the Africans, who were encouraged by the traders to neglect traditional crops and to plunder, sometimes irreversibly, natural resources such as the rubber vines, and the hardwoods of the Ivory Coast. Feeling themselves to be the key-stone of the colony's prosperity, the merchants behaved as if they were the source of wealth instead of merely its middlemen. Accordingly they left production in the hands of the blacks and devoted themselves to collecting products, which they strove to buy as cheaply as possible at the risk of ruining the trade. Faced with the necessity of penetrating farther and farther into the interior, they enlisted an increasing number of commercial travellers to whom they extended credit in the form of goods that they were expected to barter in the bush. This system bore witness to the high degree of trust that existed between the firms and their African agents. But it also led to many abuses. Some agents disappeared without ever repaying their loans, and thereby encouraged businessmen to raise their prices by between 100 and 200 per cent of the cost price. Others tried to add to their commission at the expense of the producers, who were thus exploited in a more insidious fashion than they had been by other Africans. These latter were mostly Diula traders. After about 1920 these itinerant Moslem merchants who had dominated the pre-colonial economy in the nineteenth century were supplanted by Syrians and Lebanese, who arrived *en masse* in the country between 1900 and 1914.

The colonial trade did supply Africans with a whole new range of consumption goods. But these were acquired at a high price. The peasant was bullied by the administrator and subjected to obligatory labour. Hence his lot at first worsened in these early days while the modern economy advanced. The country was as yet barely pacified, and not in a state to benefit from the end of local wars. In the early colonial period, nearly all the money earned by Africans had to be used for paying the tax. Where imposts were levied in kind, the workers were deprived of goods without compensation. Taxes in kind con-tributed to the prevailing misery because the administrator would seize goods stored for the taxpayer's own use.

In the period between the two world wars, the first great plantations, public works and lumber mills were more conspicuous for their labour-hunger than for their contribution towards the extension of cultivation and the encouragement of trade. The Africans were able to distinguish less and less between labour services due to the government and 'volunteer recruitment' for private companies, inasmuch as the district officer, for all that he tried to brake the demands of private employers, was often the only person capable of recruiting on the companies' behalf—a *de facto* situation which was made lawful by decree of 22 October 1925. By the destruction of the power of the traditional chiefs, the inhabitants had been deprived of all means of protest. Their sole weapons were inertia, deceit or flight; and they did not hesitate to make use of them.

The French at length perceived, in the aftermath of war, that an authoritarian policy all too often led to defeat. The sharp indictment drawn up by the agronomist Cosnier, who had been sent in 1919 on an official mission, bore witness to a new attitude of mind.

Economic development in French Equatorial Africa

In French Equatorial Africa, the poor relation of the French colonies, the system of concessions was soon found to be a failure. Hence efforts were made from 1910 onwards to formulate a new economic policy. In 1898 the state had in effect abandoned the greater part of the territory to businessmen, in the mistaken belief that they would by themselves undertake the necessary investment. However, the businessmen contented themselves with extracting from the jungle the maximum of advantage in the minimum of time, when they did not confine themselves merely to speculating on the stock exchange.

THE POLICY OF CONCESSIONS. The idea of a concessionary policy went back to P. Leroy-Beaulieu, an economist who played a major role in the genesis of French imperialism. The policy was defended enthusiastically by Eugène Etienne, who was Under-secretary of State for the Colonies in 1891. Etienne proposed to concede to giant companies for ninety-nine years 'the fruits of the soil, of hunting and fishing ...the rights of police and of justice', the privilege of levying taxes and even that of making treaties with neighbouring states.[1] This idea, inspired more or less by the chartered companies of the *ancien régime*, meant imitating the Royal Niger Company, Cecil Rhodes's Chartered Company, and above all the Congo Free State. The latter, however, was still in financial difficulties, and Prime Minister Freycinet did not dare to create states within a state by simple decree. The project therefore fizzled out in the Chamber.

The Colonial Party was to gain an unexpected ally in the person of

[1] Henri Brunschwig, *La colonisation française du Pacte colonial à l'Union française* (Paris, 1949), p. 101.

Brazza. The Commissary-General had no connexions or interest in the world of colonial capitalism. It was no accident that the year of the decree of concession was also the year of his resignation, which showed how far he disagreed with the mercantile community. But he was largely responsible for the illusions that were prevalent in French Equatorial Africa about 'its riches in men and its economic future... false notions that did a lot of harm'.[1] Brazza believed that a régime of free competition would bring about disastrous overbidding. He therefore favoured prematurely, and before French interests were ripe for it, the formation of great companies: the C.P.K.N. and the S.H.O. (C° Propriétaire du Kouilou-Niari and Société Commerciale, Industrielle et Agricole du Haut-Ogooué).

From the time of his second voyage (1880-2) Brazza had dreamed of a railway that should link Stanley Pool with the sea. When the state refused to pay the very considerable cost, he made an agreement, in 1890, with the Governor of the Crédit Foncier; but Belgian pressure caused the enterprise to be abandoned. The idea was taken up again in 1892 by A. Le Châtelier, a businessman, who obtained a concession to 'study the means of communication between the sea and the Congo across French territory'.[2] The funds available for the purpose, a total of 600,000 francs, appeared ridiculously small compared to the 25 million francs raised at the same time by the Belgian Thys-Urban group. Although the building of the Belgian railroad meant the ruin of these projects, the company nevertheless had a brilliant future before it. Under the name of C.P.K.N. it passed in 1899 into the hands of Lever Brothers of Liverpool and was to become one of the component parts of the powerful firm of Unilever.

The failure of this initiative might well have served as a warning. But Brazza, and with him many sincere colonialists, believed in the primary role of trade as a weapon of penetration and a means of 'civilization'. The exaggerated nationalism of the Commissary-General made him believe that only a company that was powerfully protected by the state could drive out the dominant foreign traders, be they Dutch or Belgian as in the Congo, or English or German as in

[1] R. Pasquier, 'Chronique d'histoire d'outre-mer: l'Afrique noire d'expression française', *Revue Française d'Histoire d'Outre-Mer*, 1963, no. 178, p. 78.

[2] Alfred le Châtelier was the son of an engineer and the brother of a famous chemist. Himself an unsuccessful man of affairs but well educated, he published the first notable work on black Islam (*L'Islam dans l'Afrique occidentale*, Paris, 1899), and from 1903 onwards occupied the chair of Moslem sociology at the Collège de France.

the Lower Ogooué. About 1882 he sent to Marius-Celestin Daumas, the only businessman of real substance in the colony, a plan for a vast monopolistic company that would cover the country with a close network of its factories.[1] But it was not until 1893 that he succeeded in getting Delcassé to grant him the concession of a large quadrilateral in the Upper Ogooué, including 11 million hectares of jungle and 700 km of river. The exorbitant powers of the company, to which the state had delegated sovereign rights of police and of patronage, aroused its competitors and public opinion. The concession was withdrawn in 1896, but this decision was reversed on appeal to the Conseil d'Etat.

The S.H.O., which began its activities in 1897, was the first and the greatest of the concessionary companies, and also the best endowed. Complete master in its domain, it was not constrained in the matter of native reserves, nor was it obliged either to pay rent or to make plantations. Envied and soon imitated, it contributed powerfully towards developing in the Congo a new and exclusive system of monopolistic commerce.[2]

In the following year the Colonial Party triumphed. Forty-one companies shared 70 per cent of the territory. The state issued decrees giving the companies for a period of thirty years all rights of enjoyment and exploitation, with the exception of mining, in return for a fixed annual rent and payment to the state of 15 per cent of the profits. The smallest of these concerns, the Nkémé-Nkéni, received 1,200 sq. km, the largest (the Company of the Sultanates of the Higher-Oubangui) 140,000 sq. km. In relation to the immensity of these territories, the capital investment was insignficant—varying from 300,000 francs (for the Compagnie Bretonne du Congo with 3,000 sq. km) to 3 million (for the Compagnie Française du Congo with 55,100 sq. km). The Company of the Sultanates with a capital of 9 million francs was an exception.

If the state had hoped to develop the country at the least possible expense by eliminating competition, its hopes were doomed to disappointment on several counts. In order to encourage investment on the part of the companies, the decree granted them freehold rights over any territory they developed, but the definition of 'development' was derisory. It amounted, for example, to a harvest from rubber trees at the rate of twenty trees to the hectare, or buildings on one-tenth of the area.

[1] Brouillon, undated, *Fonds Brazza*, 3rd mission, IV.
[2] *Concessions A.E.F.* I, Archives Nationales, and Archives de la Société.

The domestication of an elephant would give a right to 100 hectares! Hence the companies did nothing except to engage in commerce.

The greater part of the territory belonged to the conventional basin of the Congo, where free trade was guaranteed by the powers. Thus the government could not use customs duties as a device for driving out foreigners. A subterfuge was resorted to in the creation not of companies with a commercial monopoly such as the S.H.O., but of companies that would have exclusive use of the products of the soil. Nevertheless, the trade of the metropolitan country did not gain a decisive advantage from this device. Most foreign firms concealed themselves under cover of a company registered in Paris. The Dutch company N.A.H.V. (Nieuwe Afrikaansche Handels Vennootschap) became the 'Brazzaville' company and stood behind the C.C.C.C.F. (Compagnie Commerciale de Colonisation au Congo Français), which received a concession of 12,400 sq. km. Moreover, a number of French administrators lent their names as cover for foreign enterprises: the Alkélé group (Lefini, Nkémé-Nkéni, and Alima) was in fact under Belgian control.[1]

THE WRETCHED CONDITIONS IN FRENCH EQUATORIAL AFRICA. The companies, whether French or foreign, met with the same disappointments: the country was poor and the government ineffective. The savannah in the north was barely known and out of reach. It might take three months to reach Chad, and development was impossible as long as transport depended on human porterage. In the south there was jungle, impenetrable as far as the eye could reach, inhabited only along the waterways, an insalubrious region where many whites died of fever. The rain-forest zone proved little healthier to Africans who were weakened by malaria or decimated by sleeping-sickness that spread with the extension of trade.

The country produced practically nothing but ivory and wild rubber. Ivory production, worth 1·4 million francs in 1896, was declining. The stores laid up in the villages were exhausted, and the elephants were being wiped out. The height of the trade was reached in 1905, when 210 metric tons worth 4 million francs were exported; by 1920 exports had fallen to 97 metric tons. As for wild rubber, the record export of 1906 (1,950 metric tons, equal to half the production of French West Africa) was unequalled before the war. In 1920, for want of any product to replace it, the export exceeded 2,000 tons. The export

[1] *A.E.F.* XI, B (2).

of wood had barely started. For a long time the only species sought were ebony and a red wood used for dyestuffs. However, since 1893 Daumas had set great hopes on *okoumé*, 'this new business which has just started and which is not yet in the hands of everyone'.[1] An initial sample of 7 or 8 tons sent to the metropolis sold well, but the Havre merchants, who were accustomed to the northern woods, ganged up against it. Hence trade in *okoumé* wood was for a long time retarded in France, while in Hamburg it suffered from a glut on the German timber market. Nevertheless, production rose from 7,000 tons in 1905 to 91,000 tons in 1911. It was a kind of rosewood, but soft and close-grained, whose low specific gravity made it float easily. It served first as a cheap substitute for mahogany, but did not come into its own until after the war, when the sheet and plywood industry was set up. Although the total exportation of wood jumped from 2,000 metric tons in 1898 to nearly 150,000 tons in 1913, a survey of the forest riches of Gabon remained to be made.

French Equatorial Africa was the poor relation among the French colonies. Its total trade in 1920 was estimated at only 146 million francs, compared to 1·2 billion francs for French West Africa and 2·2 billion for Indochina. The country found itself in this invidious position not so much because of the poverty in resources, but because of its economic system. The concessionary companies limited themselves to trade even more rigorously than in French West Africa. They considered themselves to be proprietors of the product, and paid the grower only a paltry price for gathering and transporting the product. They paid for merchandise preferably in kind, or even in a private currency accepted only in their own stores.[2] They charged more for their merchandise than was justified even by the high risks and considerable distribution costs of the colonial trade. The Company of the Sultanates, for instance, exchanged a kilogram of salt (whose cost price amounted to 25 centimes in France and to 1·25 francs after delivery to Oubangui) for goods worth 5 francs. The general manager of the S.H.O. calculated his sale price by adding a preliminary profit of 40 per cent to the cost price. The heads of the trading stations then tacked on another 40 to 60 per cent, according to the distance involved; in

[1] Daumas to Sajoux, resident director in Africa, 9 Feb. 1893, *A.E.F.* L (1).
[2] The S.H.O. imposed the so-called *neptunes*, large plates of copper used for the payment of dowry; the Compagnie Française du Haut Congo used pieces minted with the effigies of their directors, the brothers Tréchot, a method comparable to the British truck system.

addition they charged still another 25 per cent for their private profit. The traders in turn took their cut. Hence it is not surprising that 1 kilogram of rubber (worth about 15 francs in Europe) should have been exchanged for 1 kilogram of salt or two needles. The trade goods included powder and flintlock (until the protocol of 1909 definitely stopped the sale of these items), cloth, salt, canned goods, knives, beads, and spirits in abundance. The S.H.O. alone boasted of having forbidden the entry of spirits into its territory.[1]

Control by the state was nonexistent. The native reserves envisaged around the villages were never delimited. A circular in 1902, which stipulated a reserve amounting to 25 hectares per person on the average, aroused a general outcry. The minister himself had to give an assurance that these restrictions 'had nothing absolute about them'.[2] The Colonial Inspectorate, which was in charge of a special commissary, appeared illusory. From time to time tours of duty would reveal some crying abuses. An inspector in 1906 described a company of native carriers of the S.H.O. as 'unfit, puny, eaten up with ulcers…some moved along on their knees, others could not stand upright…children had large bald patches as a result of carrying loads; [out of] twenty men, the group had lost, in the course of its first voyage to Haut-Scoi, four men dead of fatigue, weakness and privation'.[3]

But the government had no power to punish or to control these abuses. In 1905, in the whole of the Middle Congo it had only 100 civil servants, of whom 54 were at Brazzaville and 12 at Loango. It was obliged to leave to the companies not only the policing of the territory but also the collection of taxes. On the very eve of Brazza's mission, the authorities were about to legalize a system whereby the agents of the concessionary companies received contributions in kind and turned over the proceeds to the colonial government.[4] Not surprisingly, ill-paid, ill-instructed and often unscrupulous traders committed abuses in order to secure workers, carriers or produce. There were low wages, broken contracts, camps for hostages, trails or timberyards lined with corpses. The mounting mortality among the natives and the rate of desertion diminished dividends year by year.

From the outset, some ill-informed concessionaries had been brutally

[1] Note of 3 Feb. 1913, *A.E.F.* L (3).
[2] Circular of the Commissioner-General, 7 March 1902; circular of the Minister, 11 Sept. 1902, *A.E.F.* XIII, A (1).
[3] Dec. 1906, cercle de Samba, Archives de la Société.
[4] Circular of Commissioner-General Gentil, 27 April 1905.

disillusioned: though ten companies in 1905 could count profits totalling 10 million francs since their formation, the total deficit of the other twenty-one exceeded 9 million. After 1903 there were no more than twenty companies, some of which existed only on paper. The most scandalous case was that of Ngoko-Sangha concern, which in 1908 took advantage of the frontier rectification in favour of the German Cameroon to claim an indemnity. Only energetic action on the part of a group responsible for publishing the 'Cahiers de la Quinzaine',[1] supported by the socialists, prevented the company, in 1911, from obtaining 150,000 hectares in freehold by way of compensation for fictitious damages suffered in a territory that had been left uncultivated.

THE TURNING-POINT OF 1910. After Brazza's mission of inspection in 1905 had revealed the abuses of the system, the concessionary régime stood condemned. Having decided to get rid of it, the state authorized the amalgamation of firms that were losing money. Many concerns combined with others in order to reduce their high overheads. Eleven companies merged into the Forestière Sangha-Oubangi. Another group was formed on the Gabon coast on condition that the interested parties should restore free trade in part of their territory or limit their monopoly to wild rubber. A more rigorous control was set up in the ministry, though there may be some doubt as to its efficacy in view of the fact that the departmental representative with the Compagnie Forestière entered the service of that company in 1913 and shortly afterwards became its president and director-general.

In setting up a federation on the model of French West Africa, the authorities sought to give the country the political structure required for the large-scale investments from which the concessionary régime had hitherto abstained. Having laboured for fifteen years and having expended 1·5 million francs, the S.H.O. had only managed to create a road 100 km long in Middle Ogooué, so wretched that it was soon abandoned. In 1909 parliament voted a loan of 21 million to finance preliminary studies for a great development loan. On 13 July 1914 French Equatorial Africa was authorized to borrow 171 million to pay for a series of railroads that would free the country from the burden of porterage (Congo to the ocean with branches from Ogooué to Ivindo

---

[1] A review started in 1900 by the poet Charles Péguy after his breach with the socialists; Pierre Mille and above all Félicien Challaye, a young philosopher who accompanied Brazza in 1905, campaigned in the periodical against the scandals in the Congo.

and Oubangui to Chari). This project was delayed by the war and it was only in 1934 that the scheme was partly inaugurated.

Under such conditions, the least economic disturbance was liable to bring on catastrophe. Between 1915 and 1916 a terrible famine broke out when the people, in addition to meeting habitual demands on them, had to contend also with the seizure of their food and the impressment of carriers for the use of troops attacking the German Cameroons. The system of monopolistic exploitation, brutally carried out in a poor and sparsely populated country, led to an intolerable situation. In the aftermath of the war, the companies prepared to reform themselves. From 1919 on, the S.H.O. resolved to extend its activities to 'negotiation...of all businesses or enterprises whatsoever, agricultural... financial, forestry, mining..., of importation, and of exportation... of every sort of industrial and commercial establishment...and to take in all products'.[1] The time had come for the appearance in French Equatorial Africa of great trading companies, constituted on the model of those in the neighbouring federation (S.C.O.A., C.F.A.O.).

From 1900 to 1920 French Equatorial Africa and French West Africa contrasted in every respect. The sole feature common to both was their unconditional devotion to trade; but French West Africa appeared relatively prosperous, while French Equatorial Africa suffered bitter distress. French West Africa had been able to evolve in an empirical fashion by reason of given historical or economic conditions. French Equatorial Africa, on the other hand, poor as it was in goods, in money and in men, could never do more than imitate its neighbours. French West Africa developed relatively harmoniously, around a long-standing colonial nucleus that was well-organized administratively and economically. French Equatorial Africa, made up of bits and pieces, without a model or centre of attraction, was a permanent field for abortive experiments. Its unity, tardily achieved, was always more apparent than real. French West Africa was the uncontested domain of free trade, tempered by a relatively strong administration. The conjunction of these two elements created the infrastructure necessary for its later development; in French Equatorial Africa, on the other hand, the monopolistic chartered companies managed for a long time to check any serious attempt at reform.

[1] Extraordinary general meeting of 1919, for the revision of the statutes, Archives de la Société.

On the eve of war, however, both federations had come to a turning-point. The French had begun to understand that the principle of government hitherto relied upon for developing the wealth of the country had proved ineffective. Taxes and forced labour had discouraged or even reduced the population, ignorance of natural conditions or the absence of adequate means of transport had caused the failure of the first European plantations (cotton in Sudan, bananas in Guinea, coffee or cocoa in the Ivory Coast). It was in West Africa, more attractive to enterprise and better organized, that a real effort for economic development was first made. This attempt led to the extraordinary growth of the trading economy (predominance of the companies, and extension of export crops), and rested on a thorough acquaintance with the people, their aspirations and their needs. Following the example of a few great forerunners ('The hour is past, in Africa as in the other continents of the world, where orders can be imposed and maintained against the wish of the people.'[1]), the rulers understood 'the need to understand men in order to direct their future'.[2] Native policy, less devoted to assimilation than hitherto, would now hinge on the study of local civilization, and would work for the benefit of Africans by the employment of technicians and the creation of new rural types of organization to even out the ups and downs of traditional economic society.

Revealing in this respect was an attempt made in the years after 1910 by two administrators in Senegal. By grouping peasants into *Sociétés de prévoyance*, which were at the same time buying co-operatives and credit organizations, and which the Africans administered themselves without French control, the founders attempted to ensure not only the education of the Africans, but their protection against the snares of private trade. All too often the experiment merely led to a more subtle form of exploitation. Nevertheless it did achieve considerable success. After the war the scheme developed to a remarkable degree and came to represent a turning-point in history. Hitherto the French had been content to exploit black Africa; now at last they thought in terms of accepting the local people as partners in a common enterprise.

[1] *Van Vollenhoven*, pp. 38–50.
[2] Hubert Deschamps, *Les méthodes et les doctrines coloniales de la France du XVIe siècle à nos jours* (Paris, 1953), p. 167.

BIBLIOGRAPHY

Alexandre, P. 'L'Islam en Afrique noire', *Marchés Tropicaux du Monde* (superseded by *Marchés Tropicaux et Méditerranéens*), 12 Oct. 1957, no. 622, and 19 Oct. 1957, no. 623.

'Le problème des chefferies en Afrique noire française', *Notes et Etudes Documentaires*, 10 Feb. 1959, no. 2508.

Une âme de chef, le Gouverneur général J. Van Vollenhoven: à la mémoire du capitaine J. Vollenhoven, Gouverneur général des colonies, tué à l'ennemi. Paris, 1920.

Angoulvant, Gabriel Louis. *La pacification de la Côte d'Ivoire, 1908–1915: méthodes et résultats.* Paris, 1916.

Benilan, J. 'Le statut des administrateurs des colonies.' Doctoral thesis. Paris, 1937.

Berge, F. 'Le Sous-secrétariat et les Sous-secrétaires d'Etat aux Colonies: histoire de l'émancipation de l'administration coloniale', *Revue Française d'Histoire d'Outre-Mer*, 1960, nos. 168–9.

Besse, Auguste. *Manuel de l'employé de commerce aux colonies.* Lyon, 1905.

Blanchard, M. 'Administrateurs d'Afrique noire', *Revue Française d'Histoire d'Outre-Mer*, 1953, **40**, nos. 140–1.

Bondet, Jacques, ed. *Le monde des affaires en France de 1830 à nos jours.* Paris, 1952.

Boutmy, Emile Gaston. *Le recrutement des administrateurs coloniaux.* Paris, 1895.

Bruel, Georges. *L'Afrique équatoriale française.* Paris, 1918.

Brunschwig, Henri. *L'avènement de l'Afrique noire du XIXe siècle à nos jours.* Paris, 1963.

'Colonisation—décolonisation: essai sur le vocabulaire usuel de la politique coloniale', *Cahiers d'Etudes Africaines*, 1960, **I**, no. 1.

La colonisation française du Pacte colonial à l'Union française. Paris, 1949.

Mythes et réalités de l'impérialisme colonial française, 1871–1914. Paris, 1960.

ed. *Brazza explorateur, l'Ogooué, 1875–1879.* Paris and The Hague, 1966.

Camentron, E. 'Les bois coloniaux: mesures préconisées pour accroître leurs débouchés', *La Petite Gironde*, 26 Oct. 1917.

Canu, H. *La pétaudière coloniale.* Paris, 1894.

Chailley-Bert, Joseph. *Dix années de politique coloniale.* Paris, 1902.

Charbonneau, Jean, and René Charbonneau. *Marchés et marchands d'Afrique noire.* Paris, 1961.

Charmeil, Pierre. *Les gouverneurs généraux des colonies françaises: leurs pouvoirs et leurs attributions.* Paris, 1922.

Chevalier, Auguste. *La forêt et les bois du Gabon.* Paris, 1917.

'Rapport sur une mission scientifique dans l'Ouest africain, 1908–1910', *Nouvelles Archives des Missions Scientifiques et Littéraires* (Paris), 1912, n.s., fasc. 5.

Coquery-Vidrovitch, Catherine. 'De Brazza à Gentil: la politique française en Haute-Sangha à la fin du XIXe siècle', *Revue Française d'Histoire d'Outre-Mer*, 1965, **52**, no. 186.

'Les idées économiques de Brazza et les premières tentatives de compagnies de colonisation au Congo française, 1885–1898', *Cahiers d'Etudes Africaines*, 1965, **5**, no. 17

Cornevin, Robert. 'Evolution des chefferies traditionnelles en Afrique noire d'expression française', *Penant*, 1961, nos. 686–7.

Histoire du Dahomey. Paris, 1962.

Histoire du Togo. 2nd ed. Paris, 1962.

Cosnier, Henri. *L'Ouest africain français: ses ressources agricoles, son organisation économique*. Paris, 1921.

Defauconfret, P. 'Etude économique du Sénégal, du Soudan français et de la Guinée française.' Doctoral thesis. Paris, 1898.

Deherme, Georges. *L'Afrique occidentale française: action politique, action économique, action sociale*. Paris, 1908.

Delafosse, Maurice. 'L'Afrique occidentale française', in *Histoire des colonies françaises et de l'expansion de la France dans le monde*, vol. IV, Gabriel Hanotaux and Alfred Martineau, eds. Paris, Société de l'Histoire Nationale, 1931.

Haut-Sénégal-Niger: le pays, les peuples, les langues, l'histoire, les civilisations. 3 vols. Paris, 1911.

Delavignette, Robert L. 'L'administrateur territorial en Afrique noire française', *Revue des Travaux de l'Académie des Sciences Morales et Politiques*, 1965, **118**, no. 4.

'Des "Commandants" français aux préfets africains', *Le Mois en Afrique*, 1966, no. 2.

'L'Œuvre de nos administrateurs d'outre-mer', *Tropiques*, July 1959, no. 419.

Demongeot, Antoine M. J. *Notes sur l'organisation politique et administrative du Labé avant et depuis l'occupation française* (Mémoires de l'Institut Français d'Afrique Noire, no. 6). Paris, 1944.

Deschamps, Hubert. *Les méthodes et les doctrines coloniales de la France du XVIe siècle à nos jours*. Paris, 1953.

Le Sénégal et la Gambie. Paris, Presses Universitaires de France, 1964.

Dresch, Jean. 'Les investissements en Afrique noire', in *Le travail en Afrique noire* (Présence Africaine, 13). Paris, 1952.

'Méthodes coloniales au Congo belge et en A.E.F.', *Politique Etrangère*, 1947, **12**, no. 1.

'Recherches sur les investissements dans l'Union française outre-mer, leur répartition, leurs conséquences', *Bulletin de l'Association des Géographes Français*, Jan–Feb. 1953, nos. 231–2.

'Sur une géographie des investissements de capitaux: l'exemple de l'Afrique noire', *Bulletin de l'Association des Géographes Français*, Jan–Feb. 1946, nos. 177–8.

'Les trusts en Afrique noire', *Servir la France*, 1946.

'Villes congolaises', *Revue de Géographie Humaine et d'Ethnologie*, July–Sept. 1948, no. 3.

'Villes d'Afrique occidentale', *Cahiers d'Outre-Mer*, 1950, no. 11.

Duchêne, Albert Paul André. *La politique coloniale de la France: le Ministère des Colonies depuis Richelieu*. Paris, 1928.

Forgeron, J. B. *Le protectorat en Afrique occidentale française et les chefs indigènes*. Bordeaux, 1920.

France. Agence Générale des Colonies. *Renseignements généraux sur le commerce des colonies françaises et la navigation en 1921*. Paris, 1923.

France. Ministère des Colonies. *Statistiques coloniales...1890–1914*. Superseded by France. Office Colonial. *Statistiques du commerce des colonies françaises* for 1897–1914.

France. Office Colonial. *Statistiques décennales du commerce des colonies françaises (1896–1905)...*, P. Chemin Dupontès, ed. Paris, 1910.

François, Georges, *L'Afrique occidentale française*. Paris, 1907.

L'Afrique occidentale française et ses matières premières. Paris, 1920.

Froidevaux, Henri. 'La politique indigène au Congo français', *Questions Diplomatiques et Coloniales*, 1906, **21**.

Gide, André. *Voyage au Congo, carnets de route*. Paris, 1927.

Goulven, Joseph Georges Arsène. *L'Afrique équatoriale française, ancien Congo français: son organisation administrative, judiciaire, financière*. Paris, 1911.

Hanotaux, Gabriel, and Alfred Martineau, eds. *Histoire des colonies françaises et de l'expansion de la France dans le monde*. 6 vols. Paris, Société de l'Histoire Nationale, 1929–33.

Hervet, G. *Le commerce extérieur de l'Afrique occidentale française*. Paris, 1911.

Jeaugeon, R. 'Les sociétés d'exploitation au Congo et l'opinion française de 1890–1906', *Revue Française d'Histoire d'Outre-Mer*, 1961, **48**, nos. 172–3.

Lasserre, Guy, 'Okoumé et chantiers forestiers du Gabon', *Cahiers d'Outre-Mer*, April–June 1955, no. 30.

Le Châtelier, Alfred. *L'Islam dans l'Afrique occidentale*. Paris, 1899.

Le Myre de Vilers. *Préparation aux carrières coloniales, conférences sous les auspices de l'Union coloniale, 1901–1902*. Paris, 1904.

Leroy-Beaulieu, Paul. *De la colonisation chez les peuples modernes*. 6th ed. 2 vols. Paris, 1908.

Les grandes compagnies de colonisation: conférence faite sous le patronage de l'Union coloniale française. Paris, 1895.

Massion, J. 'Les grandes concessions au Congo français.' Doctoral thesis. Paris, 1920.

Masson, Paul. *Marseille et la colonisation française*. Marseille, 1906.

Meillassoux, Claude. *Anthropologie économique des Gouro de Côte d'Ivoire: de l'économie de subsistance à l'agriculture commerciale*. Paris, 1964.

Newbury, Colin W. 'The formation of the government general of French West Africa', *Journal of African History*, 1960, **1**, no. 1.

Pasquier, R. 'Chronique d'histoire d'outre-mer: l'Afrique noire d'expression française', *Revue Française d'Histoire d'Outre-Mer*, 1963, **50**, no. 178.

'Villes du Sénégal au XIXe siècle', *Revue Française d'Histoire d'Outre-Mer*, 1960, **47**, nos. 168–9.

Person, Yves. 'La jeunesse de Samori', *Revue Française d'Histoire d'Outre-Mer*, 1962, **49**, no. 175.

'Soixante ans d'évolution en Pays Kissi', *Cahiers d'Etudes Africaines*, 1960, **1**, no. 1.

Renard, Ulysse Marie Alexandre. *La colonisation au Congo français: étude sur les concessions accordées au Congo en vertu du décret du 28 mars 1899*. Paris, 1901.

Roberts, Stephen H. *History of French colonial policy, 1870–1925*. 2 vols. London, 1929.

Rotté, Charles Robert. *Les chemins de fer et tramways des colonies: historique; organisation administrative et financière*. Paris, 1910.

Saintoyant, Jules F. *L'affaire du Congo, 1905*. Paris, 1960.

Servel, A. 'Etude sur l'organisation administrative et financière de l'Afrique équatoriale française.' Doctoral thesis. Paris, 1912.

Suret-Canale, Jean. *L'Afrique noire occidentale et centrale*. 2 vols. Paris, 1958–64.

Terrier, Auguste. 'L'Afrique équatoriale française,' in *Histoire des colonies françaises et de l'expansion de la France dans le monde*, vol. IV, Gabriel Hanotaux and Alfred Martineau, eds. Paris, Société de l'Histoire Nationale, 1931.

Thompson, Virginia, and Richard Adloff. *The emerging states of French Equatorial Africa*. Stanford University Press, 1960.

French West Africa. Stanford University Press, 1957.

Ziegle, H. *L'Afrique équatoriale française*. Paris, 1952.

CHAPTER 6

WEST AFRICAN STATES AND THE EUROPEAN CONQUEST

by JOHN D. HARGREAVES

A common though superficial view of the partition of Africa is that Europeans, having decided to impose their power, proceeded to do so, enabled by the superior technology represented by Belloc's famous Maxim gun. J. S. Keltie, author of the earliest and still the most detailed general account, believed that 'we have seen the bulk of the one barbarous continent parcelled out among the most civilized powers of Europe.'[1] In such a perspective, European occupation inaugurated such a radically new phase in African history that the methods and motivations of the conquerors seemed a vastly more important subject for study than the reactions of the conquered.

From the new frontier of African historical studies, the view is rather different. We can trace how, in the centuries before the partition, African states, entering into more or less stable relations, grew or diminished in power as a result of commerce, statecraft, war and internal changes. The nineteenth century provided in Africa many examples of what philosophic historians might earlier have called 'great revolutions ...and the rise and fall of states'. One may see what has been described as a sort of African partition of Africa, a radical reshaping of political structures and boundaries, taking place throughout the century. It is most evident in the Muslim countries of the western Sudan, with the great Fulani jihad in Sokoto, the consolidation of Bornu, the rise and defeat of Macina, the foundation of the Tukulor state of El Hadj 'Omar and later of the military empires of Samory (Samori) and Rabeh. But in coastal areas, too, many peoples were adapting their attitudes and institutions in response to the challenges presented by foreign traders, missionaries and governors. Wolof states took to peanut-growing and to Islam; the Fon state in Dahomey reorganized its economy and extended its power; the 'city-states' of the Oil Rivers perfected their mechanisms for controlling trade.

[1] *The partition of Africa* (London, 1893), p. 1.

199

Not all such states were completely wiped from the map by European imperialism. Although some, like the Muslim empires that faced the French military in Haut-Sénégal–Niger, were deliberately broken up by the conquerors, the cultural identity, institutional structure and ruling personnel of others survived not only under colonial rule but after its termination. The Tolon Na, a traditional Dagomba chief, represented Nkrumah's radical republic of Ghana in Lagos; the ancient dynasty of Mossi played active if somewhat conservative roles in Voltaic politics during the 1940s and 1950s; rulers of small Mende and Temne chiefdoms provided much of the basis for the rule of the Sierra Leone People's Party. Most striking of all was the power wielded within the Nigerian federation by representatives of the ruling houses of the Fulani empire. It is therefore relevant to many present problems to inquire how such survivals became possible, what forces or conditions determined whether African states could retain their identity, what characteristics were needed for survival through the violent mutations induced by the European partition.

Historians of colonial policy might propose a simple hypothesis: that the decisive factor was the policy and attitudes of the occupying powers, whose material superiority was such that they could reshape the continent in accordance with their national interests and ideologies.[1] British governors and consuls, their activities watched on the one hand by ministries drilled in the need to economize by administrative improvisation, and on the other by merchants anxious not to damage potential customers too badly, were unable to press so severely upon the African states that confronted them as ambitious French *militaires*, shrugging off civilian control as they sought Napoleonic conquests. One mode of expansion pointed towards the pragmatic philosophy of Indirect Rule, the other towards an integrationist ideal attainable only after French control had imposed rigorous processes of levelling and indoctrination. As a recent thesis by A. S. Kanya-Forstner emphasizes, the general outlook of the marine infantry officers who carried out the conquest of French Sudan was radically unfavourable to any policy of preserving as collaborators or subordinates the large Muslim states by which they found themselves faced.[2] Some were interested only in

[1] Whether their power was really so dominant is another matter. Much of what Professor T. O. Ranger says in Chapter 9 about the weakness of early colonial administrations in East Africa could be paralleled for parts of the west.
[2] 'The role of the military in the formulation of French policy towards the Western Sudan, 1879–1899.' Ph.D. thesis, Cambridge University, 1965.

military glory and promotion; others were moved by ideals of spreading French civilization and liberating subject pagan peoples from Muslim tyranny.

Much is no doubt explained by these contrasting attitudes; and certainly in the longer run administrative policies and doctrines developed which made it far easier for African political structures to survive, and even harden, under British rule than under French rule. Professor Hubert Deschamps recently argued that the contrast is commonly oversimplified and sharpened; nevertheless, as Michael Crowder retorted, one cannot explain away important differences in the spirit and style of colonial policy.[1] While British practitioners of Indirect Rule were led to revive political institutions which their predecessors had destroyed—or even, as in Iboland, to create state structures that earlier generations of Africans apparently neglected to develop for themselves—the French tended increasingly to turn chieftaincy into a bureaucratic hierarchy of subordinate *fonctionnaires*.

But in the earlier period, while the partition of West Africa was still taking place, the contrast between French and British policies was far less absolute. The British were led by the circumstances of their incursion to destroy many historic states as political entities, to acquiesce in the arbitrary partition of others. Professor J. C. Anene has recalled how in Southern Nigeria British officials in the later nineteenth century overthrew established authorities like Ja Ja and Nana, under pressure from trading interests or out of doctrinaire hostility towards 'middlemen'.[2] Indeed, throughout the nineteenth century British attitudes towards African authority were by no means consistent. The interest which many saw in identifying and strengthening 'strong native governments' as collaborators in the policies of 'informal empire' was in practice largely neutralized by pressures arising out of local interests and commitments, or evangelical impulses to remould the continent more nearly in Britain's image.

Towards Ashanti (Asante), for example, British officials from time to time advocated policies of coexistence and collaboration with a state which seemed to be capable of bringing tranquillity and ordered market

---

[1] Hubert Deschamps, 'Et maintenant, Lord Lugard?' *Africa*, 1963, **33**; Michael Crowder, 'Indirect rule, French and British style', *Africa*, 1964, **34**.

[2] *Southern Nigeria in transition, 1885–1906: theory and practice in a colonial protectorate* (Cambridge University Press, 1966), esp. pp. 87–92, 149–61. But on the background of merchant pressure cf. Cherry Gertzel, 'Relations between African and European traders in the Niger Delta', *Journal of African History*, 1962, **3**, 361–6.

conditions to an extensive area of the Gold Coast hinterland. Yet Britain's position in and commitments to the coastal states led to repeated conflicts, strengthening an antithetical stereotype of 'a savage and barbarous power...a constant menace to the safety of the Gold Coast Colony...a formidable hindrance to its development and the advance of civilisation...an obstacle to trade, and...a disgrace to humanity'.[1]

By January 1896 fears of advancing French influence in the Sudan, pressure from British and Gold Coast merchants interested in trade with the interior, and the failure of some half-hearted and unskilful attempts to establish a form of supervisory control led Joseph Chamberlain to authorize a military expedition. Although Prempeh, the Asantehene, offered no military resistance, his failure to satisfy inflated demands for a gold indemnity provided the occasion for his deposition and exile, and the establishment of a British protectorate in which the member states of the confederacy were placed under the direct supervision of the Resident. Here as elsewhere British attitudes towards African states seem to have been determined with characteristic British pragmatism.

But Frenchmen could be pragmatists too, quite prepared to maintain such African political structures as might fit in with their short-term programmes. This, on the whole, happened more frequently in coastal districts, where civilian officials and commercial interests could more effectively check the belligerence of military officers, and where the need to forestall the British led French officials to conclude protectorate treaties with chiefs whose territories they were not yet ready to occupy physically. In Fouta Djallon, for example, the treaty that established French protection in 1881 was made at a time when France's control of the Guinean coast was still precarious. Only after twenty-five years of progressive interference did the French begin to break up this historic Muslim state. By 1912 its provinces had been converted into administrative cantons, and traditional chieftaincy was coming to be regarded as a barrier between the French and their subjects. Because of this creeping extension of French control, the chiefs of Fouta Djallon were slow to appreciate its implications. Alfa Yaya of Labé, for example, collaborated with the French until their contemptuous distrust of chiefly power became unmistakable.

Even in the military districts of the Sudan, Frenchmen would

[1] Memo by Hemming, Feb. 1895, quoted in William Tordoff, *Ashanti under the Prempehs, 1888–1935* (London, Oxford University Press, 1965), p. 55.

maintain traditional structures so far as this might seem expedient, notably among Berber peoples of the desert marches, whose complete subjugation would have been a formidable military task. A good example of tentative attitudes by both French and Africans in the early period of contact is provided by French relations with the populous, old-established Mossi kingdoms of Upper Volta. Never visited by Europeans before the arrival of Krause at Ouagadougou in 1886, Mossi and its caravan markets quickly became an object of interest to Germans, British, and particularly to imperial-minded French officers. This meant that the Mossi, once they had learned to distinguish among these nationalities, might hope to balance one against another; and that the French had to reckon with the possible danger of being forestalled.

In 1888 Gustave Binger, the first French visitor, concluded that the Mossi state was in process of disintegration, though he does not seem very clear whether this was because of the inertia of Mogho Naba Sanum or of his oppressive acts.[1] When Binger proposed a protectorate treaty, Sanum reacted vigorously enough, ordering him to leave the country. Having recently heard reports of armed Europeans at Salaga, he feared a concerted encircling move. (The party was in fact German, under von François, though Binger assumed it was British.) Binger hoped that French overtures might make progress after the accession of the heir-apparent, Bokari Koutou, who had treated him very amicably. But two years later, when Dr Crozat found Bokari enthroned as Mogho Naba under the name Wobogo, this cordiality had been replaced by cautious awareness of the growing danger to his independence. He would welcome Frenchmen as traders, he told Crozat, but not too many of them.[2] The following year Wobogo refused to receive P. L. Monteil at all. Frenchmen tended to find these Mossi attitudes perverse and vacillating, unduly influenced by the hostility of the Muslim community towards France. But Muslim traders and *hajis* knew more about Europeans than Europe knew about Mossi; and Wobogo himself was perhaps better able to distinguish between different European nations after Lieutenant-Colonel L. Archinard's treacherous attack on the Tukulor empire in April 1890. There is no reason to suppose that he did not sign and consciously accept the treaty

[1] *Du Niger au Golfe de Guinée par le pays de Kong et le Mossi, 1887–1889* (Paris, 1892), I, 460–5, 502.

[2] 'Rapport sur une mission à Mossi', *Journal Officiel de la République Française,* 5–9 Oct. 1891, pp. 4280–3, 4835–7, 4847–50.

of friendship and trade presented to him on 2 July 1894 by G. E. Ferguson, a Eurafrican in Gold Coast service, even if the Union Jack provided was converted into a garment for Wobogo's principal wife.[1] British troops were less likely than the French to march on Ouagadougou, and the terms of the treaty did not threaten Mossi's independence.

But the very remoteness of British troops reduced the practical value of this treaty. French forces were now much closer. In May 1895 they imposed their candidate as Naba of the neighbouring state of Yatenga, and in July 1896 the imperious Lieutenant Voulet set out to occupy Ouagadougou. Having failed to keep the French away by diplomacy, Wobogo raised an army of horsemen to oppose them. Accounts differ about the effectiveness of his resistance, but the relatively small French force occupied Ouagadougou in September, and replaced Wobogo by a more pliable brother, who agreed to accept a treaty of protection. By June 1897 Mossi resistance was over. Wobogo took refuge in the Gold Coast, but the British were not prepared to risk war with France to defend their tenuous rights under Ferguson's treaty.

Although this was the end of Mossi's independence, it was not the end of the Mossi state. The French, lacking resources to impose direct administration in a populous country so remote from the base of their power, installed successors who they hoped would prove compliant. In accordance with their view of the 'decadence' of the Mossi monarchy they began by trying to weaken the political power of the Mogho Naba by supporting his vassals against him. Yet it gradually became apparent that his social and religious influence could conveniently be used to control anti-French marabouts, and that administration might be facilitated by the co-operation of a ruler acknowledged by his people as a true and legitimate Mogho Naba. Although obliged to promote onerous French demands for revenue and labour, the Nabas retained enough of their traditional authority to establish a strong position in the modern politics of Upper Volta, which was re-formed as a separate entity in 1947 largely through their efforts. Even in face of the least

[1] Ferguson's treaty is in C.O. 879/41—Conf. Print. African (West) no. 479, pp. 27–8. The covering report gives only a brief account of Ferguson's visit to Ouagadougou. The story about the flag is in 'Les missions françaises dans la boucle du Niger', Comité de l'Afrique Française, *Bulletin*, April 1897, **7**, no. 4, pp. 108–9; the allegation in this report that Ferguson did not reach Ouagadougou until December is uncritically accepted in the otherwise useful account in Elliot P. Skinner, *The Mossi of the Upper Volta: the political development of a Sudanese people* (Stanford University Press, 1964), ch. 9.

tolerant arm of French imperialism, they did not lose all possibility of bargaining and manoeuvre.

Comparisons between French and British policies need to be taken no further in this discussion. Neither side embarked on the occupation of its African empire with a fixed and monolithic policy, pointing towards a single inevitable fate for the African polities in its path. If the aims and aspirations of those Europeans who led the advance sometimes implied a need for military conquest, more often they were such as could be satisfied by some form of treaty providing access to commercial markets, denying land to rival imperialisms, laying foundations for political control. Of course, as Saadia Touval reminds us, there were treaties and treaties.[1] Some were taken seriously by both signatories, some by neither; some were far-reaching in their terms, others almost meaningless. After the onset of the scramble, and the enunciation by the Berlin Conference of the principle of 'effective occupation',[2] African signatories were usually required to make more far-reaching surrenders of their rights of independent action than in the days of 'informal empire'. Yet, since they were more liable to diplomatic challenge, these later treaties needed to be better authenticated. When the European signatory needed collaborators in policies which he was still too weak to carry out directly, there might still be genuine reciprocity of obligation. Even when imperial control had become secure, it was still necessary to find *interlocuteurs valables* within the colony; ex-employees of the postal department, however shrewd, did not make ideal 'chiefs'.[3]

Given this range of possible attitudes on the part of the European invaders, a number of options might be open to African rulers. Among the short-term advantages obtainable from treaties or from collaboration with Europeans were not merely access to fire-arms and consumer goods, but opportunities to enlist powerful allies in external or internal disputes. Why then did so many African states reject such opportunities,

[1] 'Treaties, borders and the partition of Africa', *Journal of African History*, 1966, **7**, 279–93.

[2] Strictly this principle applied to coastal territories only. (See S.E. Crowe, *The Berlin West African conference, 1884–1885* (London, 1942), pt. 2, ch. 6.) But after 1885 the powers became more conscious of the need to provide each other with documentary evidence for their territorial claims.

[3] For the career of 'Fama' Mademba Sy, see Abd-el-Kader Mademba (his son), 'Au Sénégal et au Soudan français', Comité d'Etudes Historiques et Scientifiques de l'Afrique occidentale française, *Bulletin*, April–June 1930, **13**, no. 2.

choosing to resist the Europeans in battle? In West Africa, as in East and Central Africa, it cannot be said that those who opted for resistance were less far-sighted or forward-looking than the 'collaborators'.[1] In fact they were often the same men. Wobogo, for example, first received Binger cordially; became much more suspicious of the French after his accession; but only fought them after the Voulet mission had made their hostility unmistakably clear. Lat-Dior, *damel* of Cayor, a Senegalese kingdom with much longer experience of the French, was a 'modernizer' in his acceptance of commercial ground-nut production, and adjustment to its social consequences. After resisting Faidherbe's attempts to replace him by a more compliant ruler, he co-operated with succeeding governors on the more generous terms they offered, but finally reached the sticking-point when the French began to build a railway through his country. Convinced (rightly) that this 'steamship on dry land' would erode his sovereignty, he chose to die resisting in 1886.[2] (His name, and reputation, however, live on in the Senegalese army barracks in Dakar.)

Examples could be multiplied indefinitely. Nearly all West African states made some attempt to find a basis on which they could coexist with Europeans. Virtually all seem to have had some interests which they would defend by resistance or revolt—some conception of what can only be described as a rudimentary 'national cause' anterior to, and distinct from, the national loyalties demanded by modern independent states. An analysis of the 'national cause' of any specific people would need to embrace some values deeply rooted in their own culture and not very readily comprehensible to outsiders, together with some that can be universally understood—claims to territory, freedom to settle matters of internal concern without foreign interference. On this basis they would face the problem of relations with foreigners. Whether it was judged necessary to defend the national cause in battle, and at what stage, depended on variables on both sides of the Afro–European relationship—on African statecraft as well as on European intentions.

In countries where African political structures had already been

[1] Compare Roland Oliver and John D. Fage, *A short history of Africa* (Harmondsworth, Middlesex and Baltimore, 1962), p. 203, and the comments on their thesis in Professor Ranger's essay in this volume, p. 302.
[2] Vincent Monteil, 'Lat Dior, Damel du Kayor (1842–1886) et l'islamisation des Wolofs', *Archives de Sociologie des Religions*, July–Dec. 1963, **8**, no. 16, pp. 77–104; Germaine Ganier, 'Lat Dyor et le chemin de fer de l'arachide, 1876–1886', Institut Français d'Afrique Noire, *Bulletin*, 1965, ser. B, **27**, nos. 1–2, pp. 223–81.

deeply affected by the growth of export trade, Afro-European relationships were conditioned by economic change. In the Niger delta, among the Yoruba, in coastal areas near Sierra Leone or on the Ivory Coast, political authority was diffused, and many African rulers were moved by considerations of commercial advantage or profit. Studies of 'conjuncture' may be needed to explain not only the pressures behind the European advance, but certain African reactions. Trading chiefs and heads of houses, as well as European merchants, sought to maintain the rate of profit in times of falling produce prices. The present discussion approaches the study of African resistance chiefly through rather simple cases, where centralized monarchies possessing the physical means of resistance defended national causes that can be described in fairly simple terms. To extend such an analysis to West Africa as a whole will, however, involve detailed studies of the relations between trade and politics, such as the one A. G. Hopkins is undertaking for the Lagos hinterland.

One of the classical cases of military resistance seems to be that of Samory, who between 1891 and 1898 fought the French with remarkable tenacity and military skill. Yet the record of his relations with France and Britain in the preceding decade shows many examples of his readiness to negotiate bases for genuine co-operation with either or both, provided that such bases safeguarded certain fundamentals of his independence. His early contacts with the French, beginning with the armed conflict at Keniera in February 1882, were indeed characterized by mutual mistrust and antagonism. But the French had to act circumspectly while building up their military force in the Niger valley, and it was only in early 1885 that Commander A. V. A. Combes's invasion of Bouré (whose gold was so important to Samory's economy) revealed prematurely the full extent of their hostility.

Samory's response was to develop his contacts with the British in Sierra Leone, first established in 1879–80. After occupying Falaba in 1884 he sent emissaries to Freetown to invite the governor 'to ask the Queen to take the whole of his country under her protection'.[1] The purpose of the offer was clearly to obtain British support in warding off the French, and Governor Rowe was doubtless correct in interpreting it as a diplomatic flourish not intended to alienate sovereignty. More

[1] Memorandum by Festing, 21 May 1886, of Nalifa Modu's message 25 Aug. 1885, C.O. 879/24, C.P. African 318, p. 13; Memorandum by Lawson, 8 Oct. 1886, *ibid.*, p. 25.

intent on protecting Sierra Leone's sphere of commercial and political influence among Temnes and Limbas than in seeking influence on the Niger, he did not even report the offer to London until a year later. His reply to Samory was amicable but cool, simply welcoming his promise to respect Temne country—'the Queen's garden'—and agreeing to develop friendly relations and trade.[1]

Yet this was not without importance for Samory. Commercial contacts alone gave him a vital interest in collaboration with Freetown. Until 1892, when the Sierra Leone government enforced the licensing of arms sales according to the Brussels convention of 1890, this route provided Samory with his supply of modern breach-loading rifles, which he was increasingly aware might be needed for use against the French.

Even now, Samory had not accepted armed conflict with France as inevitable. He was not leading a jihad against all Christians, nor a pan-African revolt against imperialism. He was concerned, practically, with governing and extending the empire he had conquered, with controlling its resources of gold, agricultural produce and men (including, of course, its slaves) and with enforcing the observance of Islam. It was perhaps less evident in the 1880s than later that these conditions were incompatible with the purposes of the French forces on the Niger. French relations with the Tukulor empire of Ségou remained somewhat ambivalent until 1890; and the French military, desperately anxious to forestall supposed British ambitions and chafing under restraint from Paris, were reduced to signing treaties with Samory also.

In March 1886, when Colonel L. L. Frey was obliged to divert his forces against Mamadou Lamina, Samory was able to make a French mission under Captain Tournier modify the terms which they had intended to impose upon him. He secured French recognition not only of his territories on the right bank of the Niger, but of his rights over the contested districts of Bouré and Kangaba. This left him more independence of action than the French were prepared to tolerate; and the following year, J. S. Gallieni (of all the French commanders the one most susceptible to the idea of protectorate relationships with Muslim rulers) sent Captain E. Péroz to negotiate new terms. Samory, although reluctant to damage his prestige by surrendering territory, wished to avoid further battles against French military power at a time

[1] Rowe to Granville, 19 June 1886, and enclosures, C.O. 879/24, p. 208; Rowe to Samory, 4 Sept. 1885, M.P. 1400/85, Sierra Leone Archives.

when he was about to attack his arch-enemy Tiéba, chief of Sikasso. After discussion he therefore agreed, by a treaty of 23 March 1887, to abandon the gold of Bouré to the French and to accept a boundary line on the Tinkisso river. According to the French, he agreed also to place his state and any future acquisitions under their protection.

As is often the case with such treaties of protection, it is difficult to tell how far Samory was aware of having entered into some new relationship with France under the protectorate clause. Certainly he interpreted it quite differently from the French (whose immediate concern was not to define their permanent status in his territories, but to acquire a legal title against the British). There is some evidence that Samory believed that the French had undertaken to assist him to further his own designs, in particular against Tiéba; counting on the alliance, he asked Binger for troops and artillery to help in his siege of Sikasso. But he certainly did not regard himself as having made an irreversible surrender of sovereignty. When the French refused to assist him, began to encroach on his territory, and tried to prevent his trading with Freetown, Samory 'began to doubt whether, after all, the white man's word could be thoroughly relied upon' and tried, somewhat naïvely perhaps, to reverse his policy.[1]

There still seemed to be possibilities of balancing British against French. In May 1888 Samory, while still besieging Sikasso, was visited by Major A. M. Festing, an official from Sierra Leone. This devout, garrulous and pompous man had exaggerated faith in his personal powers of persuasion and influence. He had an unrealistic vision of Samory, with Festing as adviser, making peace with his enemies, consolidating his dominions into a genuinely united kingdom, and admitting the railway which the house of F. and A. Swanzy hoped to build from Freetown. Samory was interested, accepted the principle of a railway, and promised to sign a treaty when he returned to Bissandougou; but he refused to risk provoking a French attack before defeating Sikasso.[2] In February 1889, indeed, he signed a new treaty with the French, accepting the Niger as the frontier everywhere and agreeing to direct trade towards French ports; but soon afterwards he returned this treaty (though not that of 1887) to the French. He told

[1] Thomas J. Alldridge, *A transformed colony: Sierra Leone, as it was, and as it is...* (London, 1910), p. 325 (from Garrett's Journal, 24 May 1890).

[2] Festing's journal, C.O. 879/29, C.P. African West 366, esp. pp. 23, 47, 50-1, 54, 59, 64, 120-3; also Maltby to Knutsford, 13 Oct. 1888, C.O. 879/24, African 318, no. 126.

another British travelling commissioner that he now considered himself free of obligations and ready to place his people and country under British protection; and on 24 May 1890 he signed a treaty promising not to alienate territory nor undertake obligations to third powers except through the British government. It was, however, too late. London had already decided that the French protectorate treaties must be recognized, that war with France for West Africa was excluded, and had agreed with France on a partition of influence through the middle of Samory's empire. G. H. Garrett's treaty was not ratified, and Samory's partisans in Freetown tried in vain to persuade the government to work with him.[1]

Samory's diplomacy was thus doomed to failure by the constant hostility of most French soldiers. Although some civilians wanted to avoid, or at least defer, a conflict, the ambitious and thrusting Colonel Archinard was hostile to any policy of tolerating Muslim empires. In April 1891 he again slipped the long rein of civilian control and attacked Kankan, intending to cut Samory's supply route to Sierra Leone. Thus the final period of armed resistance began. Until all of Yves Person's work has been published, assessment of Samory's personality and achievements can only be tentative. His dealings with the French were so marked by mutual mistrust and cultural incompatibility that a sober judgement is difficult; but it seems that Samory's attempts at coexistence were at least as seriously intended as those of the Frenchmen with whom he was dealing. For both sides, collaboration involved accepting restrictions of their rights, interests and prestige which came to seem intolerable.

Samory's case thus hardly supports the view of Professors Oliver and Fage that 'nothing was to be gained by resistance and much by negotiation';[2] nothing that he held important could have been permanently gained by either method. (J. Suret-Canale suggests that something might have been achieved had Samory, Ahmadou and Tiéba been 'capable of rising above their quarrels in time to present a common front to the invader'.[3] Although such a coalition might have postponed the French conquest, however, it is doubtful whether it could have averted it.)

[1] For Garrett's mission, C.O. 879/32, C.P. African 387, esp. nos. 34, 62a, 79, 99, 115, 125, 126, 136, 219; Alldridge, *Transformed colony*, pp. 320–6.
[2] *Short history*, p. 203.
[3] *Afrique noire, occidentale et centrale* (Paris, 1958), I, 211.

On the other hand, resistance—if combined at other times with willingness to accommodate and skill in doing so—could further the cause of national survival. In Northern Nigeria, most evidently, the military resistance of the emirs did much to determine the basis of the very special relationship which their successors enjoyed with the British administration. Even here, however, D. J. M. Muffett has argued that the conflict of 1903 was due less to intransigent resistance by Sultan Attahiru than to Lugard's determination that, before the British could utilize the Fulani as a 'ruling caste', the military basis of British suzerainty should be asserted by conquest. Muffett cites reports by Burdon and Temple to show that before the expedition to Kano and Sokoto Lugard was receiving 'a mounting tale of evidence of the Sultan's readiness to be amenable and of the ripeness of the time for a diplomatic approach'; and he questions the translation and the dating of the famous assertion by Attahiru's predecessor that 'Between you and us there are no dealings except as between Mussulmans and unbelievers—War, as God Almighty has enjoined on us'.[1] Lugard may indeed have hoped the conquest of Kano would make that of Sokoto unnecessary.[2] But as Attahiru saw British soldiers invading his provinces from the south, as he was joined by the stream of Tijaniyya fugitives from the French in the west, it must have seemed increasingly clear that 'the doings of the Europeans'[3] threatened the independence of Muslim Africa. It was left for his successors to discover how much could be preserved by collaboration with the British conquerors.

Ashanti, faced with ambivalent British attitudes touched on above, may have missed opportunities of profiting by a more flexible diplomacy. Even hostile officials like W. Brandford Griffith presented a less formidable menace to African autonomy than did Combes or Archinard. Anglo-Ashanti relations have been described as 'a mutual and protracted misunderstanding between peoples with fundamentally different conceptual frameworks'. The freedom which British imperialists claimed to be bringing to the peoples of Ashanti was not the

---

[1] *Concerning brave captains...* (London, 1964), esp. ch. 3.

[2] *Ibid.*, p. 109, Lugard to Chamberlain 21 Feb. 1903; Margery Perham, *Lugard*, vol. II: *The years of authority, 1898–1945* (London, 1960), II, 120, Lugard to his wife, 6 March 1903.

[3] Cf. the narrative of Hassan Keffi in Muffett, *Concerning brave captains*, p. 64: 'The first news that we in Keffi had of the doings of the Europeans was brought by a group of Tijani who had been driven out of their country by the French...Then later, men from Bida came to tell us of the war waged there by men of "the Company".'

freedom demanded by the resisters of 1900—freedom 'to buy and sell slaves as in the old time', freedom 'from demands for carriers ..', 'from the obligations of building houses and supplying thatch', and from the unwelcome attentions of 'huxters and strangers'.[1]

Yet contradictions of this sort, which existed along the whole front of Afro-European relations, did not inevitably have to be resolved by head-on conflict. Might not Prempeh have preserved more of Ashanti political and cultural autonomy by accepting, for example, Griffith's unauthorized Protectorate of 1891? He would have preserved the unity of the confederacy, its right to levy customary revenue, and some at least of the 'habits and customs of the country'; and although the Asantehene would in many respects, no doubt, have become increasingly dependent on the British Resident who was to be appointed, an adaptable Asantehene would doubtless have made the Residency equally dependent upon his own collaboration. In retrospect Prempeh's decision that 'Ashanti must remain independent as of old' seems to have led logically on to his own deposition in 1896, to Governor Hodgson's ill-advised claim in 1900 to assume the authority of the Golden Stool, and so to the final military conflict and the subjection of Ashanti to direct British administration.[2]

Yet this was by no means the end of the Ashanti nation. In 1900 some of the outlying peoples of the Confederacy, who had not always been noted for their loyal support of ruling Asantehenes, rallied to defend Ashanti against British aggression. Prempeh in exile became a more powerful focus of unity than he had been in Kumasi; British administrators in Ashanti, cherishing their separate status under the Governor of the Gold Coast, came better to appreciate the strength and complexity of Ashanti national feeling. The advice of R. S. Rattray, appointed as government anthropologist in the 1920s, furthered this reassessment. Ashanti began to seem a natural theatre for experiments in Indirect Rule. In 1924 Prempeh returned to the country; in 1926 he was recognized as Omanhene of Kumasi. The confederacy was restored under his nephew in 1935, and in 1943 crown lands in Kumasi were restored to

[1] Hodgson to Chamberlain, 16 April 1900 in George Edgar Metcalfe, *Great Britain and Ghana: documents of Ghana history, 1807–1957* (London, 1964), no. 431; B. Wasserman, 'The Ashanti war of 1900: a study in cultural conflict', *Africa*, 1961, 31, pp. 167–79.
[2] For the British offer, see Griffith to Knutsford, 19 May 1891, and enclosure in Metcalfe, *Documents*, nos. 372–3. Prempeh's reply, 7 May 1891, is at Tordoff, *Ashanti*, pp. 43–4. Tordoff, chs. 2 and 3, analyses Hodgson's aims in 1900, and the organization of British rule after 1901.

the Asantehene. One may reasonably ask whether, but for the resistance of the 1890s, Nkrumah's Convention People's Party would, over fifty years later, have faced such strenuous opposition from the National Liberation Movement, '...a Kumasi-centred Ashanti movement, which appealed for support in the name of the Asantehene, the Golden Stool, Ashanti interests, Ashanti history and Ashanti rights'.[1] References to military exploits against the British enabled the Ashanti to counter the anti-imperialist centralism of the Convention People's Party with claims to having been anti-imperialist from the first hour. In the long run, something was after all gained by resistance for the Ashanti 'national cause', if not for that of a future unitary Ghanaian nation.[2]

This conclusion is reinforced by a comparison of the experience of the Fon and the Gun during the French occupation of Dahomey. The Fon state of Abomey throughout the nineteenth century exhibited attitudes of proud resistance towards all European attempts to encroach upon its sovereign rights or to compel changes in a way of life which Europeans found particularly abhorrent. This does not imply that it was 'hostile to modernization'. King Gezo, although unable to meet fully British demands that he should cease exporting slaves and conducting the sacrificial 'customs', did much to encourage and participate in the production and sale of palm-oil as soon as Europeans showed interest in buying it. But although trade and diplomatic intercourse were welcome, the Dahomeans were uncomfortably aware that Europeans who entered African states to trade sometimes ended by ruling. Thus in 1876, Gelele preferred to undergo a British naval blockade rather than admit European interference in a commercial dispute which lay within his own jurisdiction.[3] Yet he was anxious to avoid a military conflict, for 'he who makes the powder wins the battle'. When the French sent troops to Cotonou under a treaty of

[1] Dennis Austin, Politics in Ghana, 1946–1960 (London, Oxford University Press, 1964), pp. 265–7.
[2] The important subject of what Professor Ranger, quoting J. Iliffe on p. 309, calls 'post-pacification revolts' is not dealt with in the present discussion. Resistance at this stage might help also to focus the loyalties of later generations. Note, for example, the popularity of Bai Bureh in modern Sierra Leone—not among northerners alone. (At least one eminent Creole intellectual has named his son after him.) On the other hand, the Mende rising does not appear to have had the same effect.
[3] Cf. memorandum by Ouidah cabooceers, Feb. 1876, arguing that 'this palaver is a trade palaver, and whoever thinks that we cannot [sic] capable of judging such palaver they are mistaken', F. O. 84/1464.

cession of 1878 (made in Gelele's name but probably without his consent), he confined himself to obstruction and protests.

Rulers of the Gun kingdom of Porto Novo were more ready to co-operate with Europeans, both politically and commercially. In part, this attitude reflected fear of Abomey, whose armies for much of the nineteenth century constituted an intermittent threat to this smaller Aja state; in part it was caused by the desire of one of the ruling lineages to secure external support for its dynastic and territorial claims. In 1862 King Soji made an unsuccessful attempt to preserve these interests through a French protectorate. After 1874 his son, King Tofa, revived this policy. Tofa was a shrewd politician who worked with European traders to increase his wealth and power; 'his succession', say the traditional historians of Porto Novo, 'marked the transition into modern times'.[1] At first the French could do little to protect his territories against either Abomey or British Lagos, and Tofa showed bitter disappointment with the protectorate. But when Behanzin, who succeeded Gelele at the end of 1889, took more active steps to enforce his territorial claims, the French government was drawn somewhat hesitantly into military operations against him, largely through the intrigues of their ally Tofa.

How did Tofa, the 'collaborator', fare by comparison with Behanzin, 'the shark that troubled the bar'? Although Behanzin defended Dahomean rights more vigorously than Gelele had latterly done, he, like his predecessors, at first tried to avoid fighting France. In March 1891, after the initial clashes, Behanzin received French emissaries with apparently sincere expressions of friendship and desire for peace, and agreed not to make war on Porto Novo, since the French were there. But he refused formally to renounce his title to Cotonou, or his liberty to send armies to other parts of his dominions; and he rejected as infringing his internal sovereignty French demands for the release of some of his own subjects whom he had detained during the fighting.[2] In 1892, after receiving new arms supplies from German merchants,

[1] Adolphe Akindélé and Cyrille Aguessy, *Contribution à l'étude de l'histoire de l'ancien Royaume de Porto Novo* (Dakar, Institut Français d'Afrique Noire, 1953), p. 52.
[2] Reports of the Audéoud-Decoeur mission are printed in *Etudes Dahoméennes*, 1953, **9** ('L'histoire dahoméenne de la fin du XIXᵉ siècle à travers les textes'); see especially pp. 114 and 131–4. The account in Robert Cornevin, *Histoire du Dahomey* (Paris, 1962), ch. 9, draws on material published by E. Dunglas in *Etudes Dahoméennes*. By far the best and fullest account of Franco-Dahomean relations is in David Ross's 'The autonomous kingdom of Dahomey, 1818–94' (Ph.D. thesis, University of London, 1967), a work completed after the present account was written.

he proudly reaffirmed his right to coerce all the towns which he considered as his, excepting Porto Novo, even at risk of a war with France.

I am the king of the Negroes [he wrote to the French representative], and white men have no concern with what I do...Please remain calm, carry on your trade at Porto Novo, and on that basis we shall remain at peace as before. If you want war I am ready...'.[1]

By this time the French had come to the conclusion, somewhat apprehensively and reluctantly, that war would be necessary to defend the position which their subjects had established in Dahomey. Accordingly, in 1892 the Senegalese Colonel A. A. Dodds carried out that march on Abomey which tough Dahomean diplomacy had thus far helped to postpone. But even now France hesitated to destroy the structure of the Dahomean state. During 1893 Behanzin continued to resist with much popular support; and the French, finding difficulty in identifying other *interlocuteurs valables*, contemplated accepting his offers to negotiate. In January 1894 they recognized his brother as ruler of an area corresponding roughly to the seventeenth-century rump of Abomey, and as a temporary expedient practised a form of indirect rule until 1900. Even afterwards the dynasty continued to enjoy widespread prestige, which the French acknowledged in 1928 by arranging the ceremonial return from exile of Behanzin's ashes. (One wonders how far they had considered the implications of the analogy with the return of Napoleon's ashes to France in 1840.) Nor was this prestige confined to traditionalist circles. A clandestine newspaper published by two nationalist school-teachers in 1915 took the name *Le Recadaire* (ceremonial messenger) *de Behanzin*.[2]

By comparison, Tofa's policy of collaboration won certain advantages in the short run. He remained ruler of Porto Novo under the French protectorate until his death in 1908, but with dwindling privileges and functions. He seems to have become bitterly conscious of accusations that he had sold his country to the French. With his funeral, say the traditional historians, the monarchy of Porto Novo came to an end.[3] His heirs, for whom he had sought French support, were mere

[1] Behanzin to Ballot, 10 April 1892 in Cornevin, *Histoire du Dahomey*, p. 340.
[2] John A. Ballard, 'The Porto Novo incidents of 1923: politics in the colonial era', *Odu*, July 1965, 2, no. 1, p. 64.
[3] Akindélé and Aguessy, *Porto Novo*, 89; Colin W. Newbury, *The western Slave Coast and its rulers...* (Oxford, Clarendon Press, 1961), pp. 184–5.

French clients, their influence among the Gun eclipsed by others. On 28 November 1965 the author of this essay visited Tofa's successor in Porto Novo. Elsewhere in the town revolutionary manifestations were taking place on behalf of the Gun President of the Dahomean Republic, who had been declared deposed by a Fon prime minister. Even though this constitutional conflict clearly reflected old antagonisms of Fon and Gun, however, the royal palace had become an irrelevant backwater. President S. M. Apithy, representative of the Gun 'national cause', had begun his eventful political career as a young intellectual associated with the Catholic mission. But Justin Ahomadegbe, leader of the Fon, spoke not merely as a trade unionist, but as a member of the house of Behanzin.

Until more research has been done on the policies and aims of individual African states, a survey of this kind must be superficial and tentative. It is hardly profound to conclude that the most important element making for the survival of African polities under colonial rule was simply a strong sense of ethnic or political identity—the attachment of their subjects to what has been called the 'national cause'. This sense of identity tended to be strengthened when the rulers who represented it could point to some record of resistance to imperialism. This does not mean blind or reactionary opposition. Those leaders who achieved most for the national cause, whether immediately or in the longer run, combined military action with more or less discriminating attempts to find some basis for coexistence or collaboration. Indeed, their success in keeping old national causes alive has sometimes presented problems to modern leaders who seek to represent a broader form of nationalism.

BIBLIOGRAPHY

Akindélé, Adolphe, and Cyrille Aguessy. *Contribution à l'étude de l'histoire de l'ancien royaume de Porto Novo.* Dakar, Institut Français d'Afrique Noire, 1953.
Alexandre, P. 'Le problème des chefferies en Afrique noire française', *Notes et Etudes Documentaires*, 10 Feb. 1959, no. 2508.
Alldridge, Thomas J. *A transformed colony: Sierra Leone, as it was, and as it is, its progress, peoples, native customs, and undeveloped wealth.* London, 1910.
Anene, J. C. *Southern Nigeria in transition, 1885–1906: theory and practice in a colonial protectorate.* Cambridge University Press, 1966.

Austin, Dennis. *Politics in Ghana, 1946–1960*. London, Oxford University Press, 1964.

Ballard, John A. 'The Porto Novo incidents of 1923: politics in the colonial era', *Odu*, July 1965, **2**, no. 1.

Binger, L. G. *Du Niger au Golfe de Guinée par le pays de Kong et le Mossi, 1887–1889*, 2 vols. Paris 1892.

Coquery, Catherine. 'Le blocus de Whydah (1876–1877) et la rivalité franco-anglaise au Dahomey', *Cahiers d'Etudes Africaines*, 1962, **2**, no. 7.

Cornevin, Robert. *Histoire du Dahomey*. Paris, 1962.

Crowder, Michael. 'Indirect rule, French and British style', *Africa*, 1964, **34.**

Crowe, S. E. *The Berlin West African conference, 1884–1885*. London, 1942.

Crozat, Dr. 'Rapport sur une mission à Mossi', *Journal Officiel de la République Française*, 5–9 Oct. 1891.

Deschamps, Hubert. 'Et maintenant, Lord Lugard?' *Africa*, 1963, **33.**

Etudes Dahoméennes, 1953, **9** (special memorial issue dedicated to Edouard Dunglas).

Fyfe, Christopher A. *A history of Sierra Leone*. London, Oxford University Press, 1962.

Ganier, Germaine. 'Lat Dyor et le chemin de fer de l'arachide, 1876–1886', Institut Français d'Afrique Noire, *Bulletin*, 1965, ser. B, **27**, nos. 1–2.

Gertzel, Cherry. 'Relations between African and European traders in the Niger Delta', *Journal of African History*, 1962, **3**.

Hargreaves, John D. 'The evolution of the Native Affairs Department', *Sierra Leone Studies*, n.s. 3, Dec. 1954.

Prelude to the partition of West Africa. London, 1963.

'The Tokolor Empire of Ségou and its relations with the French', in *Boston University papers on Africa*, vol. II: *African history*, Jeffrey Butler, ed. Boston University Press, 1966.

Herskovits, Melville J. *Dahomey: an ancient West African kingdom*. New York, 1938.

'L'histoire dahoméenne de la fin du XIXe siècle à travers les textes', *Etudes Dahoméennes*, 1953, **9**.

Kanya-Forstner, A. S. 'The role of the military in the formulation of French policy towards the Western Sudan, 1879–99.' Ph.D. thesis, Cambridge University, 1965.

Keltie, J. S. *The partition of Africa*. London, 1893.

Legassick, Martin. 'Firearms, horses and Samorian army organisation, 1870–1898', *Journal of African History*, 1966, **7**, no. 1.

Mademba, Abd-el-Kader, 'Au Sénégal et au Soudan français', Comité d'Etudes Historiques et Scientifiques de l'Afrique Occidentale Française, *Bulletin*, April–June 1930, **13**, no. 2.

Méniaud, Jacques. *Les pionniers du Soudan, avant, avec et après Archinard, 1879–1894.* 2 vols. Paris, 1931.

Metcalfe, George Edgar. *Great Britain and Ghana: documents of Ghana history, 1807–1957.* London, 1964.

'Les missions françaises dans la boucle du Niger', Comité de l'Afrique Française, *Bulletin*, April 1897, **7**, no. 4.

Monteil, Parfait-Louis. *De Saint-Louis à Tripoli par le Tchad: voyage au travers du Soudan et du Sahara accompli pendant les années 1890–91–92.* Paris, 1895.

Monteil, Vincent. 'Lat Dior, Damel du Kayor (1842–1886) et l'islamisation des Wolofs', *Archives de Sociologie des Religions*, July–Dec. 1963, **8**, no. 16.

Muffett, D. J. M. *Concerning brave captains: being a history of the British occupation of Kano and Sokoto and of the last stand of the Fulani forces.* London, 1964.

Newbury, Colin W. 'A note on the Abomey protectorate', *Africa*, April 1959, **29**, no. 2.

The western Slave Coast and its rulers: European trade and administration among the Yoruba and Adja-speaking peoples of south-western Nigeria, southern Dahomey and Togo. Oxford, Clarendon Press, 1961.

Oliver, Roland, and John D. Fage. *A short history of Africa.* Harmondsworth, Middlesex and Baltimore, 1962.

Perham, Margery, *Lugard.* 2 vols. London, 1956–60.

Péroz, Marie Etienne. *Au Soudan français: souvenirs de guerre et de mission.* Paris, 1889.

Person, Yves, 'Les ancêtres de Samori', *Cahiers d'Etudes Africaines*, 1963, **4**, no. 13.

'L'aventure de Porèkèrè et le drame de Waïma', *Cahiers d'Etudes Africaines*, 1965, **5**, no. 18.

'Correspondances de la résidence du Kissi relatives à l'affaire de Waïma (1893)', *Cahiers d'Etudes Africaines*, 1965, **5**, no. 19.

'La jeunesse de Samori', *Revue Française d'Histoire d'Outre-Mer*, 1962, **49**, no. 175.

'Samori et la Sierra Leone', *Cahiers d'Etudes Africaines*, 1967, **7**, no. 25.

Samori: une revolution Dyula. Dakar, Institut Fondamental d'Afrique Noire, 1968.

Ross, David. 'The autonomous kingdom of Dahomey, 1818–94.' Ph.D. thesis, University of London, 1967.

Skinner, Elliott P. *The Mossi of the Upper Volta: the political development of a Sudanese people.* Stanford University Press, 1964.

Suret-Canale, Jean. *Afrique noire, occidentale et centrale.* 2 vols. Paris, 1958, 1964.

Tordoff, William, *Ashanti under the Prempehs, 1888–1935*. London, Oxford University Press, 1965.

Touval, Saadia. 'Treaties, borders and the partition of Africa', *Journal of African History*, 1966, **7**.

Wasserman, B. 'The Ashanti war of 1900: a study in cultural conflict', *Africa*, April 1961, **31**, no. 2.

CHAPTER 7

NIGERIA: THE COLONIAL EXPERIENCE FROM 1880 TO 1914

by JOHN E. FLINT

When the British began to extend colonial rule over Nigeria in the 1880s, they had no thought of creating a colony that would one day become a nation-state. Such a concept had existed in the earlier nineteenth century; it had formed part of the anti-slavery policy of 'legitimate commerce', and as developed by Henry Venn and Bishop Crowther,[1] it had become specifically Nigerian in character. The Church Missionary Society's all-African Niger Mission was seen not simply as a means to Christian conversion, but as a training-ground in responsibility and organization. The Niger river was regarded as a great artery of commercial and cultural development, along and around which a new African élite of educated, Christian and individualistic freemen would revolutionize the country's social, political and economic institutions. Eventually there would arise 'a kingdom which shall render incalculable benefits to Africa and hold a position among the states of Europe'.[2] But this vision was confined almost exclusively to the missionaries, though the British government could at times be sympathetic, even to the extent of annexing Lagos in 1861 to control the seaport for missionaries in Yorubaland.

Among the British these ideals had faded by the 1880s almost to the point of extinction. The growth of racial theories in Europe after 1860 had undermined the concept of a true imperial partnership. Even in the C.M.S. Niger Mission, the 'brotherhood of man' had been disrupted by a nasty and debasing struggle along racial lines between black and white clergy. If this was so in the missions, it was even more in evidence in

[1] Henry Venn was Lay Secretary of the Church (of England) Missionary Society from 1841 to 1872. Samuel Adjai Crowther, a Yoruba liberated from a slave-ship by the Royal Navy, was consecrated in 1864 as the first African to become a bishop of the Church of England.

[2] Henry Venn to H. Robbin, 2 Jan. 1857 (C.M.S. Archives, CA 2/L2), quoted in J. F. A. Ajayi, 'Nineteenth century origins of Nigerian nationalism', *Journal of the Historical Society of Nigeria*, Dec. 1961, **2**, no. 2, p. 199.

secular life. After 1880 it became almost impossible for Africans in the colonial administration to rise to positions of authority (as they frequently had in the 1850s and 1860s).

In commerce the alliance between white capital and technical skill and black commercial initiative, exemplified earlier in Macgregor Laird's African Steamship Company, came to an end after 1875 with the intense competition between white and black traders and the growing monopolistic tendencies of the white firms. In 1879, when the United African Company was formed by George Taubman Goldie, the new company dismissed all the senior African managers and agents of the firms it took over. The C.M.S., on the advice of Bishop Crowther, sold the shares allotted to it in respect of its previous shareholding in one of the firms that joined the amalgam. The company's obsessional concern for a monopoly led to its quest for administrative powers to exclude its rivals. In 1886 it received a Royal Charter to administer the Niger and Benue area, changing its name shortly afterwards to the Royal Niger Company. Goldie, its driving personality, had no sympathy for the older doctrines of 'Christianity and commerce'. Himself neither a Christian nor a free-trader, he had nothing but contempt for educated and semi-educated Christian Africans, whom he regarded as hypocrites in religion and dangerous rivals in commerce.

By 1880 the old ideal of racial partnership had soured. The British not only had put nothing in its place, but lacked even a coherent policy. All that remained in British attitudes of the earlier Victorian moral fervour was a continuing, if attenuated, sense that Britain had a special role in opposing slavery, and a declining conviction that commerce was the strongest weapon against slavery and the slave-trade.

By the 1880s the morale of the British in Nigeria had reached its lowest ebb. British officials had as yet hardly felt the quickening excitement of the new imperialism. Since their posts—being most dangerous to health—were the least desirable in the entire public service, the quality of recruits was low. Able men, if posted to West Africa, hoped to secure promotion elsewhere as quickly as possible. British civil servants moreover received little inspiration from their non-official compatriots in West Africa. The white missionaries were, by this time, usually men of limited vision, with petty obsessions, much concerned with questions of Sunday observance, opposition to the liquor trade, and personal rivalries. The white trading agents, though often picturesque characters, and sometimes men of real ability with

more understanding of the realities of African life than many missionaries,[1] wielded little real power; their decisions were made for them in
London or Liverpool. In the acute depression of palm-oil prices that
occurred in the 1880s, such decisions came to be increasingly dominated
by short-term considerations of immediate profit, and long-term
policies directed towards monopoly by amalgamation. The objective
of white traders' policies after 1880 was simply to reduce prices paid to
Africans for their produce—hardly an inspiring programme.

It is a historical irony that the only people who on the eve of the
scramble for Africa possessed a sense of a British 'imperial mission'
were the educated or semi-educated Africans. Most of these were
'liberated Africans'[2] or their descendants, mainly, though not entirely,
Yoruba with strong Lagos connexions. These men, with varying
degrees of coherency, inherited, preserved and extended the original
concepts that had lain behind the African agency ideas of the Niger
mission. Emancipated from the demanding conservatism of traditional
tribal[3] life, considerably involved in the cash nexus, and often organized,
albeit in a small way, along capitalist lines, they saw the future as theirs.
They looked to a time when enlightened Christian views, an expanding
English-language educational system, and increasing cash trade would
steadily erode the traditional tribal social structure, the obscurantism of
chiefs and traditional rulers. They despised what they regarded as the
absurd superstitions of old Africa. In their view the ancient mode

[1] This is not the general view of historians, who usually characterize the white trading
agents as 'palm oil ruffians', little better than their slave-trading precursors. Most of
these men were in fact hard-drinking and hard-swearing characters, who would flog
and even kill Africans without compunction. To the missionaries they were anathema;
and being recruited from the lower classes in Britain, they were often despised by
officials and naval officers. But some of them, through long residence on the coast,
did gain an impressive and unique insight into African life which could not be rivalled
by that of officials and white missionaries. An outstanding example was Charlie
('The Count') de Cardi, whose appendix to Mary Kingsley's *West African Studies*
(London, 1899) now forms a major historical source for the history of the Niger Delta
city-states.
[2] I.e., Africans liberated at sea from slave-ships by the West African squadron of the
Royal Navy, and landed at Freetown, whence some of them eventually returned to
Nigeria.
[3] See Colson, pp. 28–32, for problems arising from use of the term 'tribe'. To many
readers 'tribe' usually signifies a small group of people. In Nigeria the Ibo of the south-
east, the Yoruba of the south-west, and the Hausa of the north each number several
million souls; and even the smaller groups, such as the Ibibio-Efik of Ijo, can be
counted in hundreds of thousands. These 'tribes' are thus in reality the ancient 'national'
groups of the country.

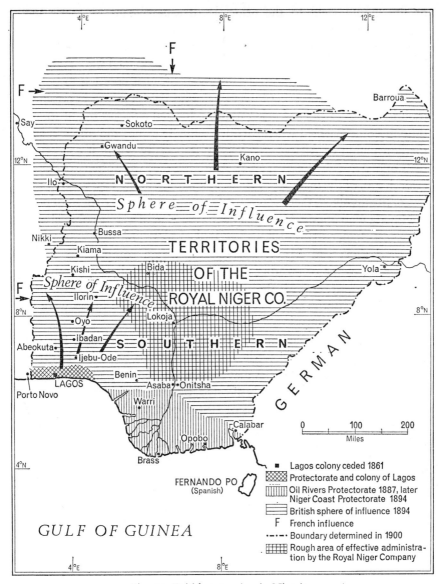

Fig. 12. British expansion in Nigeria.

of life should yield to the principle of achievement by merit and effort.

Though usually angered by hardening racial attitudes of white men in church and state, the new Africans were thick-skinned and pragmatic enough to control their hostility in favour of what they felt to be the greater good, the assertion of overwhelming British power in crushing traditional forces and enforcing unity. Educated Africans might sometimes become alarmed when partition actually came; and might resent the destruction of African sovereignty (especially where it concerned their own particular town or area). Although they were often extremely critical, too, of the methods of British expansion in the 1890s and of the loss of life involved, there was scarcely a single educated African of note in Nigeria who opposed in principle the creation of a large colonial unit in Nigeria under British rule. They looked to British sovereignty as a historical short cut. British intervention would complete in a few decades the work of creating a single territorial unit, comparable in size and population with the nation-states of Europe, a process that would take centuries to achieve if economic and social forces were to operate alone and unaided.

Herein lay a basic conflict in Nigerian history after 1880. For the British acquisition of the territories that came to be called Nigeria, and the administrative policies that Britain subsequently adopted, were not prompted, or even seriously affected, by these African aspirations—indeed, as time passed, the goals of British policy shifted farther away from them.

The motives behind British policy in the 1880s were pragmatic and practical. There was during that period no question in the minds of British politicians of building anything, least of all an empire, in Nigeria. The motives of British actions were entirely defensive, designed simply to retain existing areas of British commercial predominance. The acquisition of British political control over the Nigerian coast and the banks of the Niger in 1884-5 took place in a spirit of anti-imperialism and financial parsimony; and control was thus essentially minimal. The British meant only to prevent France from obtaining control of the British palm-oil trade on the Niger and in its delta.[1]

[1] See John E. Flint, *Sir George Goldie and the making of Nigeria* (London, Oxford University Press, 1960), chs. 3 and 4; John D. Hargreaves, *Prelude to the partition of West Africa* (London, 1963), chs. 6 and 7; and J. C. Anene, *Southern Nigeria in transition, 1885–1906*: ... (Cambridge University Press, 1966), ch. 2. All these writers argue that the basic motivation of British moves was the need to protect trade. Ronald E. Robinson and

This spirit was revealed clearly in the machinery by which British authority was extended. The Colonial Office resolutely refused to become involved in the new expansion. British policy-makers argued that they could not carry any more administrative costs, that the mortality rates for colonial officials were too high to contemplate, and that the implementation of the abolition of slavery (which would be obligatory if the territories fell under British colonial jurisdiction) would raise social problems which a Colonial Office régime could not solve.[1] The extensions of authority that took place in 1884–5 were therefore undertaken under the curious fiction that no additions were being made to the British empire. Expansion was carried out by the Foreign Office, using consular officials, under the theory that the establishment of protectorates was essentially diplomatic work. This fiction was maintained by the concept that areas brought under British control voluntarily passed over to Britain by treaty certain portions of sovereignty.

The essential power that the British needed was control over the foreign relations of African rulers. In all the treaties with the city-states of the Oil Rivers the kings and chiefs thus agreed 'to refrain from entering into any correspondence, Agreement or Treaty with any foreign nation...' and to submit all disputes with other neighbouring states for settlement by the British Consul. In negotiating these treaties the British also attempted to insert convenient clauses guaranteeing freedom for missionaries, and 'free trade'.[2] But when a local ruler became difficult, the British were prepared to reduce their demands to the essential minimum. Ja Ja of Opobo, a shrewd king, was thus able to remove from his treaty the clause granting free trade, and he promised freedom only to white, not to black-skinned, missionaries.[3] Ja Ja was

John Gallagher, with Alice Denny, in *Africa and the Victorians: the climax of imperialism in the Dark Continent* (New York, 1961), ch. 6, regard the territorial partition of Africa as a 'repercussion' of the British occupation of Egypt in 1882. This view, however, would not be acceptable to most scholars who have worked in the West African documents in detail; they would regard it as an oversimplification.

[1] For Colonial Office resistance to the idea of a colonial régime see F.O. Conf. Print no. 4824, no. 22, p. 28, where the Colonial Secretary in 1882 (Lord Kimberley) catalogues the various objections for the cabinet.

[2] The texts of the protectorate treaties in the Oil Rivers are printed in *Hertslet's commercial treaties: a collection of treaties and conventions, between Great Britain and foreign powers, and of the laws, decrees, Orders in Council, &c....* (London, 1909), XVII, 158–258. The Opobo treaty is printed as an appendix to Anene's *Southern Nigeria*, pp. 333–5.

[3] Art. VII of the Opobo treaty, an interesting example of the way in which traditional rulers regarded the African clergy as more dangerous to the social order than white

moreover suspicious of the implications of the word 'protection', and demanded a written definition of its meaning from the consul before he would sign the treaty. The answer he received was a good indication of what the British meant at the time:

I write as you request with reference to the word 'protection' as used in the proposed treaty that the Queen does not want to take your country or your markets, but at the same time is anxious that no other nation should take them. She undertakes to extend her gracious favour and protection, which will leave your country still under your government.[1]

The official instrument establishing the protectorate régime (the West African Order in Council of 1885) expressed the same concept. The Order merely conferred upon the consul the right to establish consular courts with jurisdiction over British subjects (i.e., not over the local inhabitants) and to make regulations for securing the observance of the treaties. Even the consular courts were not new. The old courts of equity, which had hitherto been run by the merchants and chiefs together under the consul's supervision, were simply given a new name and a legal basis. In practical terms also, the new administration was little different from the old consular system though two (later three) vice-consuls were appointed to assist the consul. Three or four British officials could hardly aspire to 'rule'.

Ideally, the Foreign Office at first would have liked to rid itself even of these responsibilities. Thanks to Goldie, Britain had succeeded at the Berlin Conference of 1884–5 in maintaining its predominant position on the Niger against the French. Subsequently, by issuing a charter to Goldie's company, the Foreign Office fulfilled the administrative obligations incurred at Berlin without cost to the British taxpayer or without assuming any direct responsibility.[2] The Royal Niger Company's territories bisected the consular protectorate, and the company was allowed to control the Nun mouth of the Niger upon which

missionaries. Ja Ja regarded Christianity as a dangerous phenomenon. He sent his sons to England to be educated by traders, on condition that they received no religious instruction and were not allowed to read the Bible.

[1] Consul Hewett to King Ja Ja, 1 July 1884, enclosed in Ja Ja to Salisbury, 5 May 1887, F.O. 84/1862, quoted in Anene, *Southern Nigeria*, p. 66.

[2] Goldie, by bankrupting the French Niger traders and buying them out on the eve of the Conference, had ensured the preservation of British preponderance on the Niger. The Berlin Conference had laid down rules in the Niger Navigation Act for free navigation of the Niger. After the issuance of the charter in July 1886 the chartered company became responsible for administering those rules. See Flint, *Goldie*, ch. 4.

was situated its commercial headquarters at Akassa. The boundaries between the company's territories and the consular protectorate were not clearly defined—despite fierce protests from the African middlemen of Brass and New Calabar, and their Liverpool backers, who were shut out of their old markets by the Niger Company's monopolistic practices. The Foreign Office hoped that the Niger Company and its Liverpool opponents would join forces. The British wanted the larger amalgamated concern to control the Oil Rivers and the Niger through a single chartered company régime, thereby releasing the Foreign Office and the British government from all responsibility and expense for the new protectorate.

It might appear at first sight that the Niger Company was a great deal more effective and expansionist than was the consular régime of the coast; indeed Goldie used all his not inconsiderable skill as a propagandist to create this impression. On paper, the company established an elaborate government, with a supreme court at Asaba under a chief justice, a commandant of constabulary in charge of a small military force, and an agent-general at the head of an administration. The territory was divided into large areas under the control of senior executive officers, who in turn controlled the district agents. The company claimed much wider powers than the coastal protectorate. Its treaties with Africans on the Niger were made directly with the company, not with the crown, and claimed complete and perpetual 'cession' of territory to the company. The Niger Company thus purported to be the complete sovereign ruler of the area, and the British protectorate granted to the company was simply a recognition by Britain of the company's claims. Moreover the company put forward elaborate claims to control the interior and the hinterland of the Niger. In 1885 the explorer Joseph Thomson made treaties with the Sultan of Sokoto and the Emir of Gandu; on the strength of these Goldie argued that all the emirates of Northern Nigeria fell under the company's protectorate.[1]

Most of these claims, however, lacked any basis in reality. The company's administration was little more than its old commercial

[1] For the administration of the Royal Niger Company see Flint, *Goldie*, ch. 5. The Sokoto and Gandu treaties are discussed on pp. 89–90. These treaties did not in fact grant the company a protectorate over Northern Nigeria, but 'entire rights' over the banks of the Niger and Benue. The two rulers also agreed not to trade with other foreigners. Whether the sultan and the emir were given an adequate translation of their treaties is doubtful—none has yet come to light.

organization, with the trading agents given new names. The constabulary, it is true, was an innovation, and was an effective fighting force. But it was not used for police work proper. Its real function was to undertake punitive expeditions against towns and villages that disobeyed the company's regulations, giving the company a monopoly of trade. Though the company's régime undoubtedly bore heavily, indeed oppressively, upon the Africans under its jurisdiction, its effect was thus almost totally negative. Little or nothing was done to change society, to alter beliefs, or even to develop the economy. In fairness to the company it may be said that the company did attempt two new economic developments. A botanical garden was established and attempts were made to begin rubber planting, but these were not very successful. The company also began prospecting for tin in the Bauchi area, and this eventually resulted in the development of tin-mining after 1900 under the colonial régime. But the monopolistic policies of the company, by excluding rival European and African traders, undoubtedly had the result of limiting commercial development to the level made possible by the company's own limited capital. By reducing prices paid to African producers the monopoly may well have dampened African initiative; and by harsh policies directed at excluding small African traders coming from Lagos and Sierra Leone, the company excluded from its territories the influence of the dynamic 'new Africans'. As for the claim to vast territories in the north, later events were to demonstrate how completely false these were.

Educated Africans had little to celebrate over these first timid assertions of British power in the Niger and Oil Rivers. They rightly regarded the grant of a charter to the monopolistic Niger Company as a betrayal; and from 1886 the African traders of Lagos joined with African clergy in denouncing the company and demanding that the charter be revoked and a direct British administration established. Their attitude to the consular régime in the Oil Rivers was less unfriendly, but hardly enthusiastic. Archdeacon Crowther (a son of the African bishop) had lent the consul the support and influence of his clergy in negotiating the treaties. He had indeed forestalled a French attempt to secure a treaty with the city-state of Brass, and there was general relief in Lagos that neither the French nor the Germans had secured a foothold west of Calabar. But Consul Hewett was not friendly to educated Africans; he did nothing to share power with them, nor was he able to win their support by social reforms, as slavery and the 'house-system' continued unmolested.[1] Worse still, Africans in 1887 began to hear rumours of the negotiations for amalgamation between the Niger Company and the Liverpool firms, and feared that an extension of the charter over the Oil Rivers might ruin their local trade and influence.

But nowhere were educated Africans disappointed as much as in the Lagos region and its hinterland. If proof were needed that the basic motivation of British policy lay in fear of the foreigner, and not in any wish to reform African states or conditions, the contrast between British policy in the Oil Rivers and in Lagos was sufficient. In the Oil Rivers the city-states had responded well (from the British commercial point of view) to the stimulus of contact with Europe. Trade flourished under the régimes of the local kings. No one could seriously argue that British intervention was necessary because African rulers were incapable of protecting trade.[2] Nevertheless, under the stimulus of French pressure a protectorate was established.

In contrast, the great Oyo empire in Yorubaland behind Lagos empire had crumbled in the 1840s because of internal dissension and Fulani intervention from Ilorin. Oyo overlordship had been replaced by a complex power struggle in which Ibadan, Abeokuta, Ilorin and Ijebu formed shifting alliances with the lesser powers of Ife, Ilesha, Ekiti, Ijesha and smaller states. Interstate warfare became endemic, and the trade blockade became a constant weapon used by those who controlled routes to the sea coast and Lagos. The effects of these stoppages on the trade and revenues of the colony of Lagos could be disastrous, and Yoruba rulers tried several times to enlist governors of Lagos as

[1] The 'house' was the basic unit of social and commercial organization in the city-states. It was essentially an African adaptation of traditional family and clan structures to suit commercial conditions in which these ties of blood were no longer valid. The head of the house was thus selected for his commercial ability, but revered like a clan head as a father. All slaves were attached to these houses, and disciplined by them, as well as being given the chance to rise by merit within them. Slaves frequently became house heads.

[2] This is not to say that there were no economic motives behind the establishment of the protectorate. The desire to prevent the creation of a French régime with protective duties and discrimination against the British was itself an economic motive. In addition, Anene, *Southern Nigeria*, argues that the desire to break the middleman system and trade directly with the producers of palm-oil was important. This seems to me an undue stress. Once the protectorate had been established, traders began to see it as a means to break the middleman system; but in the actual events of 1884–5 the French danger was uppermost. Hence Consul Hewett agreed to Ja Ja's terms in which his treaty actually recognized his middleman position.

mediators. But Colonial Office coolness towards such moves shows how little government circles at this time were influenced by humanitarian feelings. (It also undermines the view that the need to check 'slave trading and inter-tribal warfare' was an important motive in the partition.)

In 1881 the Colonial Secretary, Lord Kimberley, rebuked the Governor of Lagos for suggesting mediation in the Yoruba wars. Kimberley argued that whilst the wars undoubtedly affected the prosperity of Lagos, the government 'could not approve any measures involving direct interference with the inland tribes. Such a course would not fail to involve the Colonial Government in dangerous complications, and would entail on this country an extension of responsibilities which Her Majesty's Government are not prepared to undertake.'[1]

Reluctance to intervene was not overcome by the French threat of 1884–5 which had brought about the Oil Rivers protectorate. When Yoruba rulers asked the British to mediate in 1884, it was the missionaries who attempted unsuccessfully to step in. The British were much more concerned to keep the French out of Yorubaland than to resolve the country's internal problems. Lagos responded to the beginnings of the scramble by limiting its activities entirely to the coastline. It replied to the French protectorate over Porto Novo with counter-moves that eventually established British claims to the whole coastline, up to the Foreign Office protectorate in the Oil Rivers. The whole coastline from Odi to Benin was declared a part of the Lagos protectorate in February 1886.

British policy, however negative, soon went beyond the principles formulated in Consul Hewett's letter to Ja Ja quoted above. Several factors played their part in undermining the internal sovereignty of the chiefs. There was what historians have called 'the influence of the man on the spot', a phrase often used, but seldom discussed in precise terms. The very assertion of a vague British overlordship created a situation in which British officials could extend their powers and territorial influence. Civil servants might be motivated by the desire for promotion, by a genuine wish to 'do what was obviously necessary', by a sense of patriotism extending itself into imperialist ambitions, by a practical need to collect more revenue, or by a mixture of all these considerations. The Foreign Office scarcely understood the meaning

[1] Kimberley to Governor of Gold Coast and Lagos, 26 Aug. 1881, Parliamentary Papers 1887, vol. LX, C. 4957.

of its own policies; and officials in the Oil Rivers therefore received no guidance whatsoever on the legal limitations of their actions. For this reason the forthright man, exploiting the difficulties of communications, tended to present the British government with a *fait accompli*. If in the process local revenues were increased, few questions were asked.

The actions of the man on the spot were invariably influenced by demands from British traders. Merchants welcomed the new protectorate as an escape from the difficult conditions created by the fall in palm-oil prices in the mid-1880s. The Niger Company had apparently shown the way by trading directly with the producers at lower prices and by amalgamation. Even if such devices should fail, the protectorate, surely, could be used to break the middleman's profits. To this ambition the Foreign Office was in general sympathetic; the policy seemed modern and progressive. Indeed, officials and traders entirely failed to appreciate the valuable services rendered by African middlemen in transporting and collecting tiny quantities of produce into consignments that Europeans could handle economically. Neither did the Europeans allow for the middlemen's knowledge of complex creeks and waterways, or for the traditional goodwill that the middlemen supplied. After 1885, therefore, consular officials were under pressure from the British traders to enlarge the British merchant's scope at the middleman's expense. Yet it was precisely on the middlemen that the political and social strength of the city-states depended. An attack on the middlemen's privileges implied a sapping of indigenous authority in the Delta states. Opening the routes to the interior, therefore, meant enlarging British authority both in terms of governmental and administrative powers, and in territorial extent.

Such pressures, and the opportunity for British officials to respond to them, were naturally greater in the Foreign Office protectorate of the Oil Rivers than in the more formal sphere of the Lagos colony and protectorate. The trade of the Oil Rivers was much larger, the middleman system of the city-states was much more thoroughly organized, and the Foreign Office officials were under much looser control from London. Thus from 1885 to 1892 there was a paradoxical contrast in the two areas. While the colony of Lagos attempted to build its influence in Yorubaland by essentially restricted diplomatic means, the Oil Rivers protectorate transformed itself into an increasingly colonial régime not averse to using force to achieve its ends. A colonial administration, in other words, was acting as though it were the administration of a protectorate, and a protectorate administration as though it were that of a colony. In this process the original concept of retaining 'native sovereignty' was altered beyond recognition.

In some of the city-states of the Oil Rivers the growth of British power was assisted by a failure of indigenous institutions to provide stability. In Bonny, for example, there was a long history of civil strife. The growth of trade had produced a situation in which the monarchy had become poor in relation to other houses. The heads of important houses, in fact, actually commanded the resources to put more fighting men and armed canoes onto the river than did the king. Ja Ja's defection and his foundation of Opobo in 1869 had been symptomatic of this development. Like Ja Ja, the overmighty subjects in the Bonny of the 1880s were often of slave origin, and this fact alone created difficult social tensions. In 1886, when Bonny was on the brink of civil war, the powerful heads of houses virtually nullified the authority of the king, and were yet incapable of providing alternative government. Consul Hewett therefore intervened, established a governing council of five chiefs, and reserved to himself the right to veto objectionable laws. This was an important departure from the original conception of the protectorate. The Foreign Office officials were uneasy; but the Bonny people, anxious for settled institutions, made little objection. Since the scheme paid for itself through taxation, it was allowed to continue.

Intervention of a more forceful kind followed at Opobo, where the situation was quite unlike that of Bonny. King Ja Ja had no difficulty in controlling his own subjects. Despite his slave origins, he was a properly installed monarch invested with all the respect due to rulers among Africans. He was truly the founder and the father of his kingdom. At the same time he controlled the greater part of the commerce and wealth of the kingdom through his own trading-house. If in 1884 the British had been intent on adhering to Hewett's definition of protectorate status in Ja Ja's case, Opobo would have been the ideal testing ground—a state that was clearly stable, under firm rule, prospering and expanding its trade. Britain needed only to keep out foreign intruders. Ja Ja was genuinely grateful for such protection, and voluntarily refused to deal with French or German traders. Before the days of the protectorate, he had demonstrated his loyalty to Britain in even stronger form by sending a contingent of troops to fight in the Ashanti campaign of 1875-6, and proudly displayed to visitors the engraved sword presented to him by Queen Victoria.

Ja Ja's real sin, in the eyes of those who plotted his downfall, was his commercial acumen, for he was a brilliant businessman. Determined to monopolize contact with the producers, he was adept at exploiting the rivalries between British firms. By 1885, with the offer of preferential contracts, he had attached to his cause the Glasgow firm of Miller Brothers—this to the enormous chagrin of the Liverpool men, who had tried for decades to keep out the non-Liverpool traders. Above all, Ja Ja, from the 1870s, had cherished ambitions of competing in the seaborne trade by shipping oil direct to Liverpool. Though his fingers had been burned by dishonest brokers in England, he was intelligent enough to see that this should be his ultimate ambition. Thus did the greatest African middleman of all time plan to remove the European middleman![1]

To the Liverpool men, therefore, Ja Ja was a menace. As early as 1882 Liverpool traders had begun to challenge him. In that year George Watts began trading directly in the Qua Ibo river, which the king claimed as one of his markets. The affair touched off a series of disputes in which Consul Hewett took Watts's side, only to find himself forced to compromise in order to secure Ja Ja's agreement to the 1884 treaty. By removing the article securing free trade, the British consul had apparently lost the battle. But the struggle was soon resumed, however, on the ground that the disputed markets were outside Ja Ja's sovereignty, and that the Opobo treaty could not possibly bind areas outside Opobo. This issue raised the impossible question of whether a market which was in essence a protectorate of an African state fell under the rule of that state.

Ja Ja then appealed directly to the Foreign Office; he revealed for the first time that he had secured the definition of protectorate status from Hewett, with its unequivocal statement that there would be no interference with his country 'or your markets'. The British answer altered the whole basis of Britain's relationship with the city-states. The Foreign Office stated, over the secretary of state's signature, that a protectorate must be construed as

the promotion of the welfare of the natives of all these territories *taken as a whole* [italics added] by ensuring the peaceful development of trade and facilitating their intercourse with Europeans. It is not to be permitted that

[1] Information based mainly on a reading of Ja Ja's private papers, preserved in the Nigerian National Archives at Ibadan.

any chief, who may happen to occupy a territory on the coast should obstruct this policy in order to benefit himself.[1]

By this statement the British abandoned the narrow legalistic concept of protectorate and introduced what was in essence a doctrine of *raison d'état*. In effect they now claimed sovereignty, for the criterion of 'the welfare of the natives...taken as a whole' implied an overriding judge, superior to the individual city-states, with power to put in abeyance individual stipulations of the treaties conflicting with the greater good.

As yet, however, the Opobo situation remained unresolved. Hewett fell ill and at the end of 1886 was invalided home. His place was taken by Vice-Consul Harry Johnston, a man of a new stamp. Young and ambitious, Johnston lacked the normal accepted background of public school and university for direct entry to the higher echelons of the foreign or colonial services. He was convinced that the partition of the African continent was at hand, and determined to use his humble vice-consulship as a stepping-stone to higher things. Because he felt that history was moving towards the assertion of European authority, a bold and successful stroke appealed to him. The pleas of the Liverpool traders for the breaking of African middlemen and for direct access to the interior seemed to him a part of that historical process.

Johnston therefore carried forward the quarrel with Ja Ja. His first step was to demand a stoppage of trade with Opobo. Then he requested permission from the Foreign Office to deport the refractory monarch. The confused situation provided a classic case of the influence of the man on the spot in the early phase of partition. Lord Salisbury, the Prime Minister and Foreign Secretary, was clearly opposed to a peremptory deportation of Ja Ja. Salisbury wished instead for a proper judicial inquiry by naval officers (whom he regarded as less partial to the Liverpool traders than Johnston) in order to determine the precise extent of Ja Ja's powers and exact legal rights. But Salisbury went on holiday to the south of France. Delays and difficulties of communication caused a telegram to be sent to Johnston which was intended to approve the stoppage of trade, but was so vaguely worded that Johnston took it to mean approval for Ja Ja's deportation. Johnston therefore invited Ja Ja to a conference on board a British man-of-war; and though he had given Ja Ja a safe-conduct, he then offered him the

[1] Rosebery to Hewett, 15 April 1886, quoted in Anene, *Southern Nigeria*, p. 74.

alternative between deportation and war. Ja Ja chose the former, was taken to the Gold Coast, and was subsequently exiled to the West Indies.[1]

Lord Salisbury disapproved of Johnston's actions, but nothing was done to reverse his *fait accompli*; and the protectorate was henceforth steadily transformed into a real administration under Johnston and subsequent consuls. Johnston immediately used the deportation of Ja Ja for a show of naval strength throughout the rivers. In Opobo he imposed an essentially alien system based on a Governing Council, with himself as president and a majority of six British traders as members with three Opobo chiefs. The council was given executive, legislative and judicial powers. Most important of all it secured the right to collect the 'comey' or customs duties hitherto collected by the king. This system was extended to Bonny early in 1888; and though the Foreign Office pointed out that the measures were illegal, as 'Her Majesty's Government have not assumed the administration of the Territories in question', the new system continued to function.[2]

The Ja Ja affair began the process whereby the scheme to extend chartered company rule was wrecked, for Ja Ja's allies, Miller Brothers of Glasgow, continued to espouse his cause after his deportation. Millers were a part of Goldie's Niger Company,[3] and their agreement was essential to amalgamation. As prospects for amalgamation lessened, the Liverpool men formed the African Association Ltd., and hoped to secure an independent charter. But by 1888 opposition to this project was growing on all sides. The Niger Company was not keen on the prospect of a rival chartered company that would dispute its boundaries. In addition the German government began to oppose the plan, fearing its traders would be excluded from the Oil Rivers as they had been on the Niger. Elder Dempster, the steamship company, began mobilizing the powerful British shipping lobby in opposition, fearing that the Liverpool men planned to run their own vessels once they held a monopoly of trade. In order to placate all hostile agitation, the British

---

[1] For contrasting views of the affair see Roland Oliver, *Sir Harry Johnston and the scramble for Africa* (London, 1957), pp. 93–121 *passim*; and Anene, *Southern Nigeria*, pp. 77–92.

[2] F.O. to Johnston, draft, 10 Feb. 1888, F.O. 84/1881.

[3] Miller Brothers had become part of the United African Company in 1879, and were thus a part of the Royal Niger Company's directorate at this time. However, the firm continued to exist as a separate entity in the Oil Rivers, competing with the Liverpool traders. They thus played a key role in the negotiations, for their assent was necessary both within the directorate of the Royal Niger Company and as an independent and large Oil Rivers concern.

government decided to send Major (later Sir) Claude Macdonald as Special Commissioner to investigate the form of government most suitable for the Oil Rivers.

Macdonald's report[1] represented a watershed in local British administrative policy. Hitherto the consuls or their deputies like Johnston had gradually, and largely illegally, transformed the nature of the protectorate. The Foreign Office, whilst not always accepting what had been done, had allowed matters to drift steadily in the direction of closer administration and control, hoping that chartered company rule would soon take these matters out of their hands. Macdonald brought a refreshing and honest forthrightness to his inquiry. He wanted to find out what the inhabitants really desired. He tried to see, either in public meetings or private consultations, all the various interest groups in the city-states, not only the British trading-agents, but also the kings and heads of houses. Through consultations with the African clergy of the C.M.S. Niger Delta pastorate, he even attempted to obtain a view of the feelings of the ordinary people and slaves.

To each of these groups he put forward three alternatives: a continuance of the *status quo*, the establishment of a proper colony, or chartered company rule. Every group vehemently rejected chartered company rule. Some of the Liverpool agents even privately warned Macdonald that it would be disastrous, despite instructions from their firms, to press for the scheme. In general, most of the kings and chiefs advocated 'Queen's government', and at the same time asked for assurances that the government would not interfere with traditional social institutions, including slavery. The African clergy wanted a straightforward colonial régime, for they knew that a colonial status would bring the area under the act of 1833 abolishing slavery in all British colonies. Macdonald therefore recommended the establishment of a crown colony in the Oil Rivers.

To Lord Salisbury this was oversanguine; he felt that Macdonald had underestimated the difficulties which the ending of slavery would create.[2] The result was a compromise between the colonial and protectorate concept. Macdonald was appointed Consul-general and Commissioner to establish an effective administration. The territory would in effect be a colony, though legally a protectorate, outside the

[1] The report was never published. It is to be found in F.O. 84/1940. Macdonald's report on the Royal Niger Company is filed separately in F.O. 84/2109.
[2] Lister to Salisbury, 18 June 1889, with Salisbury's minute, F.O. 84/1997.

British empire. Its people would not be British subjects, and not therefore subject to British legislation affecting all colonies.

The new administration nevertheless seized the reins of power. From the very beginning it gained control of the two essentials of government—revenue and military force. The kings and chiefs were deprived of their power to levy 'comey' and other taxes on trade; instead they were given subsidies from the protectorate revenues, derived henceforth from regular customs duties levied on a uniform scale on trade at all ports. A small but effective constabulary of African troops was organized, and regularly paid from these resources. The trade of the area was in fact sufficiently large so as to yield a revenue of £96,000 in the first year and £169,000 in the second.

In Macdonald the British had found the ideal administrator for the day. Though an imperialist, determined to expand British authority and to establish efficient institutions, he was also a man of great humanity, averse to bloodshed, who believed in making gradual progress through adequate consultation with African opinion. He thus continued the policies he had advocated during his inquiry, and gave the impression that these were a reflection of local wishes. Even the establishment of customs duties was accomplished by agreement. Steadily the institutions of a colony emerged; and by 1895 small but effective customs, marine, medical and postal departments were in operation. By his cautious policy, Macdonald was able to secure the co-operation of traditionalist kings and house-heads. His genuine sense of mission and humanity also secured him the support of the new Africans, who expected his policy to produce more opportunities in trade, wider professional careers and better schooling.

An essential element in gaining the support of educated Africans was Macdonald's neutrality in the racial struggle between black and white clergy. This occurred after the death of Bishop Crowther in 1892 over the appointment of a white bishop as Crowther's successor. When the African clergy in the Niger Delta broke away to form a separate self-governing pastorate, Macdonald surprised the white community by agreeing to become the patron of the new congregation and by granting to it a small educational subsidy from protectorate revenues.

Above all Macdonald was concerned for the value of human life, and it was perhaps this quality more than any other that endeared him to Africans. Two major violent episodes, for neither of which Macdonald was responsible, marred this record. The first was a crisis analogous to that of Opobo in 1887. It involved Nana, the chief of the Itsekiri people, who controlled the trade of the Urhobo oil-producers and also acted as middlemen in the trade from Benin. In 1894, whilst Macdonald was on leave in England, his deputy, Ralph Moor, brought to a head quarrels with Nana over access to markets. Moor invaded Nana's country and forced Nana to flee to Lagos, from where Nana was exiled.[1] In the following year came the revolt of the Brass people against the régime of the neighbouring Niger Company, which had excluded the Brass from their traditional markets. For several years Macdonald had unsuccessfully pressed for some redress of Brass grievances. The Brassmen had then taken the law into their own hands and had destroyed the company's headquarters at Akassa. The inevitable punitive expedition followed, but even here Macdonald characteristically attempted to secure a proper inquiry into the Brass grievances and to mitigate the severe measures against them.

Meanwhile, Lagos began to abandon the older policy of noninterference in the Yoruba hinterland. In January 1886 the administration of Lagos was detached from that of the Gold Coast. The separate administration naturally began to concentrate on the problems of the war-torn Yoruba interior that so profoundly affected the colony's revenues. Almost immediately the new Governor, C. A. Maloney, sent peacemakers into the interior, of whom the most successful were the two African clergymen, the Reverend S. Johnson and the Reverend C. Philips. The two patched up bilateral settlements between various factions; these agreements enabled the Lagos governor to call a conference in Lagos of all the hostile parties (except Ilorin, a Muslim Yoruba state nominally under the protectorate of the Niger Company, which refused to negotiate). Up to now, these activities had been entirely diplomatic; the British had made no attempt to control the country by establishing protectorates. But all the same, the British became more involved in the situation by the dispatch of a small force of African troops to supervise the dismantling of camps and fortifications.

It was the threat of French intervention that pushed the British into full-scale intervention. In 1888 a French mission arrived in Abeokuta, the capital of the Egba state (which controlled one of the vital access routes to Ibadan and the interior). The French obtained certain railway

[1] The deposition of Nana is dealt with in detail in a Ph.D. thesis by Obaro Ikime, 'Itsekiri-Urhobo relations and the establishment of British rule, 1884–1936' (Ibadan University, 1965).

privileges. The Lagos governor replied by making a treaty with Oyo, now a feeble power that none the less still pretended to overlordship of Yorubaland. The new agreement did not establish a protectorate, but bound the Alafin of Oyo not to interfere with trade or to levy tolls without Lagos agreement, and to cede no territory to foreign powers.[1]

Little immediate result came of this treaty. The French expedition in Abeokuta lacked official sanction, and the French government repudiated the treaty. The French had worries enough on the Dahomean coast: their hinterland was blocked by the powerful kingdom of Dahomey, which they meant to conquer. Just as the British feared French inroads in Yorubaland, so the French dreaded British interference in support of Dahomey. Hence the French in 1889 agreed to a compromise whereby a line was drawn between the spheres of influence of Lagos and Porto Novo up to the ninth parallel of latitude.

With Yorubaland free from French encroachments, Lagos could afford to limit its ambitions. Between 1889 and 1892 Yoruba rivalries thus began to reassert themselves. These struggles resulted in frequent closing of the trade routes to the interior. Lagos finances remained in a parlous state, but almost nothing was done from Lagos to assert its overriding authority. Indeed, the British presence in the Yoruba interior at this time was largely dependent on the missionaries, mostly Africans, who by virtue of their alienation from traditional ties and loyalties emerged as arbitrators, respected for their impartiality. Lacking effective sanctions to enforce peace, it is small wonder they often longed for British intervention.

In 1892 came a sudden, dramatic coup that resulted in the rapid establishment of a virtual British protectorate over the whole of Yorubaland. The process was set off by events in Ijebu, the state north of Lagos controlling one of the routes to Ibadan and the interior, but was determined by the wider conflict between the British and the French in the area. In 1891 relations between France and the King of Dahomey came to an open breach, and throughout 1892 the French openly prepared to invade Dahomey. Once they had succeeded, they could move north of the line agreed on in 1889, and swing down into Yorubaland. Thus, when the ruler of Ijebu in 1892 demanded from Ibadan the heads of two missionaries (one of whom was an African), the British in

[1] The most up-to-date scholarly account, based on British Archives, is A. A. B. Aderibigbe's Ph.D. thesis, 'The expansion of the Lagos Protectorate, 1863–1900' (London University, 1959).

Lagos responded in a hitherto uncharacteristic manner. A military expedition was mounted, the Ijebu forces scattered, and their territory occupied.

The Lagos educated group hailed this as the dawn of a new era. The Reverend Samuel Johnson wrote: '...it was like the opening of a prison door: and no one who witnessed the patient, long-suffering, and toiling humanity...could refrain from heaving a sigh of gratification on the magnitude of the beneficial results of the short and sharp conflict'.[1] Governor Carter of Lagos exploited the psychological advantage of the Ijebu war to the full, and in 1893 set off on a grand tour of Yorubaland. He concluded treaties which, whilst often preserving the fabric of existing African government in considerably more detail than the earlier arrangements made in the Oil Rivers, nevertheless established virtual control over Yorubaland. The governor obtained control over routes, the right to build railways and power to settle interstate disputes.

The establishment of British control in Yorubaland was in many respects a phenomenon unique in the partition of Africa. It certainly differed radically from the way the British extended their power in the rest of Nigeria. The Yoruba were exhausted by futile interstate warfare, their rulers were demoralized and desperate, and there is little doubt that the masses of the people, their minds prepared by the influence of African Christians, wanted British rule. Ijebu, where Christians had been excluded by the ruler, was the exception; but once Ijebu had fallen, the rest of Yorubaland offered no resistance to the British. A small rebellion in Oyo in 1895 might be regarded as another exception.

The effects were dramatic. The colony of Lagos was at last stirred into activity. In 1892 its revenues had been £68,421; with the virtual cessation of the interior wars they rose in 1893 to £115,317, and to almost £180,000 in 1896. These figures reflect a steady increase in trade, which increased by over 50 per cent between 1892 and 1896.[2] Educated Africans, by acting as middlemen or direct employees of the European firms in the interior markets, shared in this development. Their activity and buoyancy of spirit in turn led to great advances by the missions, especially in the Ijebu country. Even the growing racialistic tendencies

[1] Quoted in Michael Crowder, *The story of Nigeria* (London, 1962), p. 188.
[2] W. N. M. Geary, *Nigeria under British rule* (London, 1927; reprinted New York, 1965), p. 49. Geary's book still provides the best published collection of statistics relating to Nigeria.

in Colonial Office appointments policies, and the increasing reluctance to put Africans into the highest administrative posts, was temporarily offset by the immediate demands for junior officials and clerks brought about by extended government.

Moreover, the active policies of Lagos at last seemed to secure support from the British government. In 1894, with the retirement of Gladstone and the appointment of the Liberal imperialist Lord Rosebery as Prime Minister, the Colonial Office at last discussed plans for ambitious public works, including a deep-water harbour and a railway to Ibadan, as feasible propositions. A railway survey was authorized. Joseph Chamberlain, who in 1895 became Colonial Secretary in Salisbury's Conservative government, announced his platform of 'developing the imperial estates'. The railway survey was begun, and the first tracks were laid for a line to Ibadan.

The railway was greeted with tremendous enthusiasm by Africans. To the educated group it symbolized their national yet Lagos–centred ambitions. They saw the iron road as an agent of progress that would push into the hinterland, across the Niger, into the Muslim feudal north, binding the country together, and centring its cultural, economic and social life on Lagos. The governors of Lagos shared these aspirations. Regarding themselves as the senior British representatives in the Niger region, they looked to the time when the Niger Company's rule would end, when the Colonial Office would take over the Niger Coast Protectorate and a single colonial unit would come into being.

The days of the Niger Company were clearly numbered, for by 1895 its administration contrasted feebly with that of Lagos or the Niger Coast Protectorate. Sir John Kirk's report on the Brass[1] disturbances had exposed the monopolistic nature of the company. Chamberlain refused to implement a scheme of reform suggested by Kirk (but prompted by Goldie) whereby the company would cease to trade, and become nothing but an administrative organization. Chamberlain preferred to avoid tinkering, and to abolish the company altogether.

The company's worst sin, however, had been its failure to meet the challenge from the French. In 1894 the French, having subdued Dahomey, began to move into Borgou on the company's frontier, with

[1] Kirk's report was published in a much edited form as Great Britain, *Parliamentary Papers*, vol. LIX, C. 7977, p. 361, *Report by Sir John Kirk upon the disturbances at Brass* (London, 1896). The original manuscript version is to be found in F.O. 83/1382, under Kirk's covering letter of 25 Aug. 1895.

the object of securing Bussa and access to the navigable Niger, whence they could move into the Fulani empire itself. Goldie attempted to forestall them by employing Frederick Lugard to make treaties in Borgou, but the French scorned these scraps of paper and started to occupy Borgouan towns with small parties of troops. The company clearly could not compete with France in effective occupation. Chamberlain thus appointed Lugard in 1897 to organize an imperial army of African soldiers (which shortly became the West African Frontier Force). The British taxpayer thereby paid for operations designed to protect a chartered company, and the company accordingly lost its *raison d'être*. And it was only because Chamberlain feared a possible French contention that the company's liquidation would cause its treaties, and therefore British claims, to lapse, that the company's régime lasted until the end of 1899. Once the Anglo-French agreement of 1898 had settled the boundaries of Northern Nigeria, all that remained was to compensate the company and to take over administration of the territory. On 1 January 1900 Lugard, as High Commissioner for Northern Nigeria, inaugurated direct administration.

In these years the imperialist mood in Britain, the expanding revenues of the territories and the temperaments of British officials all conspired to create more aggressive policies with a definite militaristic tinge. After the Ijebu war the British posted garrisons in many Yoruba towns, and augmented the forces of Lagos and the Niger Coast Protectorate. In 1896 attempts by Niger Coast Protectorate officials to force the ruler of Benin to allow contact with Europeans led to the murder of British officials and African soldiers. In the following year a large British expedition crushed the ancient kingdom and exiled its ruler. In 1897 the Colonial Office compelled the Niger Company to undertake its only major military campaigns in wars against Nupe and Ilorin designed to stop Ilorin's interference in the Lagos protectorate. Armed intervention continued in the early 1900s, until the vast open areas of Northern Nigeria and the Ibo heartlands of the south-east were under firm control.

By 1898 it was clear that the new imperialism would lead to effective occupation. The British had by then also started to create the substructure of a modern transport system. While the abolition of the Niger Company's charter and the question of future administration in the north were being considered in 1898, the British established the Niger Committee, the first official body to discuss the broader questions involving Nigeria as a whole. Its chairman was Lord Selborne, the Colonial Under-Secretary; Goldie represented the Niger Company, Sir Clement Hill the Foreign Office, Sir Reginald Antrobus the Colonial Office. Sir Henry McCallum, the Governor of Lagos, and Sir Ralph Moor, Commissioner of the Niger Coast Protectorate (transferred to Colonial Office control in 1898), were also members.

Naturally, the views of Moor, McCallum and Goldie, the men most closely in contact with local affairs, carried great weight. All agreed that they should aim at eventual unification. But they felt that the poor state of communications rendered this impossible for the moment. They therefore recommended the creation of two provinces; the northern one would consist of the area roughly to the north of a line drawn through Idah, including the Yoruba state of Ilorin; the southern province would be an amalgam of the Niger Coast Protectorate, Lagos and its Yoruba hinterland and the lower Niger below Idah hitherto ruled by the Niger Company. The committee also favoured an administrative policy for both provinces that would utilize the existing African states, with their traditional political, judicial and social institutions. Such a course would obviate a costly and overstaffed direct British administration, and would prevent interference by headstrong, young officials who might provoke African opposition and even violent resistance.[1]

Joseph Chamberlain, whilst accepting the main lines of the committee's report, decided that the creation of a single southern province was premature. In December 1899 the Crown issued a formal unilateral (and in the strict sense, illegal) declaration of protectorate over the Lagos interior. At the same time the Niger Company's territory below Idah was taken over by the Niger Coast Protectorate, now renamed the Protectorate of Southern Nigeria, under Moor as High Commissioner. The Protectorate of Northern Nigeria, with Lugard as High Commissioner, assumed charge on 1 January 1900 over the Niger Company's territories north of Idah.

Despite the new imperialism, this reorganization was strictly pragmatic. Though the British were now prepared to administer, and even to develop, the Nigerian economy, they stressed administrative economy and efficiency. There was no discussion of long-term goals, and the deeper purposes of British governance were not considered at all. The fundamental question of the African relationship to British control

[1] Report of the Niger Committee, 4 Aug. 1898, C.O. 446/3.

and of the Africans' future share in economic, political and administrative life remained open.

In the absence of an overall policy, such fundamental issues were determined in succeeding years by impersonal forces scarcely understood by the men on the spot. Everything now tended to destroy the aspirations of educated black people, and the alliance between Christian Africans and British power began to weaken. Important medical advances, assisted by Chamberlain's sponsorship, led to an influx of European officials. Ross's discovery in 1897 of the way in which malaria was transmitted, the consequent spread of mosquito-control and the use of mosquito netting soon enabled British officers to bring their wives to Nigeria. Englishwomen demanded higher standards of housing and neighbours of their own race, so that after 1900 the British developed segregated residential areas for themselves, usually on choice hillsides. This policy was always justified on sanitary grounds. (One wonders whether an open admission that Europeans preferred to live detached from everyday African life would not have placated African opinion more effectively!) Easy, unofficial contact between educated Africans and British officials became rarer; hence educated Africans lost influence on day-to-day policies.

Besides, the very speed of British expansion after the 1890s was bound to reduce the influence of educated and Christian African opinion. As long as the British confined their activities to the coastal cities and towns, the new Africans were numerous and important enough to demand a voice both in commerce and in politics. But the vast territorial acquisitions in the Ibo interior and the north changed the whole balance of power and made the Christian group entirely unrepresentative. This was especially true in the Muslim north, where the memory of Usman dan Fodio's jihad[1] led the British to placate Islam. Traditional African rulers were not slow to make known their dislike of Christian Africans; black Christians were everywhere associated with the slave or ex-slave status, and the facility with which some of them used their literacy and knowledge of English to secure personal advantages did not win them favour.

The years from 1898 to 1904 thus produced a reversal of alliances in the Afro-British relationship in Nigeria. During these years British

[1] This was the religious war of the Fulani, led by Usman, which had created the Sokoto-Gandu empire in the first decade of the nineteenth century. See M. R. Waldman, 'The Fulani jihād: a reassessment', *Journal of African History*, 1965, 6, no. 3, pp. 333–56.

expansion and authority were without exception opposed by traditional rulers or ruling groups, who in general fought for their independence, only to be crushed by military means. This process was expensive; and the British, seeking to keep costs down, limited conquest to the simple assertion of overall political sovereignty; they restored to office traditional overlords, or their relatives. African chiefs lost much power, including their command of military force, their authority to conduct affairs with other states, and the greater part of their judicial and taxation rights. But they undoubtedly gained in security once they began to realize that British arms would be used to support co-operative rulers.

In the decade from 1904 to 1914 the traditional dignitaries of Nigeria thus swung into close alliance with the British colonial régime. The old rulers became increasingly dependent on British support for their authority against the erosive influences of economic, commercial and educational development. The very forces that had most fiercely contested the establishment of colonial rule now became its closest allies. Educated Africans, on the other hand, became ever more critical of British policies; for the British now seemed more concerned with maintaining those elements of traditional life that literate black people wanted to destroy through colonial rule.

The British method of ruling through chiefs has come to be known as indirect rule. This general term, however, embraces many different policies. In the three separate British administrations that governed Nigeria in the early 1900s, for instance, the emphasis differed in each, and reflected the way in which British officials responded to local influences. These differences, and the impossibility of foreseeing which of these policies really embodied British long-term intentions, did a great deal to mute the criticism of educated Africans, and indeed delayed the emergence of organized political nationalism in Nigeria.

This was especially true in Lagos and in the Yoruba interior. Here, educated and Christian Africans continued to maintain their influence even under indirect rule. For ever since the 1840s liberated Africans from Sierra Leone had penetrated into Yorubaland, as they had not done in any other portion of the Nigerian interior. They had established positions for themselves within traditional communities. They had been constantly reinforced by local converts and by newcomers from the Lagos community. In some states they had reformed the original African political institutions to such an extent as to become a powerful political factor. The presence of these literate groups had also affected the character of the British protectorate. When the treaty system was established during and after Carter's tour of 1893, the African negotiators had a real grasp of British demands. The local Africans thus ceded fewer powers than elsewhere, and could afterwards maintain internal independence on a firmer legal basis. British control did develop steadily after 1893. There was more interference in the internal administration of the states, but this was generally achieved by peaceful means and by genuine negotiations.

The success of British policy in Yorubaland owes much also to Governor Sir William MacGregor, who held office from 1899 to 1904. MacGregor was prone to petty jealousies, pomposity, and a feeling of insecurity caused by his background of professional life as a doctor and by his lack of influential connexions in Britain. But though the Colonial Office was unable to realize it, he was the right man in the right place at the right time. MacGregor was, like his colleagues in the north and east, an indirect ruler; but he could work with Africans of many kinds, not merely with traditional authorities. He was proud of the pacific aspects of his policies, and spoke of indirect rule as a means to avoid military ventures (a theme designed to emphasize failure of his counterparts elsewhere!). Describing his system in 1904, MacGregor argued that the Lagos system

takes native character, native customs, and native susceptibilities into account, and the native authorities are allowed and required, to take such a large share in their own government that punitive expeditions, or plots against the government, are unknown.... Under such a system a great chief is a very valuable possession; his authority is an instrument of the greatest public utility, which it is most desirable to retain in full force.[1]

The situation in the Egba state illustrates in extreme form the problems faced by the British in Yorubaland, and the influence of the educated. The Egba state had a long history of Christian evangelization and of settlement by liberated Africans. In the nineteenth century the Egba country had attained great symbolic importance among British Christians as the 'sunrise within the tropics', as the example of an African polity that managed spontaneously to modernize its institutions. In the 1860s and 1870s this vision faded. There were bitter conflicts between the Egba and the British at Lagos when the Egba were drawn into the Yoruba wars. The Egba state nevertheless survived the parti-

---

[1] From a speech given before the Royal African Society.

tion; and under the British protectorate its internal sovereignty was more faithfully preserved than in any other Yoruba state (even to the extent of the word 'independence' being used in the Egba treaty). The Colonial Office thus disliked this instrument as a legal anomaly, but MacGregor dealt patiently with Egba affairs. When he needed increased powers, particularly because of railway building, MacGregor conducted private negotiations; and in 1904 the *Alake*, in return for a renewed recognition of Egba independence 'in its internal administration', agreed to the setting up of a mixed court under the British Railway Commissioner. These concessions were the result of steady British support for the *Alake*'s authority, including the use of troops to put down rebellions in 1901 and 1903. Egba government in fact had been republican; the *Alake* had never been a true monarch. But now the *Alake* used British predilection for 'a great chief' to transform his authority.

In 1900 the new railway reached Ibadan. This might by itself have been enough to shatter the basis of the traditional Yoruba states. The cash revenues of these states had heretofore been almost entirely collected from tolls and duties on transit trade. Such mediaeval taxes could not be levied on railway trains, and the issue provided strong ammunition for opposition from British traders to all internal taxation. Such cases led to constant minutes in the Colonial Office stressing the importance of 'ending independence' in these states. Yet MacGregor could see that the states must collapse without an income of their own. He patiently discussed the question with Yoruba rulers; he systematically defined the extent of such duties; he obtained the chiefs' agreement to reforms in collecting procedures and to the publication of accounts. By the end of 1904 he had succeeded in abolishing all tolls on the railway route. For his patience with African rulers he suffered unpopularity at the hands of European merchants, and irritated his superiors at home.[1]

Such policies undoubtedly aimed at bolstering up traditional society in the interior, but the criticism that they might have provoked from the educated groups in Lagos was severely blunted by MacGregor's own attitude. Unlike the classic indirect rulers, he exhibited little of the contempt they usually showed for 'gentlemen of colour', a term used in the early nineteenth century as a polite and genteel expression, but which by the 1890s was beginning to contain a note of sarcasm.

---

[1] Sir William MacGregor still awaits an adequate biography. The only detailed study of his policies in Nigeria is the London Ph.D. thesis of 1963 by S. M. Tamuno, 'The development of British administrative control of Southern Nigeria, 1900–12'.

MacGregor acted as if Lagos were the capital of Nigeria, assuming that the railway would first bind together Yorubaland and later the whole country. According to his local speeches, the country's future unity would make southern civilization spread to the north. MacGregor mixed easily with educated Africans, and was willing to admit them to positions of trust within the administration. In 1900 he promoted Henry Carr, a Nigerian graduate, already an inspector of schools, to the post of Assistant Colonial Secretary with special responsibility for native affairs; and, even though this appointment was not a success, Carr rose to be Director of Education in the Colony. MacGregor appointed several Nigerians to the Legislative Council also. This body was already regarded by the educated elements as an embryonic national parliament, even though it contained no elected members. In 1901 the Nigerian medical doctor, O. Johnson, and the lawyer, C. Sapara Williams, joined the Legislative Council, and MacGregor continued the appointment of C. J. George, an African trader.

British policy in the Protectorate of Southern Nigeria, though it, too, came under Colonial Office control after 1898, strongly contrasted with that of Lagos, although its High Commissioner, Sir Ralph Moor, theoretically believed in indirect rule. In Southern Nigeria British penetration was largely military in character. Negotiation played little part; and the effect, if not the intent, of policy, was destructive of traditional institutions, except on the coast. Here the long history of contact with Europe, the existence of kingship and the house system, the use of pidgin English as a *lingua franca*, the presence of an educated element at Calabar, and the labours of African clergy of the delta pastorate throughout the coast towns, had permitted steady accommodation of African institutions to British demands. The same conditions were true of the larger towns on the Niger river below Idah.

Away from the waterside, however, among the Ibibio behind Calabar, among the variegated peoples in the Cross river basin, or the Ibo interior, there were no institutions of kingship or chieftaincy that could be utilized for administrative purposes. Each village or town was a sovereign power ruled under a complex system whereby age sets carried out certain customary tasks, and elders exercised judicial powers. One of the few unifying institutions was the great oracle of Aro-Chuku. This was respected throughout the south-east as the dwelling of the Supreme Being, and operated as a kind of supreme court.

Had the Aros been ruled by a centralized monarch, the British might well have come to utilize them as intermediaries for the penetration of the interior. Instead, Aro rule, with colonies scattered at strategic points along trade routes, was simply dismissed as a vast system of trade monopoly, inimical to progress. In November 1901 a British expedition of nearly two thousand men began a three-months' campaign that crushed the Aro power. The British naïvely assumed that intervention would liberate the interior and allow the producers of palm-oil joyfully to accept beneficent British rule. Instead, almost every village received the white men with suspicion and hostility, and by 1903 the British had to accept a policy of occupying the area by military columns. This took years to complete, and in the northern Ibo areas several important towns were not effectively administered until the eve of the First World War.

Despite the conspicuous absence of chiefs in this area, the British tried to enforce indirect rule. In practice this resulted in the somewhat naïve and ill-advised extension into the interior of policies designed for the coastal city-states. From 1 January 1902 the protectorate authorities abolished all slave-dealing; and in order to prevent a drying up of labour, and to prop up the house system, the administration in 1901 passed the Native House Rule Proclamation, which attempted to bind labour to the heads of houses and maintain the taxation rights of houses. These provisions were often mistakenly extended later into the interior, where the house system did not exist in its coastal form, and where they caused great resentment. Similarly, the administration set up 'native courts' supposedly consisting of 'influential natives', and 'chiefs' began to be appointed. In reality this was a system of direct rule. The British utilized whoever appeared to command influence or power. There was accordingly opportunity for arbitrary and corrupt justice, and this undoubtedly caused considerable suffering.

Opposition to these policies came, however, mainly from traditional sources. The educated and Christian groups of Calabar and the coast found little to criticize (except perhaps the House Rule Ordinance). In any case, many of them were as ignorant as the British about the nature of inland society. Some educated Africans shared in the commercial and political opportunities provided by British penetration. From the Lagos Africans there were more complaints, especially concerning the military aspects of penetration and of the authoritarian nature of a régime where the high commissioner was all-powerful and where there was no legislative council to watch his activities.

In any case, the Southern Nigeria Protectorate soon fell under the sway of Lagos, as recommended by the 1898 committee. In 1904, when Moor and MacGregor both left Nigeria, Sir Walter Egerton succeeded to their posts. A senior provincial commissioner was appointed to Calabar in 1905, thus marking its subordination to Lagos. In 1906 the two areas were formally amalgamated as the Colony and Protectorate of Southern Nigeria, with the seat of administration in Lagos. The colony was divided into three provinces, western, central and eastern, each under a provincial commissioner. The Legislative Council in Lagos now became responsible for making laws and imposing taxes throughout the colony. (The Council consisted of ten officials, three European unofficials, and three African unofficials, Dr O. Johnson, Sapara Williams and K. Ajasa.)

Among Lagos educated elements there were signs in 1906 of dissatisfaction with amalgamation. Sapara Williams demanded more than three African representatives on the Legislative Council, a request that was refused. There was more popular backing for the first manifestation of real hostility to the British régime in the north. Many Yoruba were disappointed that Nigeria as a whole had not been unified, and meetings were held demanding that the Yoruba Muslim state of Ilorin and the related northern province of Kabba should become part of Southern Nigeria.

The British system in Northern Nigeria indeed completely negated all the aspirations of the educated and Christian groups. In no other part of Nigeria was British pragmatism carried to such negative extremes, despite the impression of positive energy created by the writings and theorizings of northern officials. What was worse, the northern régime from its early years began to bid for dominance over the whole country. In comparison with the southern administrations, the northern régime was a failure, whether judged in terms of administrative efficiency or of economic development (the normal criteria for assessing the progress of a colony). Yet the northern administration displayed a vehement defensiveness, asserting that it alone had discovered true principles of African administration. In reality the British had done little more than make themselves the overlords of an existing feudal system. This feudalism, being of a highly developed and strongly Islamic type known only in the savannah belt of West Africa, was quite foreign to the rest of tropical Africa, and had almost no relevance to the general principles of African administration.

The British essentially balked at the gigantic task which a real colonial policy would have imposed in Northern Nigeria. Their course was implicit in the whole history of British contact with Nigeria. It was but a continuation under new circumstances of the older nineteenth-century reluctance to make large commitments, especially financial ones, in colonial ventures. In Southern Nigeria this unwilling-ness to shoulder risks was overcome by the profitability of the palm-oil trade, by the growth of revenues, by able and sometimes imaginative officials, and by the presence of an intermediary group of westernized Africans. In the north, only the Niger trade and the C.M.S. mission played a similar part, but they were weaker; and official reluctance to become involved was symbolized by the chartered company régime. Joseph Chamberlain's new imperialism was sufficient to secure direct Colonial Office governance in 1900, with Lugard as High Commis-sioner, despite the fact that the military costs of occupation were high and revenues almost nonexistent. But overall political control repre-sented the limit of British ambition, and the task of integrating the north into a single developing colonial unit could only be considered once revenues had begun to grow.

In fairness to the British it should be stressed that the matter of governing the north posed huge and forbidding problems encountered nowhere in the south. The north was more than twice the size of the southern provinces. Its indigenous political constituents also appeared more formidable. The Fulani empire, with its twin heads, the sultan of Sokoto and the emir of Gandu, was the greatest indigenous 'state' in tropical Africa except Ethiopia. Its rival Bornou, lying to the east around Lake Chad, was also one of the largest. The Fulani had estab-lished their feudal overlordship over the Hausa population by a jihad in the early nineteenth century. This alone made the British circumspect, for the death of Gordon in the jihad of the Mahdists was regarded by the British as a national disaster. In the purely military sense also the British needed to be cautious, for transport was difficult and reinforce-ments from Britain or Southern Nigeria were subject to serious delays on the Niger followed by long journeys overland.

Even after 1900 the Colonial Office would have preferred peaceful penetration, but Lugard was determined to found the British title on the right of conquest. Accordingly he forced the pace several times, and succeeded in presenting the Colonial Office with *faits accomplis*. Nevertheless he could not hope to establish a direct administration without large sums of money, especially in view of his small establishment (this amounted to only 200 officers in 1900, rising to about 300 in 1906).

Even had he wished, Lugard was thus in no position to initiate a social or political revolution while he served as High Commissioner (1900–6). He concentrated instead on removing, by force where necessary, those Fulani emirs who refused to submit to the control of British residents; but he was careful to replace them with men of the same ruling families. Muslim law and courts were retained. The entry of Christian missions was carefully controlled, and Christian Africans from the south were kept out of the administration, except for subordinate clerks. Lugard, however, was not at this time a dogmatist. He regarded these measures as temporary expedients 'in gradual course of development'; where necessary he would centralize power in his own hands, and allow his residents to collect taxes. He was much interested also in the prospects of commercial development, and was not as opposed to missionary activity and education as is often supposed.

A dogmatic concept of northern indirect rule and an assertive northern patriotism began to emerge among British officials only after Lugard left Nigeria in 1906. From 1906 to 1909 he was succeeded by Sir Percy Girouard, a former Royal Engineer who was an expert on railway construction, appointed mainly to deal with the urgent communication problems of the area. There was now a basic divergence between northern and southern Nigerian policies. The south had always assumed that the railway from Lagos, via Ibadan, would eventually cross the Niger and attract the northern trade. In 1904 the extension from Ibadan to Oshogbo had been sanctioned, and in 1906 the Colonial Office accepted plans for pushing the line to Ilorin in the northern region. But in 1907 Girouard recommended that, since the Lagos railway would take years to reach the north, a local northern railway should run from Baro on the Niger to Kano. Baro would thus become a river port, and Lagos would receive none of this commerce. Since the north lacked financial resources for the project, the Colonial Office raised a loan on the security of Southern Nigeria's finances. Governor Egerton tried to resist this expedient, but in the end had to be content with the promise that the Lagos line would eventually cross into Northern Nigeria and link up with the Baro–Kano line.

Both Girouard and his successor from 1909 to 1912, Sir Hesketh Bell, admired the principles of indirect rule, but lacked experience of supervising its workings. Lugard's developing administration thus ossified into what became the classic indirect rule system. The new governors were forced to rely on the experienced Residents in the emirates. These began to stress the need to preserve the emirs' prestige and sphere of independent action (which in fact meant leaving the Resident freer from central control). During this time British administrators also elaborated the characteristic institution of Northern Nigerian indirect rule, the native treasury. These treasuries were set up to utilize traditional taxation systems and to alleviate thereby the desperate shortage of revenues in the Protectorate. The system also preserved some initiative to the emirs by leaving in their hands a share of the revenues (ideally one-half). The Residents were responsible for the assessment, and naturally exerted a powerful influence with the emirs over the ways in which the money was spent. Thus real authority was virtually transferred from the Governor to the Residents.

The extent to which this development was idealized and rationalized can be seen in its most extreme form in the views of Charles Temple, a Resident from 1901 to 1910, who was afterwards promoted to Chief Secretary and in 1914 to Lieutenant-Governor of Northern Nigeria. Temple, a well-connected young man, became a devotee of the north. He spoke fluent Hausa and flirted with Islam. He admired aristocracy, despised individualism, and regarded European industrial capitalism as a decadent form of society. He became a fanatic for the northern indirect rule system, turning the traditional paternalism of colonial morality upside down. For him the duty of colonial trusteeship lay not in bringing European 'progress' to 'savages', but in protecting the virtues of northern aristocratic life and its communal economy from the 'barbarizing' effects of European capitalism, democracy and individualism. He was willing to accept the implication of these attitudes to the full. His policies in fact negated the *raison d'être* for the colonial presence, for he was ready to pass back sovereignty to natural rulers within one or two generations, perhaps within a federal structure controlled by the African princes. Trusteeship for him thus meant teaching the traditional rulers the craft of preserving their societies intact, despite the pressures from the outside world. His views, like those of so many of the northern Residents, were not limited in application to the Fulani emirates, for he believed that the *obas* of Yorubaland could be moulded into feudal potentates by the application of the northern system.

Temple's views were extreme, but most of the northern Residents shared his conviction of the uniqueness and rightness of their system.

Moreover, government by Residents gave wide scope for individual policies and initiative. It thus attracted able officials with a speculative and intellectual cast of mind whose views were listened to with interest at the Colonial Office. The impact of these unusual and exotic ideas was naturally greater than those of the more humdrum southern officials, who were more concerned with augmenting their customs revenues, or increasing cotton or cocoa under cultivation.

The brilliance of the northern administration, however, could not obscure one fact—the northern system could not pay its way. For this the northern administration could not be blamed. Lacking a sea coast it had no appreciable sources of customs revenue, the normal stand-by of all African colonies at this time. But even with such sources the position would have been little better, for the north had its own closed economy, and its imports and exports were very limited. Its external trade contributed slightly to Southern Nigeria's customs revenue; but from 1900 the southern administration contributed to northern finances (£34,000 per annum from 1901 to 1903, £50,000 from 1904, rising to about £70,000 from 1906 to 1912). The southern subsidy, however, remained small in relation to northern needs. From 1904 the north's annual expenditures could not be kept below £500,000; it was this lack of northern resources which helped to bring about direct taxation and the institution of native treasuries. The government's share of these direct taxes rose from £8,433 in 1903–4 to £274,078 in 1913. But total local revenue in the north never approached even fifty per cent of administrative costs, except after 1911–12 when local revenue was listed as £545,291 by including the share of revenues kept by the native authorities! As a result the imperial government was involved in heavy subsidies. Nor were these substantially reduced as the administration developed.

Year	Imperial Grant-in-Aid (£)	Year	Imperial Grant-in-Aid (£)
1900–1	88,100	1906–7	315,000
1901–2	280,000	1907–8	295,000
1902–3	290,000	1908–9	290,000
1903–4	405,000	1909–10	237,000
1904–5	405,500	1910–11	275,000
1905–6	320,000		

The Colonial Office, constantly harassed by the Treasury on this topic, naturally began to advocate amalgamation of the north and south in order to end imperial grants in aid. The years after 1906 saw a phenomenal increase in trade and revenues in the southern protectorate; from 1906 to 1912 imports and exports doubled, and the revenue rose from just over £1 million to £2·2 million. Despite the need to service large railway loans, the administration at last accumulated useful reserves. The surpluses on Southern Nigerian revenues were not enough to carry the whole of Northern Nigeria's annual deficits; but if the two areas were amalgamated, the southern surplus could be used for a substantial reduction of the imperial subsidy.

A second factor was the progress of railway building. In 1909 the Lagos railway reached Jebba, on the Niger, and the line to Kano opened in 1911. In the same year a narrow-gauge line was begun to link the main line with the tin mines in the Bauchi plateau. There was also a need for a railway in the south-east, to tap the palm-oil trade of the Ibo, and to exploit coal resources discovered in the Udi area. An amalgamated Nigeria could co-ordinate the planning and financing of an overall railway system.

Such were the main motives in Colonial Office thinking; and once again their *ad hoc* and pragmatic character is striking. There was scarcely any discussion in London concerning the fundamental significance of amalgamation. Even in 1912 imaginative men might have seen the union of north and south as a great advance in Britain's Nigerian mission, as the first step towards a new nation. But British officials never seriously discussed how conflicting policies in the two Nigerias might be harmonized, how the rapidly growing individualism of the south, with its cash crops, its rapidly expanding mission schools, its growing wage-earning and clerical class, its African entrepreneurs and petty capitalists, could be blended with northern feudal conservatism, Muslim law and self-sufficiency. Few administrators, even those from the south, argued that the northern system would now have to adapt itself to new conditions. The constant reiteration of the superior values of the northern indirect rule system had produced among many southern officials feelings of inferiority and a lack of confidence in their own unsystematic and haphazard relationships with Africans.

Once again the choice of an individual strongly influenced events. In 1912 the Colonial Office again sent Lugard to Nigeria, after an absence of six years, to devise and carry through a scheme of amalgamation. In making such a choice, the Colonial Office ensured that the northern system would be maintained, for Lugard was by background and temperament committed to the northern system, and filled with hostility for Southern Nigeria. In his report[1] he dismissed the southerners except Yoruba, as 'of a low and degraded type'. Educated Africans made him uneasy in public and irrational in private. His biographer comments that he 'looked at the government of the south with something very close to disgust'.[2] His report, whilst accepting that the south had made 'astonishing' material progress, condemned almost every aspect of the southern administration. At times he even seemed to imply that there was something immoral in southern prosperity (especially in the amount of revenue gained from taxation of alcoholic liquor). He described the northern administration as 'a native policy whose aim was primarily administrative', in contrast with the south where policy was 'commercial, and directed primarily to the development of resources and trade'.

Lugard's proposals, presented to the Colonial Office in May 1913, were in effect designed to avoid the real implications of a unified administration, to preserve the *status quo* in the north, and even to spread northern administrative ideas into the south. Lugard rejected for all Nigeria the older ideals of an Afro–British partnership whereby 'civilised men' worked towards Christian and liberal ideals.

Indeed the 'Amalgamation Report' discounted amalgamation in practice. Lugard proposed the complete amalgamation of only the railways, the marine department and the customs service. As the whole purpose of amalgamation from the Colonial Office point of view was to unify finances and transport, he could hardly have done less. Lugard proposed also that medical, postal, telegraphic and survey departments should each have an all-Nigeria head of department, and that the West African Frontier Force should be put under one command; but in these cases he wanted a separate northern and southern establishment under the single head. The only other unifying administrative office was to be that of Governor-General. Lugard himself meant to fill this post. He would thus occupy a strongly authoritarian position, and would control the government under a scheme of continuous administration, even when on leave in England. Otherwise the division of the country would remain. Lieutenant-governors in the north and south would prepare separate budget estimates for inclusion in the whole.

[1] The report is enclosed in Lugard to Harcourt, 9 May 1913, C.O. 583/3. It was made into a Confidential Print no. 1005. Quotations in subsequent paragraphs are taken from the MS. version.
[2] Margery Perham, *Lugard: the years of authority, 1898–1945* (London, 1960), p. 422.

NIGERIA: THE COLONIAL EXPERIENCE

Alternative schemes suggested by Bell and Temple, and an unofficial scheme elaborated by the journalist E. D. Morel, would all have created a unified central administration over several provinces (whose boundaries were intended to represent ethnic and religious divisions). But these were rejected partly because they would have reduced the area of Fulani control, and partly because Lugard regarded them as extending 'the provincial system of Southern Nigeria which... does not appear to have been a success'. The southern administration was criticized for its general lethargy, for failing to introduce direct taxation, for the fact that chiefs took 'no effective part in the administration', for the semi-autonomous legal position of some of the states and for its judicial system. The north escaped without a hint of blame on any administrative count.

Not surprisingly, therefore, Lugard proposed major reforms in the south. In essence these amounted to the introduction of northern administrative procedures. He advocated the division of the south into provinces like those of the north, and the granting of judicial and executive powers to the district officers, who would thus be stirred to keenness 'as in Northern Nigeria'. In time, chiefs would be 'found and trained' so that they could be 'entrusted to exercise control'. Native courts should be established, and the progressive expansion of British law throughout the south halted. Barristers would be allowed neither in native courts nor in new provincial courts modelled on those of the north. The jurisdiction of the Supreme Court would be limited to the coastal towns, to cases involving foreigners, or to retrials ordered by the Governor-General. Lugard meant to end the fifty-year-old process whereby English legal ideas had spread in the south, a process rightly welcomed by educated Africans (though also abused by some) as a steady extension of human freedom.

Lugard suggested special measures for the government of Lagos which he well knew amounted to an open challenge to Lagos aspirations. He declared that Lagos could never become the capital of amalgamated Nigeria, on the extraordinary grounds that its 'native population' was too large, with the result that 'Segregation is practically not feasible'. Instead, a new capital should be built in Northern Nigeria where the railway crossed the Kaduna river. Moreover, Lagos should be detached from the south, and governed separately from the Yoruba interior by an administrator, so as to reduce its influence.

Lugard favoured also what was tantamount to the destruction of the

Legislative Council, rightly regarded as the symbol of eventual African democratic participation in government. He argued that a Nigeria-wide Legislative Council was impossible on the ground that it could not adequately represent the country as a whole (though African colonial legislative councils had never aspired to more than partial representation of influential minorities). The 'intelligent emirs' in particular could not be members, as they were unable to debate in English, and the Lagos group were 'in no sense representative of the tribes of the interior'. According to Lugard, it was

a cardinal principle of British colonial policy that the interests of a large native population shall not be subject to the will either of a small European merchant class, or of a small minority of educated and Europeanised Natives, who have nothing in common with them, and whose interests are opposed to theirs

—as if it was a question of granting responsible self-government!

Lugard therefore proposed to reduce the Legislative Council virtually to the status of a municipal council. Its scope would be entirely confined to Lagos; its power to legislate for Southern Nigeria would be abolished. In its place Lugard proposed the creation of a Nigerian Council, to which African notables would be nominated, whose functions would be entirely advisory, and which would meet only three days a year.

The Colonial Office received these far-reaching proposals almost without criticism. The reduction of the status of Lagos was welcomed as 'a bold new departure' by one official, who commented also that the southern provincial system 'will die unlamented by me'. There were some doubts on the legal ramifications involved in the Lagos reorganization, and on the virtual abolition of the Legislative Council; but most of the comment in the Colonial Office was on the details of the continuous administration scheme, which was not liked, and on the exact nature of Lugard's future title.[1] In 1914 Lugard's scheme was put into operation with only minor changes.

The amalgamation of 1914 was a landmark in the history of British colonial rule. The British had apparently made a final decision: they would not aim at the creation of a new Nigerian nation. The British likewise seemed to have repudiated the humanitarian and missionary ideals of the nineteenth century. It was perhaps doubly unfortunate for

[1] Minutes on Lugard to Harcourt, 9 May 1913, C.O. 583/3.

them that they should have inaugurated this policy on the eve of the Great War. For world-wide conflict unleashed new forces of nationalism that Lugard's measures and attitudes could no longer accommodate, but simply forced into new and unfamiliar channels.

BIBLIOGRAPHY

Aderibigbe, A. A. B. 'The expansion of the Lagos protectorate, 1863–1900.' Ph.D. thesis, University of London, 1959.

Ajayi, J. F. A. 'The British occupation of Lagos, 1851–1861', *Nigeria Magazine*, Aug. 1961, no. 69.

 Christian missions in Nigeria, 1841–1891: the making of a new élite. London, 1965.

 'Henry Venn and the policy of development', Historical Society of Nigeria, *Journal*, 1959, I, no. 4.

 'Nineteenth century origins of Nigerian nationalism', Historical Society of Nigeria, *Journal*, Dec. 1961, 2, no. 2.

Ajayi, J. F. A., and Robert S. Smith. *Yoruba warfare in the nineteenth century.* Cambridge University Press, 1964.

Alagoa, Ebiegberi Joe. *The small brave city state: a history of Nembe-Brass in the Niger Delta.* Madison, University of Wisconsin Press, and Ibadan University Press, 1964.

Anene, J. C. *Southern Nigeria in transition, 1885–1906: theory and practice in a colonial protectorate.* Cambridge University Press, 1966.

Ayandele, Emmanuel A. *The missionary impact on modern Nigeria, 1842–1914: a political and social analysis.* London, 1966.

Biobaku, S. O. *The Egba and their neighbours, 1842–1872.* Oxford, Clarendon Press, 1957.

Bull, Mary. 'Indirect rule in Northern Nigeria, 1906–1911', in *Essays in imperial government, presented to Margery Perham,* Kenneth Robinson and Frederick Madden, eds. Oxford, 1963.

Crowder, Michael. *The story of Nigeria.* London, 1962.

Dike, Kenneth O. *Trade and politics in the Niger Delta, 1830–1885: an introduction to the economic and political history of Nigeria.* Oxford, Clarendon Press, 1956.

Flint, John E. *Sir George Goldie and the making of Nigeria.* London, Oxford University Press, 1960.

Geary, W. N. M. *Nigeria under British rule.* London, 1927; reprinted, New York, 1965.

Great Britain. *Parliamentary papers.* Vol. LIX, C. 7977. *Report by Sir John Kirk upon the disturbances at Brass.* London, 1896.

Hargreaves, John D. *Prelude to the partition of West Africa*. London, 1963.

Hertslet's commercial treaties: a collection of treaties and conventions, between Great Britain and foreign powers, and of the laws, decrees, Orders in Council, &c., concerning the same, so far as they relate to commerce and navigation, slavery, extradition, nationality, copyright, postal matters, &c., and to the privileges and interests of the subjects of the high contracting parties, compiled from authentic documents... London, 1827–1925. 31 vols.

Ikime, Obaro. 'Itsekiri-Urhobo relations and the establishment of British rule, 1884–1936.' Ph.D. thesis, Ibadan University, 1965.

Johnson, Samuel. *History of the Yorubas from the earliest times to the beginning of the British protectorate*. Lagos, 1921; reprinted, 1956.

Jones, G. I. *The trading states of the Oil Rivers: a study of political development in Eastern Nigeria*. London, Oxford University Press, 1963.

Kingsley, Mary. *West African studies*. London, 1899.

Muffett, D. J. M. *Concerning brave captains: being a history of the British occupation of Kano and Sokoto and of the last stand of the Fulani forces*. London. 1964.

Newbury, Colin W. *The western Slave Coast and its rulers: European trade and administration among the Yoruba and Adja-speaking peoples of south-western Nigeria, southern Dahomey and Togo*. Oxford, Clarendon Press, 1961.

Oliver, Roland. *Sir Harry Johnston and the scramble for Africa*. London, 1957.

Perham, Margery. *Lugard*. 2 vols. London, 1956–60.

Native administration in Nigeria. London, Oxford University Press, 1937.

Robinson, Ronald E., and John Gallagher, with Alice Denny. *Africa and the Victorians: the climax of imperialism in the Dark Continent*. New York, 1961.

Tamuno. S. M. 'The development of British administrative control of Southern Nigeria, 1900–1912.' Ph.D. thesis, University of London, 1963.

Temple, C. L. *Native races and their rulers: sketches and studies of official life and administrative problems in Nigeria*. Cape Town, 1918.

Waldman, M. R. 'The Fulani jihād: a reassessment', *Journal of African History*, 1965, **6**, no. 3.

Webster, James B. *The African churches among the Yoruba*. Oxford, Clarendon Press, 1964.

CHAPTER 8

THE CONGO FREE STATE AND THE BELGIAN CONGO BEFORE 1914

by JEAN STENGERS

The Congo is the archetype of a political entity brought into being on African soil completely by the will of a European. One would seek in vain for any African substructure, any autochthonous base for this state as it appeared toward the end of the nineteenth century. It had nothing in common—save the name—with the Congo of former times, the Congo that had two or three centuries earlier been an important African kingdom. Its origins are to be found entirely in the will of one man— Leopold II of Belgium. In 1884–5 Leopold traced its boundaries firmly on the map of Africa. These extended to the very heart of the Black Continent and included regions largely unexplored up to that time. These borders were recognized by the powers and thus the Congo was born.

From 1885 to 1908 the area constituted an independent state, the Congo Free State, under the personal government of Leopold. In 1908 it was annexed by Belgium and so became a Belgian colony. It retained this colonial status until 1960, when it became independent.

Strictly speaking, there was no such thing as the 'Belgian Congo' *except* from 1908 to 1960. Well before 1908, however, the term was being employed abroad to designate the Free State and had even found its way into diplomatic speech. This can readily be understood when one considers the way in which the Free State appeared to contemporaries: the sovereign of the state, they thought, was the King of the Belgians, who was, as everyone knew, ardently devoted to Belgian interests. The central services of the state were located in Brussels, and all its functionaries were Belgian. As for the Congo itself, in the administration, in the army, and in the courts, the essential role was played by Belgians, particularly by officers of the Belgian army assigned to African service. Even the religious missions—at any rate those of the Catholics, which were most favoured by the state—almost all had a markedly Belgian character. How, in such circumstances, could contemporaries have failed to come to speak naturally of a 'Belgian Congo'?

Nevertheless, the usage is improper and the historian should avoid it. It was contrary both to the situation in law and—what is much more important—to the situation in fact. In law, before 1908, Belgium and the Congo were two absolutely distinct states without any common organ; their sole link rested on the fact that they had the same sovereign. But —and this is an essential point—Leopold II distinguished very clearly between his role as sovereign of the Congo and that as king of the Belgians. In Belgium he was a constitutional monarch and played with perfectly good grace the game of constitutional monarchy in the English fashion. He submitted the texts of his speeches to his ministers beforehand, in accordance with the rules. But these same ministers could only learn by reading the papers that the Congo had leased the upper Nile or concluded a treaty with Portugal: the government of the Congo was something with which they did not interfere. Up till 1908, the sovereign of the Congo directed the policy of that country in a fashion that was in all respects independent; Belgium had no part in it. Hence reality was well expressed in the term 'Congo Free State'.

Our analysis will concentrate successively on three points. First we shall seek to point out the distinctive features of the Congo Free State; then we shall examine the reasons for them; and lastly we shall see to what extent these characteristics were retained after 1908 under the Belgian régime.

Original characteristics of the Congo Free State

Every human group, every community, every state, considered in isolation and compared to its neighbours, reveals features peculiar to itself. In the case of the Congo Free State these traits were so extraordinary as to make it unique.

(1) The Congo Free State was unique, first of all, by reason of its political organization. It was not merely an absolute monarchy in which the sovereign held all powers, but something more. It was a state that one might say was confounded with its sovereign. Sovereignty was invested in the person of the king, who considered the state his private property. Leopold II called himself the 'proprietor' of the Congo, and he disposed of it as if it were indeed his private property. In his will, which was made public in 1890, the king bequeathed to Belgium his 'sovereign rights' over the Congo just as if he were bequeathing a house

or a piece of real property.[1] As a jurist said at the time—and the remark was made in all seriousness—to find a precedent for such a situation one had to go back in Europe to the time of the Merovingian kings. Although never impugned in practice—since no one ever questioned openly the validity of the will itself—the status of the Congo rested on very weak juridical foundations. A reading of the will shows this convincingly. How did the king justify the origin of his 'sovereign rights' to the Congo Free State? They were (he wrote) 'recognized by the declarations, conventions, treaties, which have been made since 1884 between foreign powers on the one part and the Congo International Association and the Congo Free State on the other'. The conventions agreed upon with the Congo Free State do not concern us here: they deal only with frontier questions, with the territorial limits of sovereignty, not with the essence of sovereignty, for this had already been defined at the moment when the state came into existence.

Only the conventions entered into with the Congo International Association in 1884-5 are of immediate relevance. In these treaties, concluded first with the United States (April 1884), then with Germany (November 1884), and subsequently, from December 1884 to February 1885, with practically all the European powers, the sovereign character of the Congo International Association was formally recognized. The declaration of the United States, for instance, took note of 'the flag of the Association as that of a friendly Government'. Nothing in these texts, however, made allusion to any sovereign rights possessed by Leopold II himself. He was not even mentioned in the majority of the treaties; and when he did appear, it was only as the founder of the Association. The Association was represented officially by its 'president', a senior Belgian officer, Colonel M. Strauch.

In order that the sovereignty of the Congo might pass from the International Association, in the name of which it had been recognized, to Leopold II in person, it would have been necessary for the Association to relinquish sovereignty in his favour. Possibly some such act of cession did in fact take place. If so it was never made public, and nobody asked to examine it. The juridical basis of Leopold's rights thus remained in a shadow that no one tried to penetrate.

This is not really surprising. It means simply that on this occasion

---

[1] Leopold II's will, it should be noted, never came into effect because the Congo was annexed by Belgium while the king was still alive. He died in 1909, a year after the annexation.

the facts, which were perfectly clear, prevailed over the law. In treating with the Congo International Association in 1884–5, the powers were well aware that they were really dealing with Leopold. They were so little interested in the Association *per se* that they did not even seek to investigate the nature of the body whose sovereignty they were about to recognize. A simple inquiry would have disclosed that they were dealing with a fictitious entity, with a name and nothing more. Everyone knew that the worthy Colonel Strauch, president of the Association, was no more than a man of straw.

As far as the powers were concerned, what was important was to obtain from the colonel's master, Leopold II, the commitments that they required of him. Hence, wherever the word 'Association' was used in the treaties of 1884–5, everyone had read 'Leopold II'. It was really the king who had made in these conventions the capital promise that had been the basis of his success: the promise of unrestricted freedom of trade for all. In other words, he undertook to open up Central Africa at his own expense and also to put the region freely at the disposal of the commerce of all nations. As a *quid pro quo* for this gesture by a monarch who was already celebrated for his philanthropic initiative and who now showed himself the champion and the guarantor of free trade, the powers recognized the sovereignty of the Congo in his person.

In 1884 and in the beginning of 1885, Leopold II preferred not to handle these questions officially because he feared political difficulties in Belgium. From April 1885 onwards he had no more cause for concern on this account, for the Belgian Chambers had authorized him to become the sovereign of the new state, which was to take the name of Congo Free State. Thereafter the king could officially enter on the stage; the International Association of the Congo, which had served him as cover, disappeared. No one could but applaud this brilliant performance and allow the actor to benefit from what he had acquired as a result of his skill or, to employ another theatrical metaphor, from what he had acquired under a flimsy mask.

This unique instance of a modern state whose sovereignty was invested in the person of the sovereign derives from an international arrangement that was equally unique, an arrangement by which the powers had deliberately allowed one man the legal right to create a state of which he would be the master.

(2) The economic organization of the Congo Free State rested on

principles as original as those of its political organization. They were largely contrary to what was generally admitted and practised at that time.

One of the basic economic beliefs of the Western world towards the end of the nineteenth century—a belief transplanted into the colonial field—was that the prosperity of the state was directly linked to that of private enterprise. Hence, as far as positive economic policy was concerned, the principal duty of the state was to assist in the development of independent business ventures. The Congo state, created, as we have noted, under the aegis of general free trade, ought logically to have been in the forefront when it came to putting these principles into practice. On the contrary, before many years had passed, it introduced major economic measures that had the effect of hindering private enterprise by an impassable barrier of state monopoly.

These policies were embodied, from 1891–2 onward, in what has been called the *régime domanial*. The logic of the system was implacable. The state had been declared proprietor of all vacant land, which would henceforth constitute its domain. Vacant land, it was decreed, consisted of all the land which was neither occupied nor being exploited by the natives. It happened that almost everywhere in the country the two most remunerative wild products, ivory and wild rubber, came from lands decreed vacant and so might be regarded as products of the state's domain, to be collected by the state alone. As a consequence of this system, a trader might not buy ivory or wild rubber from the Africans without becoming a receiver of stolen goods—stolen, in effect, from the state.

The *régime domanial* was not applied with equal severity throughout the territory. In certain districts, notably those where trading companies had already been solidly established before the advent of the régime, the state graciously 'abandoned' to private individuals or concerns the exploitation of the domanial products. The companies concerned might remain in existence. But in the great majority of the areas rich in wild rubber (a commodity which, thanks to its economic importance, would soon eclipse ivory as the domanial produce *par excellence*), the state strictly reserved to itself the right to all crops obtained from vacant lands, which is to say practically all the wild rubber.

The state authorities took solemn oath that they were not attacking free trade. Everywhere, they declared, exchange remained entirely unimpeded. But as the state had laid hands on virtually the only marketable products, a contemporary critic was right when he dryly observed that it had in effect made a law with two articles: '*Article* 1: Trade is entirely free. *Article* 2: There is nothing to buy or to sell.'

Although it practised a monopolistic policy in matters of trade, the state refrained from applying the same policy to other sectors of the economy. For the construction of railroads, for instance, it continued, as it had from the beginning, to look to private enterprise. In 1889 the Congo Railroad Company had been constituted to build the line from Matadi to Leopoldville, a vital artery on which the whole economic future of the country depended. In 1902 the concession for railroads in the eastern Congo was granted to the Compagnie des Chemins de Fer du Congo Supérieur aux Grands Lacs Africains (CFL). The state consistently relied on private enterprise also in the sphere of mining, in which a salient date was 1906—the year the Union Minière du Haut-Katanga was founded to exploit the Katanga copper.

Sectors that the state left to private enterprise were those that called for heavy capital investment and presented the greatest risks. Railroads are expensive; the line from Matadi to Leopoldville called for company expenditures on a scale that for several years exceeded the entire expenses of the state itself. The capital invested in it was on more than one occasion in danger of being lost. In the same way the Union Minière, before it became successfully established, had to surmount difficulties that brought it to the verge of bankruptcy.

If private capitalists were willing to invest, not indeed without hesitation, in such relatively hazardous ventures, it is clear that they would have done so far more readily in the commercial sector where conditions were markedly more favourable. Activities in that field were less risky, called for much less capital, and brought much quicker returns; but it was in that very sphere that the state set up its monopolistic barriers.

(3) A third feature peculiar to the Congo Free State was that, in order to get the maximum profit from the monopoly of the domanial products, it established a system of exploitation that inevitably led to great abuses in the treatment of Africans.

In the history of almost every colony there are pages filled with brutality. The celebrated saying that 'one does not make colonies with choirboys' applies all but universally. The colonial expedition (in the classical sense of the term), the occupation of hostile territory, the repression of native revolts, are rarely carried out in a manner pleasing to humanitarians. The case of the Congo, however, presents a special aspect. The occupation of the territory was accomplished more peacefully than in most other colonies. Stanley, who directed its first stages, made it a point of honour not to use force. As an explorer he had often been rough-handed and had been reproached for brutality; but as chief of the occupying expedition, he avoided violence so far as he could. Those who came after him did not always exercise the same restraint; but since in their progress towards the interior they did not usually meet much resistance on the part of Africans—for Stanley's successors rarely encountered groups large enough and well enough organized to be capable of resistance—they succeeded in subduing the people without great bloodshed. The sharpest struggles were those that had to be undertaken not against the Africans, but against Swahili slave-traders (often called 'Arabs' but rarely of pure Arab descent) and their followers in the eastern Congo. Moreover, once the conquest had been completed, there was no subsequent revolt of any consequence.[1]

Violence in the Congo occurred not so much in the occupation period as in the subsequent era of economic exploitation. And—a situation not found anywhere else—the abuses were due less to men or circumstances than to a system in which men were caught as in a trap. How, then, did these things come about after 1891–2? The state, in accordance with the principles of the domanial régime, required the harvesting of the wild rubber in its domain. This duty fell to the native population in the form of a tax in labour. Local officials were charged with seeing that the work was done and with collecting the crop.

The instructions sent to officials were simple and were incessantly repeated and emphasized: production must be pushed to the maximum. Officials were aware that they were dealing with a matter of major state concern, and that it was essentially in terms of the production level attained that their work would be judged. Judged and even paid: their pecuniary interests were directly affected inasmuch as they obtained a bonus proportionate to the quantities collected. On the other hand, the labour services exacted from the Africans were for a long time left to the officials' discretion; they were not defined by law. It was not

[1] The only dangerous revolts during the period of the Congo Free State were those that took place in the Congolese army. The two most important were those of Luluabourg in the Kasai, in 1895, and that of the Dhanis expedition, in the north-east of the Congo, in 1897.

until after 1903 that the duration of the forced labour rendered by workers was gradually subjected to regulation.

To obtain these labour services, officials employed numerous means of constraint and repression. They could cause villages to be supervised by soldiers posted for the purpose—these were called 'sentinels'; they could inflict floggings by means of the *chicotte*; they could take hostages. When a village showed itself recalcitrant, they could call upon the army to send a punitive expedition.

Although constraint and repression were foreseen, violence was in principle proscribed. The penal code provided for its punishment, and courts existed to enforce the code. The Congolese courts were far from being inactive, and Europeans guilty of violence towards the Africans were regularly brought before the tribunals and condemned. But though the magistracy was well-intentioned and in part at least well-staffed, its numbers were absurdly small in relation to the territory it had to control. In practice the individual official usually managed to escape any effective surveillance by the courts. The supervision exerted over him by the administration was even more lax. The whole administration was bent upon the major objective assigned to it—the gathering of rubber. An official who was somewhat heavy-handed knew that he would not be called to account so long as he obtained a high output. Only a fall in production was unpardonable.

The consequences of this system for the people living in the rubber-growing areas are readily foreseen and may be summarized in a word. The inhabitants were subjected to a degree of forced labour that often reached inhuman proportions and caused intense physical suffering. The Commission of Inquiry sent to the Congo in 1904–5 described in detail the life of a man subjected to forced labour:

In the majority of cases, he must every two weeks make a journey on foot of one or two days, perhaps more, to reach the heart of the forest where he can find the rubber creepers in sufficient abundance. There the gatherer leads a miserable existence for several days. He has to construct an improvised shelter, which clearly cannot replace his hut; he does not have the food to which he is accustomed; he is deprived of his wife and exposed to an intemperate climate and to the attacks of wild beasts. He has to take his harvest to the post of the State or the company, and it is only then that he may return to his village, where he cannot stay more than two or three days, for a fresh stint presses on him. The result is that, whatever the extent of the work rendered in the rubber forest, the native, by reason of the numerous journeys he is obliged to make, finds the greater part of his time taken up with the rubber harvest.[1]

To these sufferings was added the misery occasioned by coercive methods. If the European, at the post he directed, was content in general with the *chicotte* and with taking hostages, the 'sentinels' went much further: in the villages where they were posted, and where they reigned as despots, they maltreated, even killed people. Africans also lost their lives when military expeditions were dispatched—as they frequently were—against villages 'refractory to taxes'. It was from these expeditions that soldiers in certain regions brought back hands cut from the dead or dying, with the aim of proving to their officers that they had made good use of the cartridges issued to them.[2]

Roger Casement, in his capacity as British consul to the Congo, carried out a direct inquiry on the spot (it was this investigation that he subsequently incorporated in the famous Casement Report), and in a letter to the vice-governor general of the Congo in September 1903 he pointed to the sources of the profound evils that he had observed:

I cannot conceal from Your Excellency that, to me, the responsibility for the dreadful state of affairs prevailing in many parts of the country I have visited is not to be attributed to the meaner instruments of crime and the savage agents of extortion I have seen at their dirty work, but to the system of general exploitation of an entire population, which can only be rendered successful by the employment of arbitrary and illegal force.

That population is supposed to be free and protected by excellent laws; those laws are nowhere visible; that force is everywhere. Well-nigh each village has its gang of armed and unscrupulous ruffians quartered upon it; and where they are not actively present, the shadow of the public forces of this Government in the background, ready to be impelled into any district failing or unwilling to comply with the excessive demands continuously made upon it by the public officials of this country, serves as an ever-impending reminder of the doom awaiting the recalcitrants.

Communities that fail to satisfy the unceasing demands made upon them, either for india-rubber, food-stuffs, or some other local want of the European establishments in their neighbourhood are then said to be 'in a state of revolt',

[1] Congo Free State, *Bulletin Officiel*, Sept.–Oct. 1905, pp. 191–2.
[2] These mutilations, it should be noted, were not inflicted by way of punishment. The popular version, which made, and still makes, the cut-off hand the symbol of the Leopoldian régime, has in this respect deviated from the truth.

and the entire population, men, women, and children, are treated worse than the worst criminals in any country I have knowledge of.[1]

It would be a gross overstatement, however, to say that this dark picture applied to every part of Leopold's Congo. Casement himself avoided making this charge, although in the letter just quoted he speaks of 'many parts of the country'. Casement's feelings of horror, on the other hand, were the more lively because he could compare the situation to the one he had known during the first years of the Free State, at a time when the system that brought about the abuses did not yet exist.

The system of domanial exploitation was not introduced until 1891–2, and in some regions considerably later. Moreover, from 1906 the state limited more and more strictly the recourse to coercive methods that had brought about most of the violence (that is to say, essentially the system of 'sentinels' and the military expeditions), and this had the effect of eliminating the worst abuses. In addition, only the regions rich in wild rubber where the domanial régime was applied, principally those in the centre of the Congo basin, passed through these sombre years. Even in these zones, a number of officials were able to obtain in a humane fashion and with a minimum of pressure the labour services demanded from the workers.

Hence the picture can often be varied or mitigated. This was not true, however, in the case of the concessionary companies. Although the state most often exploited its domain directly in the manner already described, it also made use, in two regions in the Congo basin, of the system of concessions. The concessionary companies, the Abir and the Anversoise, received at once the right of collecting the products of the domain and that of collecting taxes—in effect, the right to exploit the African's labour for their own private profit. The state, in exchange, got half the shares of the companies and thus half the dividends. The Abir and the Anversoise reaped unheard-of profits, but their concessions can only be described as veritable hells-on-earth. The officials of these companies had but one law: that of profit. Their conduct in not a few cases was no better than that of the African 'sentinels' whom they employed.

In general terms, wherever the domanial régime was applied, the lot of the workers depended partly on what the European officials were like as individuals. If they were at their worst, as in the concessionary

[1] Casement to Fuchs, 12 Sept. 1903 (copy in the E. D. Morel Papers, British Library of Political and Economic Science, London School of Economics and Political Science).

companies, the lot of the Africans was tragic. But the officials, whoever they were, whatever their virtues and their vices, were ground down by the system, which brought irresistible pressure upon them. It was the system itself that, inevitably, was bound to engender grave abuses.

This became clear when the system was abolished. Those who denounced the abuses in the Congo had declared emphatically that not until the perpetrators were eliminated from the administration would the evils cease. Such a mass purge, however, never became necessary. The Congo State, as mentioned earlier, introduced important reforms after 1906 without actually giving up forced labour. Subsequent to the annexation by Belgium in 1908, forced labour itself was suppressed. Improvements in working conditions were immediate and rapid, although most of the former staff of the Free State retained their jobs. However, these were people who had escaped the pressure of the system.[1]

(4) The Congo State offers also the unique spectacle—unique at any rate at the beginning of the twentieth century—of a poor overseas country part of whose public resources were put at the disposal of a rich European country. The Congo in effect made a financial contribution to Belgium, a country considered its virtual metropolis.

Here again, the originality is striking. According to the rules of the colonial game as played at the end of the nineteenth century and at the beginning of the twentieth century, an imperial power might cause metropolitan interests to prevail over those of its colonies; but it might not attempt to take direct financial advantage of its dependencies. There was practically unanimous agreement in principle that colonial finances ought to be managed in the sole interest of the colonies themselves. Only the Congo Free State, in its time, broke this tacit agreement.

When the state was created, no one could have foreseen that things

---

[1] The British consul to the Congo, W. J. Lamont, observed this well in 1912. He wrote: 'A good deal of stress has been laid on the question of the removal of officials who under the old régime had acquired a reputation for ultraseverity in their dealings with the natives. It should not be overlooked, however, that the harshness of officials was, in many cases no doubt, born of the system under which they were obliged to produce certain quantities of rubber every month; now that this forced collection is finished, the relations of the official to the native are quite materially altered; he is no longer under the, often to him, painful necessity of driving the natives to the forest to bring in the required tale; the necessity for pressure no longer exists. Under these circumstances the attitude of most men, not endowed by nature with temperaments tending towards cruelty and inhumanity, would be likely to undergo radical changes in respect of the native' (Great Britain, *Parliamentary papers*, vol. LIX, Cd. 6606, *Correspondence respecting the affairs of the Congo* [London, 1912–13]).

would turn out that way. The young state appeared, at the time of its foundation, not as a source of funds but as a frail creature that needed aid. During the first ten years of its existence, help was indispensable to it, even for its very survival. From 1885 to 1895 its normal revenues —customs duties, taxes, etc.—remained extremely limited; they sufficed to cover only a small portion of its expenditure. In 1887-8, receipts still represented only a tenth of the expenses; in 1893-4, thanks mainly to ivory, they reached just about one-third. All the rest of the country's revenue had to come from outside. That meant, in the first place, remittances from the king, who covered most of the deficits from his privy purse. Secondly, there was the yield of a lottery loan, issued in Belgium for the benefit of the Congo, which brought in several millions. Lastly, there was direct aid from Belgium, avowed to be indispensable if the Congo were to be saved from bankruptcy. In 1890 Belgium agreed to grant the Congo a loan of 25 million francs, spread out over ten years. In 1895, when bankruptcy was still looming on the horizon, a supplementary loan of nearly 7 million francs was added.

Kept alive by these successive shots of adrenalin, the Free State would almost certainly have gone under but for a timely miracle—in the form of wild rubber. Although the domanial régime had reserved both ivory and rubber, hopes at first rested mainly on ivory. The wealth of the country in rubber was not yet suspected. When the existence of this product was revealed, however, the methodical manner in which the harvests were organized caused production to skyrocket within a very short period. In 1890 the Congo exported only a hundred metric tons of rubber; in 1896, exports reached 1,300 metric tons, in 1898, 2,000 metric tons, and in 1901, 6,000 metric tons.

The state itself, because of the domanial régime, was to be the principal beneficiary of this manna from heaven. Financially speaking the change was a momentous one. In 1890, the state took from its domain around 150,000 francs; in 1901 the domanial products—with rubber rating first—brought it more than 18 million francs. From that time on, the financial difficulties of the Congo were ended. Indeed, thanks to the domanial resources, and thanks also to the proceeds of loans—for now that its credit was solid, it could raise loans without difficulty—the Congo soon began to have budgetary surpluses. These surpluses, from 1900, it began to use in Belgium, for the advantage of Belgium.

Curiously enough, the Free State did not repay the capital of the two

Belgian loans. Its generosity toward Belgium took another form; a grandiose policy of public works and urban improvements was to be undertaken, on Belgian soil, with funds supplied by the Congo. After 1900, work began everywhere: the construction of the Arcade du Cinquantenaire at Brussels, the building of the Tervuren Museum, enlargements to the castle of Laeken, public works at Ostend, various works of urban building. These numerous undertakings redounded to the advantage of the Belgian State, which became their proprietor without having spent a penny on them.

After 1901 the transfer of funds from the Congo to Belgium even took on an institutional form. A special organization created in that year, the celebrated Fondation de la Couronne (which was first called Domaine de la Couronne), was set up. Its mechanism was simple: the Foundation was granted domain lands of enormous extent—around 250,000 square kilometres, or more than a tenth of the total area of the state, equal to half the area of France. The products collected from these lands—mainly, of course, wild rubber—brought in a very high annual income. The Free State, moreover, gave the Foundation part of the yields from its loans. It was these substantial resources that the Foundation applied to the programme assigned to it, which had as its almost exclusive object great public works in the metropolitan country.

From 1901 to 1908, the Foundation was able both to build on a large scale and to plan its future activities. The projects that figured in its programme were of a long-term character and truly magnificent in scope. Urban developments were proposed that would completely change the face of Brussels. To put these works into effect called for advance acquisitions of land on a large scale, and between 1901 and 1908 the Foundation made many such purchases, especially in Brussels.

The whole of this policy, undertaken out of Congo revenues, was conceived—let us repeat—for the advantage of Belgium, and Belgium rapidly obtained direct benefits. It was to gain, in the first place, from the buildings completed by the Foundation, because these buildings immediately became part of the patrimony of the Belgian State. But it was to benefit also from the Foundation's acquisitions of land. In 1908, after the annexation of the Congo, the Foundation was dissolved (this to be explained presently). But all the property that it had acquired in Belgium was taken over by the Belgian State. In buildings and in land, the Belgian State was thus to receive property worth more than 60 million francs.

This figure has to be set off against the expenditures that Belgium made on behalf of the Congo up to 1908. These outlays—the amount of the two loans granted to the Congo in 1890 and in 1895 and the salaries of officers put freely at the disposal of the Free State by the Belgian government, among other expenditures reached a total of some 40 million francs. Thus, in the financial transactions between Belgium and the Congo—which, may we repeat, were separate states until 1908—Belgium paid about 40 million francs and received more than 60 million. For a new colonial entity to export to its virtual metropolis during the first twenty-five years of its existence a sum of this order was indeed exceptional.

(5) Finally the Congo State, both in its genesis as well as in its policy of expansion, represented imperialism in its truest form.

In the great rush of Europeans upon Africa at the end of the nineteenth century, the imperialist spirit was omnipresent. It animated the scramble for the Dark Continent from beginning to end. But behind each of the different phases of this scramble there lurks almost always some special reason that dictated the occupation of one territory or the conquest of another. In one case it might be the response to an appeal from traders who demanded the protection of the national flag; in another it might be the necessity to forestall a rival who might otherwise have seized an important strategic position; in still another case, it might be desired, by occupation of a region, to safeguard national economic interests that would have been imperilled by the establishment of a foreign power and its protectionist policy. In other instances a European power might seek to protect missionaries by ensuring that they did not fall under a foreign jurisdiction. And of course there were combinations of all these circumstances, as well as many others. The scramble can thus be explained in general by a whole series of specific motives that served to guide the imperialist push.

The Congo Free State, however, acted purely on its own initiative; none of the special motivations peculiar to other cases appears to have existed here. The sole driving force was what Stanley, writing in 1885, called an 'enormous voracity'.[1] This voracity—that is, territorial voracity—was not, of course, blind; but it was not inspired by anything other than the political or economic value of what it might absorb or attain. Its sole principles were those of greed.

[1] Stanley to Henry Shelton Sanford, 4 March 1885, in François Bontinck, *Aux origines de l'Etat Indépendant du Congo* (Louvain, 1966), p. 300.

The story of the delimitation of the frontiers of the Congo Free State at the moment of its creation is in this aspect quite illuminating. The activities of expeditions sent out by Leopold, mainly under Stanley, had from 1880 to 1884 led to the foundation of a number of stations that assured a more or less loose territorial occupation. The majority of these posts were situated in the region of the lower Congo, around Leopoldville (today Kinshasa). Beyond Leopoldville, occupation was at that time limited to a few stations along the river, sometimes hundreds of kilometres apart, of which the most advanced was that at Stanley Falls. The whole did not amount to much, but the Congo International Association contrived to make it a jumping-off point for claiming enormous territories.

As already noted, the United States, in April 1884, was the first power to recognize the sovereign character of the Association. But this recognition neither included nor implied any recognition of frontiers, for only the flag of the Association was mentioned in the American declaration. When the Association, shortly afterwards, entered into negotiations with Bismarck, its objective was twofold: it sought to have Germany recognize both its sovereignty and its territorial limits. It was with Bismarck in mind that Leopold II, in August 1884, traced on the map of Africa, for the first time, the boundaries that he wished to obtain. His sketch was a bold one. On it, his borders stretched sometimes as much as 1,000 or 1,500 kilometres from the stations occupied by the Association. In the north, the boundary followed the 4th degree of north latitude; to the east it reached Lake Tanganyika; and to the south it extended to the 6th parallel of south latitude. The territory included in the sketch corresponded to about two-thirds of the present Congo.

The king's greed for territory was thus already great. It alarmed Bismarck at first; but toward the end of the negotiations, in October 1884, he decided, apparently on impulse, to give Leopold what he wanted. Why not, he may have said to himself, give elbow room to this little philanthropic sovereign who wants to sacrifice his personal fortune in order to open up Africa to the trade of all nations?

But what followed was still more significant. In January 1885, during negotiations with France, the Association's representatives produced a new map of the frontiers. The limits on the north and east were those that had already been recognized by Germany; toward the south, however, they had been taken this time as far as the watershed between the Congo and the Zambezi. This represented, in relation to the frontiers approved by Bismarck, a movement toward the south of more than four degrees of latitude. What had happened in so short a space of time? Had the agents of the Association pushed their occupation farther south? Not in the least. Had a new reason appeared that made it necessary or useful to attach these southern regions to the new state? Not at all. The sole new fact was that Leopold wanted to obtain still more territory for the Association. The powers too, for reasons very similar in general to those that had moved Bismarck, were ready to allow Leopold a free hand.

The Congo State, which was set up in 1885 with the frontiers thus defined, would have for several years a territory monstrously disproportionate to the resources at its disposal. We have noted how limited these means were at the outset. They did not allow establishment at first of more than a rudimentary apparatus of government. In vast regions—the 'Arab' zone to the east, the Katanga to the south—the influence of the state remained negligible. Nevertheless, a feeble state, unable to occupy more than a part of its territory, became immediately an expansionist state—the most expansionist, certainly, in the whole of Africa—seeking to extend its frontiers everywhere and in all directions.

In 1888–9, the points it sought to attain were clear: they were the upper Zambezi, Lake Nyasa, Lake Victoria and the upper Nile. An elaborate policy was devised with those ends in view. The push towards the east, for instance, would depend on the alliance with the 'Arabs': it was hoped to obtain their support in order to extend the influence of the state right up to Lake Victoria.

This vast scheme, with no means of implementation, soon encountered obstacles from almost every direction. The expeditions projected toward the upper Zambezi came to nothing. No agreement was reached with the 'Arabs'; on the contrary, it became necessary to engage in war with them. But in one direction the push did persist, indeed persisted to the very end of the Free State—the push to the Nile.

The efforts deployed for this purpose, supported in Europe by large-scale diplomatic manoeuvres, were incessant. They cannot be described in detail here, but a few salient facts may be recorded. In 1890 —that is to say, at a time when, thanks to the financial aid given to the Congo by Belgium, its resources had increased a little—Leopold II organized, with the Nile as its objective, the greatest expedition he had yet mounted in Africa, the expedition of Van Kerckhoven. In 1892, the expedition reached the upper Nile, while other Congolese forces pushed in the direction of the Bahr el Ghazal. In 1894 Great Britain, bowing before what was already in great measure a *fait accompli*, agreed to Leopold's occupation of the southern Sudan. A treaty was concluded with him under the terms of which Great Britain leased to him all the Nile basin south of the 10th degree of north latitude (the latitude of Fashoda). This device would have the advantage, the British thought, of removing from the upper Nile a much more redoubtable competitor, namely France. But France, naturally, took offence and, using all available means of pressure, forced Leopold to renounce the advantage of his agreement with England. In August 1894, he undertook to abstain from any occupation of the territory that had been leased to him, keeping only the right to occupy the most southern part of it— what was later called the Lado enclave.

These checks did not put an end to Leopold's designs on the Nile. Instead, the king was shortly to renew them in a more ambitious form. In 1896 he assembled in the eastern Congo an expedition which was without doubt the greatest that nineteenth-century Africa had ever seen. This expedition, placed under the direction of Baron Dhanis, had as its official objective the enclave of Lado, a completely legitimate one since Leopold II had already reserved the right to occupy it. But we now know the real objective. After the region forbidden to Leopold under the treaty of August 1894 had been traversed, the Congolese flag was to be planted on the banks of the Nile north of that region, that is to say, north of the parallel of Fashoda, toward Khartoum.

The schemes and ambitions of Leopold II did not stop at Khartoum. Beyond Khartoum there was Eritrea, which—following upon the disaster of Aduwa in March 1896—a considerable portion of Italian public opinion appeared disposed to abandon. Here also Leopold II was ready to seize his opportunity. He entered into secret negotiations with the Italian government, from whom he offered to lease Eritrea. His African empire would thus extend from the banks of the Congo to the Red Sea.

The realization of these grandiose projects was dependent on the success of the Dhanis expedition. Leopold's hopes crashed when the expedition met with disaster. In 1897, on the borders of the Congo and Nile basins, a part of Dhanis's troops mutinied, and the whole expedition was eventually swallowed up in the revolt. Thereafter, despite the limited forces at his disposal—for the Dhanis expedition was the great gamble on which he had staked almost everything—Leopold II nevertheless succeeded in occupying the Lado enclave and with indomitable perseverance attempted to push northward. His efforts, both military and diplomatic, to obtain as large a slice as possible of the southern Sudan lasted until 1906, the date of a new agreement with Britain and of his final defeat: far from extracting further territorial concessions from London, Leopold had to agree that the Lado enclave would be evacuated after his death. It was, in his own words, his 'Fashoda'.

Search for an explanation of the Free State's unique characteristics

Whence came these special features of the Congo Free State? Is it possible to detect the influence of the African environment, of the conditions in Africa itself in which the state developed? Or, if these special features are the result of the administration of the state, are they to be attributed to Leopold personally or to the men or the groups surrounding him? Can one point to the influences derived from the special circumstances of Belgium? These are the questions we propose to ask with respect to each of the characteristics already described.

(1) As regards the political organization of the State, it may be said that Leopold II bore the sole responsibility. It was the king who wanted to make the Congo his property in order to do with it what he would. Was this the wish of an autocrat? It would be more accurate, we think, to say that the spirit animating him was that of a great captain of business who seeks to be master of the enterprise he has built up. Leopold II had created the Congo, at the price of incessant labour day after day, and he had paid for it out of his own resources. The Congo was his work; he considered it only right and proper that it should belong to him.

Moreover, his businessman's mentality did not conflict with his patriotic ideals. The king's work in the Congo was constantly directed towards the interests of his own country. He wished Belgium to profit directly from his efforts, in the first place by gaining advantage from the existence of the Free State and secondly by annexing it as a colony. But in order that the cession of the Congo to Belgium could be accomplished in an unassailable manner it was necessary, the king thought, that his rights over the country at the moment when he handed them over should also be unassailable—should be absolute.

(2) The setting up of the domanial régime also bears the personal stamp of Leopold II. The king was in the full sense of the word the originator of the new economic policy of the years 1891–2. Incidentally, he imposed this policy against the advice of those who had hitherto been his best and most faithful supporters. Men like Beernaert, Lambermont, Banning, Janssen, who in various ways had given Leopold enormous help, were reckoned among his best-informed counsellors. Beernaert as Belgian Prime Minister had been responsible for the first Belgian loan to the Congo in 1890. Lambermont and Banning, two high officials at the Ministry of Foreign Affairs, had each played a decisive role in Leopold's diplomatic successes. Janssen had been the first governor-general of the young Free State. But all these men, who formed the king's immediate entourage, were literally horrified at the idea of monopolizing the domanial products for the benefit of the state. They saw in this policy a violation of the most solemn engagements undertaken by the Free State and a guarantee of economic catastrophe.

For them it was not merely good faith that was at stake but also economic principles. To restrict freedom of trade and the development of private enterprise was, Banning wrote, 'to repudiate the principles of economic science'.[1] A system of state monopoly could only lead the Congo to ruin. For men who had imbibed economic liberalism with their mother's milk, this was almost, one might say, a matter of faith. To pretend that such a régime could not be bad—wrote Banning elsewhere—would be 'to deny that political economy can be a science, that it has certain and demonstrable principles'.[2]

For his part, Leopold II had neither doctrinaire economic convictions nor juridical scruples. In order to sustain his theories of the domain, he had consulted numerous eminent jurists. His conscience was therefore easy on that count. For the rest, he observed the immediate financial advantages that might accrue to the Free State from the establishment of the domanial régime. As a good empiricist he considered these advantages more important than principles. He therefore forged ahead, sweeping away all objections. Soon, irritated by criticisms, he pushed aside the men themselves. All his earlier collaborators, those who, along with him, had brought the Congo into being, thus disappeared:

[1] Emile Banning, *Textes inédits d'Emile Banning*, Jean Stengers, ed. (Brussels, 1955), pp. 47 and 77.
[2] *Ibid.*, pp. 78 and 105.

with Banning, the king broke brutally; with Lambermont and Janssen there was a semirupture; and Beernaert was to fall from grace a little later.

Henceforth the king would impose firmly on his new collaborators his theory of the domain. The most important of these was for several years the Secretary of State, Edmond Van Eetvelde, who directed the services of the Congolese government in Brussels. Even so, the king encountered difficulties. As late as June 1891, Van Eetvelde wrote to the king that he could not 'in spirit and in conscience, recognize that this theory was well founded'. But in the end Leopold was able to convince him.

Thus Leopold conceived and carried through the domanial policy almost alone, in spite of the opposition he met on every side—or perhaps in part because of this opposition, whose criticisms did no more than confirm his determination. When the policy, thanks to the miracle of wild rubber, had made the financial fortune of the Congo, the domanial theory would acquire a host of supporters. But in its inception, it was the work of a single man.

(3) The régime of outright exploitation to which the people of the Congo were subjected resulted both from an order and from the manner of its execution. The order, coming from the top, had been to push exploitation to the limit. The means to attain this objective had consequently been put into effect.

The initial injunction came from Leopold II personally. The corollary of the domanial theory, in his view, was that the state ought to extract the maximum profit from its domain. But, having given his instructions, the king was very little concerned with the way in which they were carried out. The king's instructions were elaborated by the administration, both in Brussels and in Africa. To this system were added on-the-spot activities of the agents charged with carrying it out. Leopold limited himself to noting that the yield was satisfactory.

However—and this is very little known—when the first accusers rose up to denounce abuses in the treatment of the Africans, the king was deeply moved. From 1896 to 1900, as his private letters reveal, he passed through several periods of agony. 'We are condemned by civilized opinion', he wrote in September 1896 to Van Eetvelde. 'If there are abuses in the Congo, we must make them stop. If they are perpetuated, this will be the end of the State.'[1] 'It is necessary to put

[1] Letter of 13 Sept. 1896 published in the Brussels daily, *La Nation Belge*, 22 May 1931.

down the horrible abuses' that had been revealed, he instructed another of his collaborators in January 1899. 'These horrors must end or I will retire from the Congo. I will not allow myself to be spattered with blood or mud; it is necessary that these villainies cease.'[1] And a year later the king repeated: 'I am weary of being stained with blood and mud.'[2]

On the occasion of each of these crises of anger and disgust, the king reiterated strict orders: cruelty to the natives should be severely punished. The Congo administration to whom he addressed these orders accepted them and then proceeded to do nothing but wait for the storm to pass. The administration in effect held the trump cards. It had elaborated a system and it stuck to it. It refused to admit that the system of itself could be the generator of abuses, since to admit this would be to recognize its own error. The administration was conscious also of the danger that altering the system might weaken it. The lessening of pressure on the workers would naturally bring about a reduction of revenue; and the administration was well aware that, if this occurred, it would have more than royal anger to face. In other words, the administration distinguished between the king's permanent and funda-mental desire—to increase the output of the domain—and his occasional crises of conscience. It modelled its action on what was permanent and fundamental.

All those linked with the régime, therefore, and desirous of excul-pating themselves, tried to convince Leopold II that the accusations against the Congo were unjust or exaggerated and were made in great measure out of ill will. The attitude of Leopold, who, unconsciously no doubt, was ready to be convinced, thus came to undergo profound modification: instead of being affected by the attacks, he began soon to react more and more violently against them. Whereas the king almost always proudly dominated his entourage, it may be said that in this case he allowed himself to be dominated by it.

As a result, the increasingly powerful campaign against abuses in the Congo, mounted principally in England, served to unite the king, the Congolese administration, and, for a time at least, the greater part of Belgian public opinion in an indignant response. In the eyes of the Congo administration and its leaders, the Anglo-Saxon missionaries

[1] Leopold to Liebrechts, 17 and 31 Jan. 1899, Edmond Van Eetvelde Papers, no. 34, Archives Générales du Royaume, Brussels.
[2] Leopold to Liebrechts, quoted in the letter from Baerts to Van Eetvelde, 18 Jan. 1900, Van Eetvelde Papers, no. 96.

who denounced the abuses, or Consul Roger Casement, who had prepared a crushing report attacking the régime, were simply British agents who sought to damage the Congo by a recital of calumnies. Belgian public opinion was no less suspicious of those who, under the flag of humanitarianism, carried on the campaign in Britain. With the recent experience of the Boer War in their minds, Belgians suspected that humanitarianism was nothing more than a mask for greed. 'I cannot associate myself', declared an eminent liberal politician in 1903, 'with a campaign whose last word appears to be: "give up what you have so that I may take it!"'[1] E. D. Morel, founder of the Congo Reform Association, was generally regarded as the agent of a group of 'Liverpool merchants' interested, for one reason or another, in the ruin of the Free State.

It is readily understandable that the Belgians, who a little while earlier had shouted themselves hoarse cheering the Boer generals and abusing 'perfide Albion', and that the agents of the state, who in the Congo were perpetually annoyed by the watchfulness of the missionaries, should experience these passionate reactions. It caused them to misunderstand completely the real situation, which was simply that the British conscience had been seized by generous and disinterested emotion. What is perhaps more surprising is that the king, who knew England and the English very well indeed and had never since his youth missed reading a single issue of *The Times*, should have relinquished his power of reasoning to a point where he could not understand the nature and meaning of the British campaign. That campaign apparently never affected him nor caused him a moment's reflection. From 1900 onward the hour of agony was passed; Leopold had eyes for nothing but the battle. His Congo was being attacked, calumniated, menaced; he would lead a fight to the death to defend it.

In sum, the king, without having a very clear idea of what he was doing, had aligned himself with the Congo administration; he had yielded to the influence of his entourage.

(4) On the other hand, the king's entourage was in no way responsible for the policy of using the resources of the Congo for the benefit of Belgium. Here Leopold II was once more acting alone.

The king's attitude derived from one of his oldest interests, one to which he remained constantly attached. In his youth Leopold had been a passionate admirer of the Dutch colonial system, which, as it func-

[1] Paul Janson, speech in the Chamber of Deputies, 13 July 1903.

tioned in the middle of the nineteenth century, caused abundant profits from the East Indies to pass every year to the Dutch treasury. The young prince, who dreamed of getting a colony for his country, saw this direct enrichment of the metropolitan country as the cardinal advantage to be gained from the well-planned exploitation of an overseas possession. The idea remained firmly with him. At the very end of the nineteenth century, the Congo became, on the model of early Java, a country from which considerable wealth might be extracted. Without hesitation, and in conformity with his lifelong aspiration, the king sought to use those resources in Belgium. As to how they should be employed, he was especially clear. Leopold II had the soul of a builder-king. It was to a policy of public works, urbanism, and grand monumental constructions that the Congo funds were to be systematically applied. He drew up a programme. He recruited his architects and builders and indicated his plans to them. He established the Fondation de la Couronne, whose organization and functioning he regulated minutely. Thanks to these measures, he declared, the Congo would take its 'just share in the embellishment of our territory'.[1]

'Just share'—these words should give us pause. They show that not only was Leopold II a builder, excited by the possibilities that lay before him, and a patriot dreaming of enriching his country, but he was also profoundly convinced of the rightness of his policy. In the eyes of the king, a nation that endowed a new country with its civilization, its labour, its capital, had the right to 'legitimate compensation'.[2] This is what Belgium had done for the Congo; it was only fair that the Congo, in compensation, should participate in the 'embellishment' of Belgium.

No one among his contemporaries encouraged the king to think in this way. The unanimous colonial doctrine, as we have noted, rejected such a theory and opposed the idea of a tribute levied by a metropolitan country on its colonies. Those in Belgium who expressed any opinion on the matter shared these views. But if the king was not praised for his ideas, was he praised for his actions? Was he, to any degree at all, supported and encouraged by any groups? Here again, search as one may, the answer is no. The Belgian government displayed conspicuous reserve about the king's bounty. To get it accepted, the king had often to resort to subterfuges. In order to give Belgium the Arcade du Cinquantenaire, for instance, he had to conceal himself behind fictitious

[1] Jean Stengers, *Combien le Congo a-t-il coûté à la Belgique?* (Brussels, Académie Royale des Sciences Coloniales, 1957), p. 551.   [2] *Ibid.*, p. 149.

donors whom he had himself recruited and whom he thanked effusively at the official opening ceremony.

The Congo administration was still more reserved, indeed frankly hostile. Those who lived in the country could see with their own eyes how poor it was, how rudimentary its 'infrastructure'; they could see the lack of doctors, of hospitals, of means of transport. They could not but be irritated by the thought that Congolese funds were being used, to the tune of tens of millions, for monumental public works in Belgium. 'For a long time', a former colonial officer noted, 'the Arcade du Cinquantenaire in Brussels was the personal enemy of all colonials.' The officials of the Congo administration in Brussels shared the feelings of their colleagues in Africa. It is now known that they even hid from the king the existence of certain receipts from the Congo, for fear that these would be swallowed up immediately in his great enterprises.

Around Leopold II there was no one, unless it were perhaps his architects and builders, to encourage him in his policy. On the contrary, he was not spared the most violent criticism. Newspaper articles denounced the 'ruinous folly of extravagant public works'. The socialist leader Emile Vandervelde, castigating the abuses of the Congo in the Chamber of Deputies, spoke of the 'monumental arcades which will one day be called the Arcades of the Severed Hands'.

None of these objections or criticisms appears to have disturbed the king for a single instant. He was to persevere until the end. Of all the institutions that he had created in the Congo, the Fondation de la Couronne was the one he defended with the greatest fervour: it constituted, towards the end of his life, the realization of his lifelong dream.

(5) We have said that the Congo was an imperialist state. But the state in this case was no more than an instrument. Its imperialism, let us repeat once more, existed entirely in the mind of a single man. It was indeed a strange spectacle to see nineteenth-century Belgium—a small peace-loving country without foreign ambitions, contented with its lot, opposed to adventures, with a culture hardly propitious for the formation of such a character—produce the purest imperialist of his time.

The strength of the imperialist spirit that imbued Leopold was twofold. It combined unshakable economic conviction with a force less obvious but more powerful—the ambition of a visionary.

The economic attitude of mind was fundamental to Leopold: he had no doubt that a well-run overseas possession ought to be made profitable. From admiration for Java in the Netherlands East Indies, the source of his first enthusiasm, from studying the balance sheet of colonies that had been successful (and these were the only ones that evoked his interest), the king as a very young man had come to the conclusion that all colonies were economically a good thing. This conviction never left him and guided all his policy. He sought to acquire as much as he could, and that as quickly as possible—the more the better. There is something strange and fascinating about this thirst for territory. In 1888, when the organization of his immense Congo had hardly been started, Leopold, as mentioned earlier, occupied himself with sending out expeditions in all directions, aimed at extending the frontiers of the state. We must act quickly, he had explained to one of his collaborators, for 'after next year there will be nothing more to acquire in Africa'.[1] The king was ready to grab everything, even when others abandoned it. Britain appeared to recoil at the prospect of taking responsibility for Uganda, so Leopold at once made an offer for it: a lease of Uganda, he wrote to Gladstone, would suit him perfectly.[2]

But the flame that burned in Leopold II would not have had the same ardour (it was to last throughout his life) if, besides economic ambitions and interests, it had not been sustained by other elements— dreams and visions. It is only for brief moments that this side of the king's character appears to us, but these moments are revealing. In international policy, for instance, one can see how his imagination worked. In 1876, he suggested to Queen Victoria that the Prince of Wales should mount the Turkish throne jointly with a daughter of the Tsar: would it not be, he said, 'a good thing for your government to entrust the Bosphorus to an English prince?'[3] In 1895, in the presence of a polite but bewildered Lord Salisbury, Leopold developed an even more ambitious plan under which Great Britain would evacuate Egypt but would be recompensed by annexing China to the Indian Empire.[4] If he imagined these possibilities for other people, the king,

---

[1] Leopold to Strauch, 17 May 1888, Papers of Col. M. Strauch, Archives of the Ministry of Foreign Affairs, Brussels.

[2] Leopold to Gladstone, 29 Sept. 1892, William E. Gladstone Papers, Add. MSS. 44. 516, British Museum, London.

[3] Victoria, Queen of Great Britain, *The letters of Queen Victoria: a selection from Her Majesty's correspondence and journals between the years 1862 and 1878*, George Earle Buckle, ed., ser. 2 (New York, 1926–8), II, 475–6.

[4] *Letters of Queen Victoria between 1886 and 1901*, George Earle Buckle, ed., ser. 3 (London, 1930–2), II, 578–9.

when he thought of what he himself might accomplish, had still more remarkable dreams. 'I would like', he told an interviewer in 1892, 'to make out of our little Belgium, with its 6 million people, the capital of an immense empire. There are means of realizing this wish. We have the Congo; China is in a state of decomposition; the Netherlands, Spain, Portugal, are in a state of decadence and their colonies will one day or another come on to the market.'[1]

Thus for the whole of his life Leopold II lived in an imperialist dream. The only case comparable with his is that of Cecil Rhodes. Rhodes in his first will also expressed a dream that obsessed him and drove him to action. There was in one respect, however, a fundamental difference between the two. Rhodes's imperialism drew strength from a profound faith in the superiority of the British race. But nothing indicates that Leopold II ever believed in a superhuman virtue existing in Belgians; on the contrary, he was apt to judge them, when he put his mind to it, with rather contemptuous severity. Nevertheless, it was precisely because Belgium was small that he had for it visions of grandeur. He drew from them the exalted feeling of being, all by himself, the creator of this splendour.

The Congo and Africa were therefore not the sole field of Leopold II's ambitions. His eyes ranged over the entire world, seeking opportunities of which he might take advantage. Almost all his efforts, outside Africa, came to nothing; but his quest was none the less incessant. In 1888, for example, one might think that his African cares would have been enough for him. Nothing of the kind. He wrote to Strauch that he was 'looking for a traveller, by preference a German, for a delicate mission in Oceania. His business would be at once to encourage a sultan [sic!] to yield his state to us and not to allow the British to get wind of it.'[2]

True, this is something of a tale; but there were other efforts that were far more important. In 1898, the king attempted to acquire the Caroline Islands. At the same time and by other means, he exerted strenuous efforts to obtain the Philippines. His activity extended also to China, where he took a major interest in a series of big schemes.

Nevertheless, Central Africa remained the centre of his concern:

[1] Conversation of 30 Aug. 1892, in Auguste Roeykens, *Le baron Léon de Béthune au service de Léopold II* (Brussels, 1964), p. 56.
[2] Leopold to Strauch, 23 Feb. 1888, Papers of Col. M. Strauch, Musée de la Dynastie, Brussels.

Central Africa, not merely the Congo. There were times when the Nile had clear priority in the king's mind. Into his determined effort to reach that river, the king proceeded with an enthusiasm that is not to be found in any other of his enterprises. To the customary motives for his imperialism, there was added in this case a special, truly passionate element. The Nile exercised a veritable fascination over him. While the Congo appeared to him, in his own words, 'prosaic', he burned with ardour at the idea of playing, on the Nile, the role of a 'new Pharaoh'. 'It is my plume', he said, 'and I will never give it up!'

The Nile policy makes especially clear how far the king's imperialism, like so many other facets of his life, was essentially a one-man policy. When the king went in for colonization in the classic sense of the word, as in the Congo, he found among Belgians, besides sceptics or detractors, a certain number of devoted collaborators and even enthusiasts. But nobody applauded an adventurous and risky push like that toward the Nile. Nobody encouraged the king. Those who thought they had influence with him tried, on the contrary, to turn him aside from the path that they judged to be dangerous. Even his own Secretary of State, Van Eetvelde, who was entrusted, much against his will, with carrying out the sovereign's policy, declared in a private conversation that it appeared to him 'little short of insanity'. In an attempt to save Leopold II from himself, Van Eetvelde went to the unheard-of length of inciting Britain, by secret representations, to put obstacles in the path of the king's projects. The most faithful servant of all betrayed his master in his master's interest. Leopold, for his part, had no need for encouragement. He wanted the Nile and, deaf to all warnings, pursued unceasingly the object he had set for himself.

All the features peculiar to the Free State thus derived their origin from the person of its sovereign. The influence of the African environment was negligible, that of the metropolitan milieu scarcely less so. Leopold, in shaping the characteristics of the Free State, frequently acted against the advice of his own entourage. In sum, there is no other example, at least in modern times, of a state whose history can be so much identified with a single man.

Annexation of the Congo by Belgium and its consequences

On 15 November 1908, the Congo Free State was annexed by Belgium and so became a Belgian colony. We are not concerned here with writing the history of the annexation,[1] but shall limit ourselves to indicating the reasons why Belgium decided upon this course. The initiative did not come from Leopold II. The king had destined the Congo to become a Belgian colony, but he intended to preserve his personal government there as long as possible. The Belgian annexation was forced upon him by outside pressure. The two basic reasons for it were the growing virulence of the anti-Congolese campaign abroad and the awakening of Belgian public opinion to the gravity of the situation in the Congo.

For a long time the great majority of Belgians had been extremely suspicious of the British campaign, which they attributed to interested parties. What opened their eyes was the report made at the end of 1905 by an international Commission of Inquiry that had been sent to the Congo. The impartiality of this commission was beyond all suspicion. Its report confirmed, in all essentials, what Casement and the Congo Reform Association had been saying: abuses there were extremely grave. The report aroused a belief in Belgian governing circles that radical reform of the Congolese régime was necessary and that Belgium alone could carry it out. Hence, the country would have to be annexed. Abroad, annexation was called for by those who denounced the intolerable situation of the workers. The campaign led in England by the Congo Reform Association had reached the dimensions of a national movement of protest. From Britain the sentiment had spread to other countries and especially to the United States. The Congo Free State was put in the dock, and Belgium was pressed to intervene. The British government itself made quite clear that it could not tolerate the persistence of the *status quo*. Therefore the very existence of the Congo would be imperilled if Belgium remained passive. From the international point of view, also, annexation was imperative. The king, in face of the mounting strength of the offensive directed against his régime, could not but agree.

The annexation of 1908 took place in a solemn atmosphere, with no enthusiasm anywhere. Belgium was conscious of the grave responsibilities

[1] This has been sketched in Jean Stengers, *Belgique et Congo: l'élaboration de la charte coloniale* (Brussels, 1963).

it was undertaking. People were expecting a new policy, breaking with the past.

The policy adopted was sound rather than brilliant. After all the original schemes of Leopold, the wise course was clearly a return to colonial normality. Very soon after 1908, if not immediately, the special characteristics of the Congo Free State disappeared or were effaced, giving way to grey-haired orthodoxy. The situation can be briefly described for each of the features we have mentioned.

(1) For the political régime of the Free State, unique in its type, was substituted in 1908 a colonial régime of a 'classical' character. Royal absolutism was uprooted at a single blow. It is true that according to the terms of the law that organized the political constitution of the colony— the Colonial Charter—the king's powers appeared to remain considerable. The charter gave the king both executive power and, concurrently with the Belgian Parliament, legislative power. But when the charter used the words 'the king', it intended this term exactly as used in the Belgian constitution, which sets forth in detail the powers of the king. In the Congo as in Belgium the king's acts would have no validity unless they were countersigned by a minister who alone would take the responsibility for them. The rules of constitutional monarchy would henceforth hold sway in the Congo, as in Belgium. The man responsible for colonial policy would be the Minister of Colonies. Leopold II yielded to this new state of things with good grace—for as the king of the Belgians he had, as we have said, a profound sense of constitutional monarchy. His absolute rule ended on 15 November 1908. For the remaining year of life that was left to him, he effaced himself behind his Minister of Colonies, Jules Renkin.

(2) Between 1910 and 1912 Jules Renkin suppressed the domanial régime successively in the different regions of the country and re-established full freedom of trade throughout the Congo. The measures taken consisted simply in abandoning to the Africans the right of gathering and selling the natural products of the domain for their own advantage. Obligatory harvesting for the profit of the State was *ipso facto* abolished.

(3) In 1913 the Congo Reform Association decided to dissolve. After annexation of the Congo to Belgium in 1908, it had not relaxed its vigilance. On the contrary, under E. D. Morel's direction it continued to follow the situation closely, assembling a great quantity of information, notably from the missionaries and from the British

consuls. Five years after the annexation, all the evidence agreed: the abolition of forced labour and the determined efforts of the Belgian colonial authorities to eliminate abuses had brought about a normal situation. The peoples of the Congo were thenceforth subject to a régime which, given the currently admitted principles of colonization —and these principles had never been put in question by those who had attacked Leopold's system—no longer gave any particular grounds for concern or for intercession.

(4) Leopold II would have liked the Fondation de la Couronne to be maintained after the annexation. Indeed, his determined efforts to assure the maintenance of the Foundation, to which he was passionately attached, were to be the principal element of complication in the negotiations for annexation. His efforts, however, were in vain: there was no parliamentary majority in Belgium for such a system of trans-fusion of resources from the colony to the metropolitan country. Leopold II was constrained to resign himself, in 1908, to what was doubtless the most bitter sacrifice of his last years—the dissolution of the Foundation. Under the new colonial régime, beginning in 1908, colonial finances and metropolitan finances were strictly separated, according to the most orthodox rules.

(5) After 1908, Belgium possessed the Congo and was fully satisfied with it. The country did not dream of acquiring other people's possessions. The acquisition of Ruanda-Urundi, after World War I—not indeed as a colony but as a mandate from the League of Nations—was in no way the result of expansionist ambitions. It was an unpremedi-tated accident. Having led victorious military operations against the German forces in Africa, Belgium refused, by a kind of reflex action, to lose the reward for them. One does not come back from a victorious war empty-handed. That also, rightly regarded, is clearly orthodox.

Leopold II created the Congo, but a Congo of his own, as original as himself; and Belgium made of it a classical colony.

BIBLIOGRAPHY

Académie Royale des Sciences Coloniales. *Biographie coloniale belge.* 5 vols. Brussels, 1948–58. (Vols. I-III, 1948–52, published by the Institut Royal Colonial Belge, Brussels.)

Anstey, Roger. *Britain and the Congo in the nineteenth century.* Oxford, Clarendon Press, 1962.

King Leopold's legacy: the Congo under Belgian rule, 1908–1960. London, Oxford University Press, 1966.

Banning, Emile. *Textes inédits d'Emile Banning*, Jean Stengers, ed. Brussels, 1955.

Bontinck, François. *Aux origines de l'Etat Indépendant du Congo.* Louvain, 1966.

Cattier, Félicien. *Etude sur la situation de l'Etat Indépendant du Congo.* Brussels, 1906.

Ceulemans, P. *La question arabe et le Congo, 1883–1892.* Brussels, Académie Royale des Sciences Coloniales, 1959.

Congo, Belgian. Force Publique. *La Force Publique de sa naissance à 1914: participation des militaires à l'histoire des premières années du Congo.* Brussels, Institut Royal Colonial Belge, 1952.

Congo Free State. *Bulletin Officiel.* Brussels, Sept.–Oct. 1905.

Cornet, René J. *La bataille du rail: la construction du chemin de fer de Matadi au Stanley Pool.* Brussels, 1947.

Katanga. 3rd ed. Brussels, 1946.

Daye, Pierre. *Léopold II.* Paris, 1934.

Gladstone, William E. The William E. Gladstone Papers, British Museum, London.

Great Britain. *Parliamentary papers.* Vol. LIX, Cd. 6606. *Correspondence respecting the affairs of the Congo.* London, 1912–13.

Keith, Arthur Berriedale. *The Belgian Congo and the Berlin Act.* Oxford, Clarendon Press, 1919.

Lichtervelde, Louis, comte de. *Léopold II.* 4th ed. Brussels, 1935.

Louis, William Roger. *Ruanda-Urundi, 1884–1919.* Oxford, Clarendon Press, 1963.

Luwel, Marcel. *Sir Francis de Winton, administrateur général du Congo, 1884–1886.* Tervuren, Belgium, Musée Royal de l'Afrique Centrale, 1964.

Morel, E. D. The E. D. Morel Papers, British Library of Political and Economic Science, London School of Economics and Political Science.

Ranieri, Liane. *Les relations entre l'Etat Indépendant du Congo et l'Italie.* Brussels, Académie Royale des Sciences Coloniales, 1959.

Roeykens, Auguste. *Le baron Léon de Béthune au service de Léopold II.* Brussels, 1964.

Les débuts de l'œuvre africaine de Léopold II. Brussels, Académie Royale des Sciences Coloniales, 1955.

Léopold II et l'Afrique, 1855–1880: essai de synthèse et de mise au point. Brussels, Académie Royale des Sciences Coloniales, 1958.

Slade, Ruth M. *English-speaking missions in the Congo Independent State, 1878–1908.* Brussels, Académie Royale des Sciences Coloniales, 1959.

King Leopold's Congo: aspects of the development of race relations in the Congo Independent State. London, Oxford University Press, 1962.

Stengers, Jean, *Belgique et Congo: l'élaboration de la charte coloniale*. Brussels, 1963.

Combien le Congo a-t-il coûté à la Belgique? Brussels, Académie Royale des Sciences Coloniales, 1957.

Stenmans, Alain. *La reprise du Congo par la Belgique: essai d'histoire parlementaire et diplomatique*. Brussels, 1949.

Strauch, M. The Papers of Col. M. Strauch, Archives of the Ministry of Foreign Affairs, Brussels.

The Papers of Col. M. Strauch, Museé de la Dynastie, Brussels.

Thomson, Robert Stanley. *Fondation de l'Etat Indépendant du Congo*. Brussels, 1933.

Van Eetvelde, Edmond. The Edmond Van Eetvelde papers, Archives Générales du Royaume, Brussels.

Victoria, Queen of Great Britain. *The letters of Queen Victoria: a selection from Her Majesty's correspondence and journal between the years 1837 and 1861...*, Arthur Christopher Benson and Viscount Esher, eds. 3 vols. London, 1907.

The letters of Queen Victoria: a selection from Her Majesty's correspondence and journal between the years 1862 and 1878..., George Earle Buckle, ed. Ser. 2, 3 vols. (vol. III has title *The letters...years 1862 and 1885...*). New York, 1926–8.

The letters of Queen Victoria: a selection from Her Majesty's correspondence and journal between the years 1886 and 1901..., George Earle Buckle, ed. Ser. 3, 3 vols. London, 1930–2.

Wauters, Alphonse Jules. *Histoire politique du Congo belge*. Brussels, 1911.

Willequet, Jacques. *Le Congo belge et la Weltpolitik, 1894–1914*. Presses Universitaires de Bruxelles, 1962.

Zuylen, Pierre, baron van. *L'échiquier congolais, ou le secret du roi*. Brussels, 1959.

CHAPTER 9

AFRICAN REACTIONS
TO THE IMPOSITION OF COLONIAL RULE
IN EAST AND CENTRAL AFRICA

by T. O. RANGER

The myth of the early colonial period in Africa dies hard. Scholars have challenged the old assumptions concerning the white man's overwhelming moral force and the Africans' acquiescence to the invaders' rule. But opposing assumptions concerning the overpowering military superiority of the Europeans and the despairing inability on the part of Africans to determine their own fate have all too often taken the place of these long-standing conceptions. 'The "balance of power" had moved right over into the European side of the scales', writes Basil Davidson.

The armies and expeditions of Europe could now do pretty well whatever they liked in Africa, and go more or less wherever they pleased. Backed by their wealth and increasing mastery of science, the European kings and soldiers carried all before them. In doing so they found it easy—and convenient—to treat Africans either as savages or as helpless children.[1]

Africans were not completely helpless, however, during the early colonial period in East and Central Africa. They could not avoid the imposition of colonial rule, but they were not simply objects or victims of processes set in motion outside Africa and sustained only by white initiative. Even in this period Africans helped to make their own history. Many scholars have shown how Africans necessarily participated in the early colonial administrative systems. Others have demonstrated how black men shared in the economic development of the new colonial territories. Here I wish to stress that the 'balance of power' in East and Central Africa also allowed of African political initiative during the 'pacification'.

Britain and Germany of course possessed very great technical,

[1] *Guide to African history* (London, 1963), p. 68.

manpower and capital resources. But they employed only a minute proportion of these for the colonization of East and Central Africa. In the first instance, responsibility for their paper spheres of influence was handed over by the two governments to chartered company administrations. The power of European capital was called in to transform Africa, but European capital did not respond. Every company administration was grossly underfinanced. J. Scott Keltie, commenting adversely in 1893 upon what he regarded as a confusion of official and private functions, pointed out that the British Imperial East Africa Company could only call upon something like 10 s. worth of capital for every square mile of the territory it was supposed to administer and develop. The position in German East Africa was much the same; and it was worse in Nyasaland.[1] Only the British South Africa Company, drawing upon Rhodes's private fortune and the expanding economy of South Africa, was able to mobilize more capital and employ larger numbers of men. The 700 police and pioneers who entered Mashonaland in 1890 represented an exercise of European power quite without parallel anywhere else in East and Central Africa. But the B.S.A. Company, for all its resources, was unable to establish a strong administration in Northern Rhodesia. 'In Matabeleland and Mashonaland I was one of many', wrote R. T. Coryndon of his period as North-Western Rhodesia's first Administrator between 1898 and 1902;

in Barotseland and North-Western Rhodesia I was the boss of a few.... There is, alas, no-one to testify to our Homeric battles for four years against the odds in that wide and unfriendly country—in nine months we got only one mail from the south.[2]

Even in Southern Rhodesia the Chartered Company's resources proved inadequate to the task in hand: by December 1891 Administrator L. S. Jameson was being told that

it is simply imperative that we must economise all along the line...the Bank will not advance another shilling. Rhodes has got an awful sickener of the Police. They are horribly expensive and do nothing but grumble. They must be reduced to a minimum.[3]

[1] J. S. Keltie, *The partition of Africa* (London, 1893), ch. 18.
[2] Coryndon to Fox, 26 Nov. 1907 (letter in author's possession).
[3] Currey to Jameson, 11 and 18 Dec. 1891, A 1/2/2, National Archives, Salisbury.

The latest historian of Southern Rhodesia tells us that for years 'the Company's establishment remained extremely small. Militarily the Company remained equally weak.'[1]

These company administrations have been severely criticized by historians. Freeman-Grenville has told us that 'not one' of the employees of the German East Africa Company 'appeared suitable for the task in hand'. I have myself declared that company rule in Southern Rhodesia 'was inevitably producing a society whose atmosphere was profoundly different from any conceivable crown colony, and different for the worse'. But when the company administrations were replaced in Uganda, Kenya, German East Africa and Nyasaland with official colonial administrations, the new régimes were initially not much more efficient or powerful than the old.

In Kenya, so an ex-government official tells us, the new official régime inherited 'little more than an embryonic administration in the coastal belt, a few poorly garrisoned stations on the Uganda road, and an appreciation of the difficulties which had to be overcome'. The arrival of the imperial government with all its potential resources of men and money made little immediate difference to the administration. No 'deliberate planned and directed operation of conquest' was set on foot; 'none of the Commissioners was given the forces necessary to implement such a plan had one been sanctioned. As conquest was ruled out', Matson concludes, 'and staff and forces were insufficient to establish law and order throughout the country, the handful of administrative officers had to concentrate their efforts in maintaining and improving their position in the established posts.'[2] 'Here we are', recorded Meinertzhagen in his Kikuyu diary for 1902,

three white men in the heart of Africa, with 20 Nigger soldiers and 50 Nigger police, 68 miles from doctors or reinforcements, administering and policing a district inhabited by half a million well armed savages who have only quite recently come into touch with the white man...the position is most humorous to my mind.[3]

In German East Africa the new régime was similarly short of men and money. The first Governor, Baron von Soden, attempted wherever possible to avoid further commitments in the interior. 'The establish-

[1] Lewis H. Gann, *A history of Southern Rhodesia: early days to 1934* (London, 1965), p. 127.
[2] A. T. Matson, 'The pacification of Kenya', *Kenya Weekly News*, 14 Sept. 1962.
[3] Richard Meinertzhagen, *Kenya diary, 1902-1906* (Edinburgh, 1957).

ment of military stations', he wrote, 'is impossible without increased burden to the budget.'[1] Harry Johnston in Nyasaland was weaker still. 'No other administration in what became British tropical Africa', writes Dr Stokes, 'started out with such slender financial and military backing. . . . Johnston lacked the power to subdue [and] was also lacking in the means to persuade.'[2]

If the power of European governments in East and Central Africa has been overestimated, the strength of some East and Central African societies has often been underrated. Many scholars have argued that the nineteenth-century history of the area was a 'progress to disaster' which left African societies on the eve of colonization greatly weakened and divided. Perhaps the century saw a decline in terms of agricultural production, of population growth or of life expectancy. But in terms of military strength and of the ability of the stronger East and Central African societies to defend themselves, the European colonizers probably faced a more formidable task than they would have done a century earlier. The stresses of the nineteenth century had provoked reactions. Some societies at least had developed both stronger military institutions and more centralized political machinery. There were the intrusive Ngoni military systems whose decay has been greatly over-estimated. There were other societies that responded to Ngoni pressure or to Ngoni example—the Bemba, the Hehe, the Sangu. There were the Swahili–Arab trading empires and enclaves and the Nyamwezi and other interior state systems which had risen to emulate them. The pastoral peoples of Kenya, especially the Nandi, had also been moving towards more effective and centralized action. Kingdoms, long established on different bases, like Buganda and Barotseland, responded successfully to the challenge of the nineteenth century and built up military and raiding systems. Some of these had increasing access to fire-arms; many had widespread trading or diplomatic connexions which assisted them to take the white men's measure.

There were also, of course, many small-scale societies unable either to comprehend what was involved in colonization or to offer initial resistance. In armed clashes the superiority of modern weapons generally made up for lack of numbers. In any case it was always possible to

[1] Von Soden's policy is described in Marcia Wright, 'Chief Merere and the Germans', seminar paper, University of London School of Oriental and African Studies, Jan. 1965.
[2] Eric Stokes, 'Malawi political systems and the introduction of colonial rule, 1891–1896', in *The Zambesian Past: studies in Central African history*, Eric Stokes and Richard Brown, eds. (Manchester University Press, 1966), pp. 358, 365.

supplement small numbers of whites with African 'friendlies'. Where the colonial power did suffer initial reverses, it was provoked into committing more men and more money. The resistance of African societies was bound to be broken in the end. Nevertheless, the confrontation of relatively weak colonial administrations with relatively strong African military systems did produce a practical 'balance of power' very different from that described by Davidson. There were, in fact, some African societies or peoples whom the early colonial administrators could not easily afford to fight.

We may give a few out of many examples. Harry Johnston, for instance, for all his belief that the white man was destined to take over and develop the land of East and Central Africa, had to entrench the land rights of the Ganda aristocracy in 1900. He justified this policy with the explanation that he was dealing with 'something like a million fairly intelligent, slightly civilised negroes of war-like tendencies and possessing about 10,000 to 12,000 guns'.[1] British officials in Kenya would not heed Sir John Kirk's call for the ending of Masai raids by 'an aggressive war which to be successful must annihilate every vestige of the present Masai system'.[2] The British realized that 'any premature collision could scarcely breed any but evil consequences for themselves'.[3] Administrator P. W. Forbes of North-Eastern Rhodesia subdued his desire to punish the Bemba and warned Bishop Dupont in 1897: 'I would ask you always to bear in mind that although the Company will do their best to assist you in any way, we are not at present in a position to fight the whole Awemba nation.'[4] Even Rhodes chose in the end to enter Central Africa by outflanking the Ndebele rather than by confronting them.

Europeans sometimes refused to accept these facts. Some believed that they really could go where they liked and do what they liked; but they rarely believed it for long. The German East Africa Company,

[1] Johnston's comment is cited in D. Anthony Low and R. Cranford Pratt, *Buganda and British overrule: two studies* (London, Oxford University Press, 1960), p. 94.
[2] Kirk's views on the Masai from a letter of 16 Jan. 1885 to the Foreign Office are cited in H. Alan C. Cairns, *Prelude to imperialism: British reactions to Central African society, 1840–1890* (London, 1965), p. 121.
[3] Low's valuable treatment of Anglo-Masai relations is in *History of East Africa*, vol. II, Vincent Harlow and E. M. Chilver, eds., assisted by Alison Smith (Oxford, Clarendon Press, 1965), ch. 1.
[4] Forbe's letter to Dupont, dated 17 Jan. 1897, is cited from the Kasama Diocesan Archives in W. F. Rea, 'The Bemba's white chief', Historical Association of Rhodesia and Nyasaland, local series 13 (Salisbury, Southern Rhodesia, 1964).

wrote a contemporary, 'did not care to take any steps to conciliate the natives; their policy, judging from their conduct, was to treat the latter as conquered people, whose feelings it would be absurd to consider'.[1] But the company 'was quite unable to cope with the insurrection which it had deliberately incited', and its experiences served as a warning to other East and Central African administrations. In Southern Rhodesia, too, especially after the overthrow of the Ndebele in 1893, the administration acted as if Africans did not exist as a factor in the local balance of power. But the risings of 1896–7 cost the company more than £7,000,000 and gravely endangered their charter. The British Colonial Secretary received the news of the rising in the spirit of the more cautious and more general tradition: 'Are you absolutely certain', he asked, 'that the precautions you are taking will furnish force amply sufficient? The history of war with South African natives contains several disasters both to Colonial and Imperial troops.'[2] Most colonial administrators in East and Central Africa were accordingly aware of their limitations. Colonial rule, writes Professor Oliver, spread slowly, 'very conscious of its military weakness and its financial dependence, never, if it could be avoided, taking more than a single bite at a time'.[3]

The colonizers' weakness however was by no means all to the advantage of African societies. In many ways it contributed towards making the impact of European intrusion more rather than less grievous. It could produce, for instance, exercises of force and injustice over and above those implicit in the whole process. 'Under-investment in a decent administration', Mrs de Kiewiet Hemphill tells us of Kenya, 'is sometimes worse than the most thoroughly arbitrary rule.' The officials of the British Imperial East Africa Company were led through their lack of support or resources into 'unsavoury expedients' and into penny-pinching 'where economy was unwise or dangerous'. The Kikuyu, for example, were drawn into bitter conflicts with the whites because the British attempted to make company stations in Kikuyu country self-supporting, which led to raiding and looting by company officials. Thus British financial weakness 'established a series of patterns and precedents which, for better or worse, gave direction to the

[1] Keltie, *Partition of Africa.*

[2] Colonial Secretary to High Commissioner, 9 April 1896, Colonial Office Conf. Prints, S.A., no. 520, p. 16.

[3] Roland Oliver and Gervase Mathew, eds., *History of East Africa,* vol. 1 (Oxford, 1963), Epilogue, p. 454.

subsequent history of African and European relations'.[1] In Southern Rhodesia the British South Africa Company at first tried to solve its financial difficulties by calling on unofficial white settlers and prospectors. Instead of establishing a regular machinery of native administration the company allowed unofficials to recruit their own labour, to collect taxes on the company's behalf and even to mete out 'justice', with disastrous results. This state of affairs continued until 1896, when W. H. Milton was called in from the Cape to reorganize the Chartered Company's administration in Rhodesia and to bring about major reforms.

Colonial weakness not only resulted in violence and injustice but was also liable to shatter whole African polities. Dr Stokes argues that the weakness of Harry Johnston's administration in Nyasaland led directly to the 'rapid disintegration' of African political systems. Unlike Lugard in Northern Nigeria, who possessed a force formidable by colonial standards and was able swiftly to conquer and take over a functioning indigenous political system, Johnston faced 'an initial weakness in military and financial power which made it necessary to destroy rather than preserve'. Since the more powerful units could not be quickly overcome, Stokes writes:

...it was enough to meet the day to day needs of security by reducing their potential danger. The resulting practice of detaching dependent peoples or groups not merely weakened the powerful polities but engendered in them an irreconcilable hostility. The ultimate reckoning had to be accomplished by force against an indigenous structure too weakened or too dangerous to survive the shock of conquest.[2]

Yet the colonizers' weakness was often the Africans' opportunity. Even in Nyasaland Johnston's step-by-step extension of colonial administration allowed the African peoples of the north time to come to terms with other European influences, and to escape the disintegrating effect of Johnston's policies. The great missionary Dr Robert Laws saw this in terms of successful mission initiative—'We may not get the credit for it,' he wrote, 'but there is a preparation for British rule going

[1] Marie de Kiewiet Hemphill, 'The British sphere, 1884–94', in *History of East Africa*, vol. I, ch. 11, pp. 394, 416–17.

[2] Eric Stokes, 'European administration and African political systems, 1891–1897', in Rhodes–Livingstone Institute Conference, 17th, Lusaka, Northern Rhodesia, 1963, *Conference of the History of the Central African Peoples: papers presented at the...conference...May 28th–June 1st 1963* (Lusaka, 1963), p. 4.

on in Ngoniland which may yet make it the easiest transfer of power in British Central Africa.'[1] But recent studies of the Northern Ngoni and Tonga peoples have shown a two-way process of accommodation between black and white. The mission acted as 'a foreign institution which provided certain services and which through its mere presence came to play its role in Tonga politics—a role which was to some extent independent of the intentions of the missionaries themselves'. This pattern continued, once the administration had been set up. 'There was no question of the establishment of administration in the sense of imposing it without regard to the wishes of the Tonga', writes Dr van Velsen.

It was a process of growth and reciprocal adjustment in which the Administration used diplomacy rather than force and ruled through negotiation. Each party made use of the other. In adopting this approach the Administration was no doubt influenced by the fact that the Government did not have large military forces at its disposal. The Administration could not afford to ignore the desires of the local inhabitants.[2]

To establish itself and to extend its power, a colonial authority often required native allies. Hence there was wide scope for African initiative. Of course the position varied a good deal from region to region. When the British fought against the Ndebele in Southern Rhodesia, they employed only a relatively small number of African auxiliaries. But the British position in Uganda depended on the British alliance with the Ganda aristocracy. In a very different way, British control in Kenya hinged upon an implicit pact with the Masai, who allowed and even helped British penetration into other areas of Kenya. In return, the British assiduously respected the Masai territory and way of life. The Germans in Tanganyika likewise collaborated with various African groups. In North-Western Rhodesia, the British South Africa Company based their position for many years upon agreements with the Lozi. What Africans could gain from such alliances depended

[1] Laws is quoted in J. K. Rennie, 'The Ngoni states and European intrusion', in *The Zambesian Past: studies in Central African history*, Eric Stokes and Richard Brown, eds. (Manchester University Press, 1966), p. 318.
[2] J. van Velsen, 'The missionary factor among the Lakeside Tonga of Nyasaland', *Rhodes–Livingstone Journal*, 1960, no. 26; 'The establishment of the administration in Tongaland', in Leverhulme Inter-collegiate History Conference, University College of Rhodesia and Nyasaland, Salisbury, Southern Rhodesia, 1960; *Historians in tropical Africa: proceedings of the...Conference...* (Salisbury, University College of Rhodesia and Nyasaland, 1962).

upon the extent of colonial needs. The Ganda aristocracy was able to exploit British weakness occasioned by Mwanga's rising and the Sudanese mutiny. The Ganda could thus assert themselves as virtually equal partners and gain a position of entrenched power and privilege established in law. None of the others achieved so much; some were abandoned by the colonial administration when the value of their alliance had gone. But in every case the alliance was a two-way process; each party made use of the other.

Many recent studies have concentrated upon the use made by Africans of these situations, and the skill with which African rulers exploited the need, weakness and ignorance of the colonialists. Perhaps Mrs Stahl's study of the Chagga has done this most clearly. 'The chiefs showed through the centuries', she tells us, 'a remarkable ingenuity in progressively enhancing their own powers...They made use of every new thing and every new kind of human being entering the life of Kilimanjaro to enhance their own positions.' They became adept at assessing European officers, 'utilising each new officer serving a term of his career on Kilimanjaro as another element in their stratagems...they employed a whole range of new political gambits centring on the Boma'.[1] This is a far cry from African helplessness.

Such Afro-European alliances sometimes profoundly influenced the pattern of subsequent politics. Some chiefs managed to secure more power for themselves, as well as special access to new sources of prestige and profits. Ralph Austen can thus describe the period following on the establishment of German rule in Buhaya as 'the golden age of the Haya chiefdom', when men like Kahigi and Mutahangarwa approached a power 'which had probably never been equalled in any but the legendary past'.[2] Mrs Stahl tells us that

European rule did not disrupt the ancient political game on Kilimanjaro but simply required it to be played with a few new rules...European rule was tied to supporting the chiefs. Though the chiefs lost sovereignty after 1886, those...who won the favour of the European administrators were afforded ...new opportunities.... At the zenith of their careers, it is arguable that Mangi Abdiel of Machame in 1946 enjoyed more power than the greatest

[1] Kathleen Mary Stahl, *History of the Chagga people of Kilimanjaro* (London, 1964), pp. 357, 360, 362.
[2] 'Political generations in Bukoba, 1890–1939', in East African Institute of Social Research, *Proceedings of the EAISR Conference held at the Institute, June 1963* (Kampala, Makerere College, 1963), Ph.D.

sovereign ruler, Mangi Sina of Kibosho, had done until his conquest by the Germans in 1891.[1]

In some areas, in fact, the advantages gained by co-operating ruling classes within their own society amounted to radical political change.

Advantages could also be gained by one African society over another. Some Africanists have spoken of Ganda 'sub-imperialism'. But there was also a Lozi sub-imperialism. The extension of Lozi control to Balovale and Mankoya partially compensated the Lozi for the loss of other privileges. There was a Toro sub-imperialism, a sub-imperialism exercised by the family of Chief Mumia in Nyanza, and others. In many cases the subjects of these sub-imperialists experienced colonial rule more through their Ganda or Lozi overlords than through British control. The struggle against these sub-imperialisms forms one of the dominant themes in the modern political history of East and Central Africa.

The effect of African initiative exercised through such alliances has been so far-reaching that some historians have limited their attention to African societies that chose to collaborate with the whites. Many scholars have argued that the collaborators, by influencing the pattern of pacification, helped to determine the shape of colonial administration, and also gained a pathway to the future by exploiting the colonial situation. Investigators have often contrasted such societies with those that chose to resist the whites by force of arms. Oliver and Fage's general history emphasizes this point. If African political leaders, they argue,

were far-sighted and well-informed, and more particularly if they had had access to foreign advisers, such as missionaries or traders, they might well understand that nothing was to be gained by resistance, and much by negotiation. If they were less far-sighted, less fortunate, or less well-advised, they would see their traditional enemies siding with the invader and would themselves assume an attitude of resistance, which could all too often end in military defeat, the deposition of chiefs, the loss of land to the native allies of the occupying power, possibly even to the political fragmentation of the society and state.[2]

Resisting societies or groups not only ran the risk of disintegration but of cutting themselves off from modernization, education and

---

[1] Stahl, *Chagga*, pp. 359–60.
[2] Roland Oliver and John D. Fage, *A short history of Africa* (Harmondsworth, Middlesex and Baltimore, 1962), p. 203.

economic development. Resistances, according to Ronald Robinson and John Gallagher, were 'romantic, reactionary struggles against the facts, the passionate protest of societies which were shocked by a new age of change and would not be comforted'. They are to be contrasted with 'the defter nationalisms' which 'planned to reform their personalities and regain their powers by operating in the idiom of the Westernisers'.[1]

The distinctions between the fortunes and potentialities of co-operating and resisting societies are thus held to be great. Hence attempts have been made to explain the disposition to resist or to co-operate in terms of profound differences in the structure of pre-colonial systems. 'The more urbanised, commercial and bureaucratic the policy', Robinson and Gallagher tell us, 'the more its rulers would be tempted to come to terms...On the other hand the more its unity hung together on the luxuries of slave-raiding, plunder and migration, the less its aristocracy had to lose by struggle against the Europeans.'[2] In this way Robinson and Gallagher account for the co-operation of the progressive Lozi and Ganda and the resistance of the plundering Ndebele and Ngoni.

This view of African resistance as a gallant anachronism, essentially negative and backward looking, has been challenged, especially by Soviet Africanists. 'It is impossible to understand the African past without the re-establishment of the truth about this resistance', writes Professor A. B. Davidson of Moscow.

This is the main reason why it must be re-established. And without making a study of what was the answer of one people or another to the establishment of colonial rule it is difficult to understand not only the past of that people but its present as well. It is difficult to comprehend the character of the liberation movement in the recent revolutionary years...Resistance left its mark on the most important internal processes of the development of the African peoples; in the course of resistance tendencies to change developed more quickly.[3]

Soviet historians have not provided much solid evidence to buttress these conclusions, but to my mind Russian scholars have assessed the

[1] Ronald E. Robinson and John Gallagher, 'The partition of Africa', in *The new Cambridge modern history*, vol. XI, *Material progress and world-wide problems, 1870–1898*, F. H. Hinsley, ed. (Cambridge University Press, 1962), ch. 22, p. 640.
[2] Robinson and Gallagher, 'The partition of Africa', p. 618.
[3] 'African resistance and rebellion against the imposition of colonial rule', in *Emerging themes of African history*, T. O. Ranger, ed. (Nairobi, 1968).

significance of African resistance to colonial rule in a more accurate fashion than their Western colleagues. The former have a better understanding of the 'resisters'; the latter have a better grasp of the 'collaborators'. But if we are fully to understand the nature of African reactions to colonial rule, we must take account of collaboration and resistance alike. My aim in the remainder of this essay is to show how resistance, as well as collaboration, shaped African political history.

To begin with, I disagree with many of the generalizations made by 'Western' scholars. I do not consider that resisting societies were necessarily different in structure, motive or atmosphere from co-operating ones; I do not believe that co-operating societies necessarily desired modernization more than resisting societies, or even necessarily achieved it more rapidly. The foremost among the societies engaged either in resistance or in collaboration had more in common with one another in fact than with those small-scale societies that could neither resist nor exploit colonial rule. Thus the most notable resisters had some experience of foreign contact. They were centralized, sometimes highly so, and they had some capacity for intelligent choice. Again, some communities which—according to Robinson and Gallagher—should have resisted, and were expected to do so at the time, did not, in the end, do so. In certain instances, migratory military groups or societies organized for slave-raiding and looting, successfully accommodated themselves to the whites. Such communities included the Northern Ngoni of Nyasaland, the Bemba of North-Eastern Rhodesia and the Masai of Kenya.

Some resisting societies desperately attempted to avoid the necessity of resistance. Some co-operating societies made it plain that they were ready to resist if their cherished privileges were attacked. A historian has indeed a difficult task in deciding whether a specific society should be described as 'resistant' or as 'collaborative' over any given period of time. Many societies began in one camp and ended in the other. Virtually all African states made some attempt to find a basis on which to collaborate with the Europeans; virtually all of them had some interests or values which they were prepared to defend, if necessary, by hopeless resistance or revolt.

To illustrate this point we should consider, for instance, the contrast between Matabeleland and Barotseland. The former resisted; the latter collaborated. Superficially, the distinction seems clear. Lobengula, the paramount of the Ndebele people, tried to co-operate with the

British for a time. But the Ndebele, with their raiding system, had no interest in foreign commerce. The Lozi had an elaborate bureaucracy and were strategically placed athwart the transcontinental trade routes. The Ndebele seemed fated to clash with the whites. The Lozi were likely to take from the Europeans whatever was needed to improve the Lozi bureaucracy and to further Lozi trade. But what would the Lozi have done if, like the Ndebele, they had been faced with a white invasion of their eastern raiding grounds, if their regiments had been driven back, if they had faced at long last a white column marching on their capital? They surely would also have resisted. (The white missionaries at the Lozi court certainly expected them to do so.)

An even more striking comparison may be drawn between Basutoland and Barotseland. Different though they were, the two nations had certain things in common. Both gave hospitality to missionaries of the Paris Evangelical Missionary Society. They both appealed for British protection through French missionaries. Both eagerly responded to early missionary education. Yet the Basuto fought the Boers, the British and the Cape government, while the Lozi pursued a pacific policy. The aims of the two societies were much the same—their situations and their methods differed.

Resistance on the part of an African people did not necessarily imply a romantic, reactionary rejection of 'modernity', though a lengthy war might of course occasion repudiation of European influence. Similarly, non-resistance, in the sense of abstaining from armed struggle, did not always imply a readiness to modernize. Professor Low tells us that the price exacted by the Masai for the implied alliance with the British was the preservation of the Masai way of life. 'An official report of the E.A.P. Government was later to complain', he writes, 'that "no punitive expedition has ever been undertaken against the Masai"; an omission, it said, which subsequently enabled the Masai to eschew British pressures for change.'[1]

On the other hand, some societies that did offer armed resistance nevertheless desired contact with Europeans under their own control. Gungunhana of Gazaland had Protestant missionaries at his kraal, including an African minister. Gungunhana negotiated with Rhodes and desired increased trade while preparing to fight the Portuguese. Chief Makombe of Barwe, rebelling against the Portuguese in 1917, expressed his anxiety for continued intercourse with the British

[1] Low, in *History of East Africa*, II, 14–15.

'who have enriched his subjects'. Other societies developed a driving desire for modernization after the first bitter resistance was over. In terms of their eagerness for Western education, there was little to choose between the Nyasaland Tonga, who did not resist, and the Kikuyu, who did.

I must take issue also with the standard interpretation that 'nothing was to be gained by resistance' under any circumstances. Much, of course, depended on the local situation and on the military resources and psychology of the colonizers. Herero resistance against the Germans certainly turned out to be a disaster for the Herero nation. But some societies did gain benefits by demonstrating the ability to take up arms when forced to do so. The Basuto rulers wanted mission education, economic contact with the outside world and British protection. They had to fight to achieve these. It would be hard to argue that their final struggle, the so-called Gun War of 1879–81, was futile. Arising out of Basuto resistance to forced disarmament,

it dragged on for seven months, cost the Cape Government £4¾ million, and ended in complete failure. The Gun War saw only one major engagement, which the Basuto won...It aroused echoes in the Africans of neighbouring territories, whose simultaneous risings, though limited, forced the Cape Government to deploy yet more men and money...Both sides accepted British arbitration in 1881, and the peace terms did little more than save the face of the Cape. Disarmament was to remain the policy, but the Basuto could legally retain their guns at a registration fee of £1 each. White settlers were not to be allowed into the territory...most of the chiefs neither surrendered their guns nor paid their tax. At last the Cape persuaded a reluctant British Government to take the troublesome Basuto off its hands in 1883...On March 18, 1884 the Basuto finally became British subjects directly under the Queen.[1]

The Ndebele provide another, though rather different, example. After the Ndebele war of 1893, the Ndebele state was disrupted. The new rulers no longer recognized any indigenous authority. The regimental system was broken, cattle were confiscated, land was taken —all without any machinery of complaint or redress. In 1896 the Ndebele had little to lose from further armed resistance. It turned out that they had something to gain. Their rebellion threatened to smash the whole position of the British South Africa Company in Southern

[1] Jack Halpern, *South Africa's hostages: Basutoland, Bechuanaland and Swaziland* (Harmondsworth, Middlesex and Baltimore, 1965), pp. 79–80.

Rhodesia. Suppression exhausted the company's financial resources; it also involved large numbers of British troops and a great extension of British political authority. Under these circumstances Rhodes was compelled to gamble on negotiating a peace settlement so as to prevent the war from dragging through the rainy season into another year, with back-breaking expense to the company and a probable British assumption of direct control. The High Commissioner had proscribed the Ndebele leaders; the settlers demanded unconditional surrender and condign punishment. But Rhodes dealt with the leaders and came to terms. The Ndebele did not get much—the recognition of rebel leaders as well as of loyalists as salaried indunas and spokesmen for the people; an apparatus of complaint and redress; a regular system of native administration; a new commitment to make more land available to them. But it was considerably more than they would have got without a rebellion. Resistance, far from preventing future political activity, helped the Ndebele to move into a new political era.

The Wahehe of Tanganyika seem to be a perfect example of a people broken by futile resistance. They were crushed by military might. They did not even achieve a negotiated peace. Defeat left the people in a desperate state. Alison Redmayne begins her study of the Wahehe by quoting a contemporary German observer:

The small remnant of men of pure Hehe blood who still survive will become intermingled with other tribes, and instead of remaining fearless warriors and hunters, will degenerate into mere porters like most of the other natives of our colony. Their political organisation, in particular the chieftainship, is, by and large, impossible under German rule.'[1]

But the German eyewitness's prophecy turned out to be mistaken. Memories of Mkawa's resistance dominated subsequent German and Wahehe thinking alike. Partly because of pride in these memories, Wahehe institutions, or more accurately a Wahehe sense of identity, survived so well that Uhehe became the site of the most successful Tanganyikan experiment in indirect rule. Both the Germans and the British felt respect for the Wahehe, so that in later years Wahehe objections were taken especially seriously. 'In 1957', writes Miss Redmayne,

there was a mass boycott of the compulsory cattle dipping scheme...It made a deep impression on members of the provincial administration and on many

[1] All quotations on the Hehe are from Alison H. Redmayne, 'The Wahehe people of Tanganyika' (Ph.D. thesis, Oxford University, 1964).

non-officials in other parts of Tanzania. A significant number of those leading
the boycott may have been non-Wahehe...but members of the provincial
administration knew enough about the Wahehe reputation for stubbornness
and pride to abandon the scheme.

Oliver and Fage tell us that

for the African peoples the most important factor at this stage of colonial
history was...the intangible psychological issue of whether any given society
or group was left feeling that it had turned the colonial occupation to its
own advantage, or alternatively that it had been humiliated.[1]

The Wahehe can hardly be said to have turned the early colonial
situation to their profit, but they did not come out with a sense of
humiliation. 'Today all Wahehe idolise Mkwawa', wrote a British
district officer in the early Mandatory period. 'This may be because he
actually beat the white man in battle.'[2]

These examples have shown that the fact of resistance could influence
very greatly the later political history of a particular African society.
But resistance had a wider impact. Thus it was resistance and rebellion
that provoked the most extensive theoretical debates among the
colonizers and had most impact on their attitudes. In territories like
Tanganyika and Southern Rhodesia, which had experienced the terri-
fying challenge of great rebellions, memories of war or fears concerning
new outbreaks dominated the white man's mind. While indigenous
policies of acquiescence served, on the whole, to support white assumptions of African readiness to accept white moral leadership, the rebellions
challenged all easy generalizations about African gratitude and readiness
to accept colonial rule, and all assurance that whites understood the
Africans. Rebellions instead provoked almost anguished professions of
incomprehension and disillusion. 'The Negro does not love us but only
fears our power', proclaimed the German military handbook in
Tanganyika from 1911 onwards. 'There are no tribes whatever on
whose loyalty we can with certainty depend.'[3] 'This outbreak was got
up as a matter of fact so quickly and in opposition to all our native lore,
that we feel almost unable to venture any further opinion on natives at
all', wrote Acting Chief Native Commissioner, Matabeleland, in

[1] Short history, p. 203.
[2] Redmayne, 'Wahehe'.
[3] The German army handbook is quoted in John Iliffe, 'The German administration in
Tanganyika, 1906–1911: the governorship of Freiherr von Rechenberg' (Ph.D. thesis,
Cambridge University, 1965), p. 79.

March 1896, 'except this—that they are not for one moment to be trusted.'[1] The cry of outrage reached its climax with the rebellion of the despised Shona. 'I may remark', wrote the Civil Commissioner,

> that this sudden departure on the part of the Mashona tribes has caused the greatest surprise to those who from long residence in the country thought they understood the character of these savages...with true Kaffir deceit they have beguiled us into the idea that they were content with our administration of the country and wanted nothing more than to work for us and trade with us and become civilised; but at a given signal they have cast aside all pretence.[2]

African loyalty could never again be taken for granted.

Thereafter, as Dr Iliffe has written of Tanganyika, 'the fear of rebellion became the decisive argument in any political debate'. Freiherr von Rechenberg always dreaded another rebellion. Von Rechenberg's successor, H. Schnee, 'never ceased to be afraid...he had never forgotten the files (on Maji-Maji) and always present in his mind was the thought that it could happen again'. 'The principal motivation of settler politics was fear', writes John Iliffe. 'After Maji-Maji, settler thinking was defensive.'[3]

The same was true in the Rhodesias. Officials regularly expected renewed outbreaks. In 1903 a general inquiry from Native Commissioners as to the state of African opinion found one 'firmly convinced that we are in for such a row as we have not had up here yet...the whole attitude of the natives leads one to believe that they are going to have another slap at us'.[4] Another voiced the view that

> certain Mashona tribes will again rebel...The natives, although outwardly satisfied and peaceable, object to our rule...It only requires a witch-doctor who has been fortunate in the past and has obtained a footing as a true prophet to prophesy destruction of the whites to get the majority of the tribes to rise.[5]

Similar fears were being expressed in 1915. Even in 1923, at the time of the change in Southern Rhodesia to Responsible Government,

[1] Acting Chief Native Commissioner, Matabeleland, to Acting Administrator, 30 March 1896.

[2] Report by Marshall Hole, 29 Oct. 1896, A 10/1/1 and A 1/12/36, National Archives, Salisbury, Southern Rhodesia.

[3] 'German administration in Tanganyika', pp. 79–80.

[4] Hulley to Taberer, Nov. 1903, and Report by N. C. Marendellas, 25 Nov. 1903, A 11/2/12/11, National Archives, Salisbury, Southern Rhodesia.

[5] Superintendent of Natives, Salisbury, to Chief Native Commissioner, 24 April 1915, N 3/33/3, National Archives, Salisbury, Southern Rhodesia; see also N 3/32/1.

reports of instructions to Africans by priests and prophets were causing official concern. The settlers' memories of the rebellions remained vivid. One example will suffice. In 1906 the new settler population of Livingstone called for rifles to defend themselves against any rising by the Lozi or neighbouring peoples. 'How would we stand then?' asked the *Livingstone Pioneer and Advertiser*.

Alone, and if thus isolated and inadequately equipped another dark page would be added to the already dark-enough history of Africa. Out stations would be wiped out, murder (and worse) rampant, and each man fighting desperately for his life.[1]

The consequences of white preoccupation with the possibility of black rebellions are hard to assess. There was much argument over the cause of past risings and over future policy to prevent further outbreaks. Some Europeans wanted the iron hand, others the velvet glove. Fear undoubtedly had much to do with the growing expression of white prejudices against the blacks. Marshall Hole, a former Rhodesian official, admitted in the 1930s that discrimination against black Rhodesians was more acute in Southern Rhodesia than in South Africa; he thought that memories of the rebellions accounted for the difference. Nevertheless, particular African societies did profit by resistance, and the white man's awareness that—if pushed too far—black men could strike back also gave certain advantages to Africans as a whole. Black resistance also convinced Europeans of the importance of continued alliances with co-operative black communities. In Tanganyika, according to Dr Iliffe, Von Rechenberg devised his economic policy to meet peasant demands, lest rebellion become the only outlet for Africans trapped in an unjust economic system.[2]

In Southern Rhodesia the fear of rebellion led to withdrawals of over-provocative measures. In 1903 the new Legislative Council voted to increase the hut tax from 10s. to £2 a year. This was referred for the approval of the British Colonial Secretary, who minuted on 29 July that 'as explained to the Rhodesian deputation in January I could only assent on being assured that no serious trouble is to be feared from the increased tax. I shall require definite assurance of the Resident Commis-

---

[1] *The Livingstone Pioneer and Advertiser*, 10 March 1906.
[2] John Iliffe, 'The effects of the Maji Maji rebellion of 1905–1906 on German occupation policy in East Africa', in *Britain and Germany in Africa: imperial rivalry and colonial rule*, Prosser Gifford and William Roger Louis, eds. (New Haven and London, Yale University Press, 1967).

sioner to this effect before I assent.'[1] Such assurance was not forthcoming.
The Resident Commissioner expressed the view that the tax increase
would have an 'unsettling effect on the natives calculated to endanger
security and good order in the country'. Acting on the principle that
the 'governing consideration is that there should be no risk of native
disturbance', the Colonial Secretary refused to sanction the increase.
(He set the tax at only £1 a year with a delay in collection.) Fear of
native risings, occasioned by excessive fiscal demands, profoundly
affected British official thinking. In 1904, for instance, Colonial
Secretary Lyttleton remarked that in future tax questions of this kind,
'the attitude of the natives will have to be taken into account'. To this
High Commissioner Milner assented. Africans still hoped, he wrote, that
'the white man has not come to stay and that the day will come when
they will regain their country and their independence. This emphasizes
the expediency to avoid giving the natives of the territory any common
grounds for considering themselves wronged or unjustly treated.'

Secondly, African resistance sometimes stimulated important changes
in the structure of African societies. It is already well established that
such changes could be brought about by collaborating groups. Through
collaboration a society, or its leaders, could gain better schools and
greater economic opportunities. Historians have, in fact, distinguished a
number of so-called 'Christian Revolutions' in which key collaborators
tried to solve some of the weaknesses of nineteenth-century African
state systems, to make their bureaucracy more efficient through literacy
and to render the central power independent of traditional sanctions and
limitations arising out of kinship or regional groupings. 'Christian
Revolutions' of this kind were effected in Barotseland, Bechuanaland
and Buganda. They were not, of course, identical in character, but they
all tried to apply what historians have called the Christian 'great tradition' to solve problems of scale and effectiveness.

I would not deny the importance of these 'Christian Revolutions'
which did effect substantial changes. But they had serious weaknesses.
They provided opportunities for minority groups only. They rested
upon alien sanctions and did not achieve mass commitment. They
broke with traditional restraints and often weakened the mass sense of
belonging. Even internal reforms designed to improve the popular lot

[1] The hut-tax correspondence may be found in Colonial Office, Conf. Prints, nos. 717
and 746; see also A 11/2/13/11 and A 11/2/12/12, National Archives, Salisbury,
Southern Rhodesia.

by abolishing serfdom, forced labour and tribute may have weakened the feeling of identity between the rulers and ruled. Derrick J. Stenning's comments on Nkole bring this out well. Having described how the king and his court turned to Christianity and renounced traditional religious belief, he continues:

A phase in which more direct attacks on the traditional religion occurred was to follow. These were directed against rituals, particularly those of the ancestors and of the tutelary spirits...aided willingly by the Protestant chiefs, shrines were torn down, cult objects confiscated and cult leaders discredited, fined or imprisoned...The C.M.S. Mission played an important part in public life, and in so far as the BaHima had been the vehicles of that life in pre-Protectorate days, its concern with them had enabled some of them to make an effective transition into the modern world. But the majority of BaHima, the pastoralists...had had their cults proscribed, their shrines and sacred objects destroyed, the logical and institutional basis of their mystical relations to king and state diluted.[1]

Thus was created a spiritual vacuum, filled in Nkole only by the later Revival movement.

Like these 'Christian Revolutions' the modern nationalist movements of East and Central Africa attempt to erect effective bureaucratic and other institutions for a territorial state. But they also have to try to modernize at a more profound level by achieving mass commitment to reform. We can see the experiments of the 'Christian Revolutions' as forerunners of one part of modern nationalism. But if we seek forerunners in the attempt to commit the masses to an effective enlargement of scale, we have to turn rather to the resistance movements.

We must distinguish, of course, between short wars fought against the incoming whites and later protracted rebellions. In many instances the initial war was fought with the traditional military system. Little attempt was made to modify it, or to involve in the struggle wider social strata or neighbouring African peoples. But a long-drawn-out rebellion was a different matter. The insurgents faced new problems and had to search for new solutions. The distinction made by Dr Iliffe between initial tribal wars waged against the Germans in Tanganyika and the Maji-Maji rising is of great significance. 'Maji-Maji', Dr Iliffe says, was 'a post-pacification revolt, quite different from the early

[1] 'Salvation in Ankole', in International African Seminar, 3rd, Salisbury, Southern Rhodesia, 1960, *African systems of thought: studies presented and discussed at the...* *Seminar...* (London, Oxford University Press, 1965), p. 266.

resistance. That had been local and professional, soldiers against soldiers, whereas Maji-Maji affected almost everyone...It was a great crisis of commitment.'[1]

The point can be well illustrated for the Southern Rhodesian rebellions. The Ndebele had fought the 1893 war using their old military system. The subject peoples and the lower castes had taken no part in the fighting; neither had there been any attempt by the Ndebele to ally themselves with the peoples of Mashonaland or farther afield. The result had been disaster. The Ndebele then faced colonial pressures of greater intensity than anywhere else in East and Central Africa, except perhaps in the plantation areas of German East Africa. They desired to rebel—and this presented problems of organization and of scale. In 1896 not only the surviving members of the regiments and the adults of the royal family but also the subject peoples of Matabeleland and the tribes of western and central Mashonaland all joined to fight the whites.

The problem for the Shona was different. Their political fragmentation had prevented them from putting up any co-ordinated initial resistance to the arrival of the whites. As the implications of white rule were realized, individual paramounts began to refuse demands for taxes or labour, always ineffectively. Thus to 'rebel' effectively, the Shona had to discover a principle of solidarity and to recover at least some degree of the political unity which they had once possessed. The Maji-Maji rebels faced similar difficulties. It is not certain that their rising was in any sense planned. But once it had broken out, the insurgent leaders had to effect some co-ordination between the militarized Ngoni and the original rebels. This had to be achieved without any tradition of political centralization. Risings therefore led to political experimentation. Some rebels attempted to revive older centralizing institutions. But at the same time 'new men' came to the front with new ideas. (The Shona, for instance, tried to revive the ancient Rozwi kingship. But younger men also elbowed aside aged paramounts.) Above all, such insurgents developed the notion of charismatic as distinct from bureaucratic or hereditary leadership.

In considering what this involved I have found helpful a recent article by M. A. Doutreloux on prophets in the Congo.[2] He argues that the prophet cults which have been a feature of the history of the

[1] 'German administration in Tanganyika', p. 76.
[2] 'Prophétisme et culture', in International African Seminar, 3rd, Salisbury, Southern Rhodesia, 1960, *African systems of thought: studies presented and discussed at the... Seminar...* (London, Oxford University Press, 1965).

Congo from at least the early eighteenth century onwards have their roots in an essential weakness of Congolese society. This society could not find a solution to the problem of fragmentation and instability. What stability existed was given by religions of the ancestors or cults of land and fertility. But these were always operative on too small a scale and were undermined by witchcraft belief. The prophet movements rose in order to remedy this situation. These movements were assaults not only on witchcraft but also on traditional limitations; they proclaimed a church or creed for all Africans and imposed their own regulations and codes of conduct upon believers; they endeavoured to provide an indigenous Great Tradition to rival the alien Great Tradition used by the Christian revolutionaries. They pre-eminently involved the masses.

The most striking resistance movements of East and Central Africa were clearly led by prophetic figures. Among the Nandi one may trace the rise to authority of the *Orkoiyot* prophets in face of British pressure. I have pointed out the key role of the oracular priesthood of Mwari in Matabeleland, and of the spirit mediums in Mashonaland in the Southern Rhodesian rising of the 1890s. Prophets also played a major part in the Maji-Maji rebellion. In the last two instances especially, we can discern the features described by Doutreloux. The prophets imposed new regulations and new instruction on the faithful; they brought believers into the congregation by dispensing 'medicine'; they promised immunity both from witchcraft and from bullets; they promised success in this world and a return from death. They spoke to all black men. This was true in Southern Rhodesia even though the leaders involved were members of traditional religious systems with roots deep in the past. Under the stress of the rebellion situation what L. H. Gann has recently described as a 'theological revolution' took place. The officers of the old cults were able to appeal to the centralizing memories with which they were associated, but they enjoyed too an extension of power and function; they asserted a new authority over chiefs and indunas; and they imposed new obligations on their followers. For a time the charismatic leadership of the prophets brought together Ndebele aristocrats, subject peoples, deposed Rozwi, Shona paramounts. As L. H. Gann puts it, 'The proud Matabele chieftains now agreed to operate under the supreme direction of an ex-serf, a remarkable man who in "normal" times would hardly have acquired much political influence.'[1]

---

[1] Gann, *Southern Rhodesia*, pp. 129, 135.

There were many other upheavals on a smaller scale. A list of risings allegedly led by 'witch-doctors' in East and Central Africa amounts to some thirty-five to forty instances. These prophetic leaders appealed to notions of past unity but also attempted to reconstruct society. Religious leaders of resistances often came from outside the societies concerned and appealed for co-operation with peoples who had formerly been their rivals. Sometimes the religious leader claimed to speak in the name of a long-dead hero figure who had established a now-vanished unity; sometimes he claimed to be the bearer of a new divine commandment that black men should unite. The spirit medium of the Wabudya people of eastern Mashonaland, for instance, was overheard by Native Commissioner Armstrong in May 1897 rebuking his countrymen for having served as allies of the whites against their old rivals of central Mashonaland. The Budya chief, he said,

had now been killed for taking the *impi* to fight with the whites, although against the wish of the witch-doctor...There were very few white men left in the country...If it were not for the black men who were fighting for the whites, the Mashonas would easily kill the few whites left...let them be killed and Mtoko's people would no longer be slaves to the white man.[1]

Or there is the letter from Chief Songea of the Ngoni to Chief Mataka of the Yao, an old enemy, after the outbreak of the Maji-Maji rising in 1905:

We received an order from God to the effect that all White Men had to quit the country. We are ready to fight them...I wanted to send you cattle as a present, but I was unable to send them. This war ordered by God must come first. Send 100 men with guns. Help me in taking the Boma...Let us forget now our former quarrels.[2]

Thus resistance movements of this sort can hardly be regarded as tribal-conservative ones, involving as they did calls to recognize new authorities, new injunctions and co-operation on a new basis. Neither were they completely reactionary and anti-modernizing. The situation gave scope for the 'new man' with specially relevant skills—like the trained Ndebele policeman in 1896. Gann has pointed out that among the followers of the chief Shona religious leader in 1896, Kagubi, were

[1] N. C. Armstrong to Chief Native Commissioner, 26 May 1897, N 1/1/7, National Archives, Salisbury, Southern Rhodesia.
[2] Songea's letter is given in Fr. Elzear Ebner, 'History of the Wangoni', Peramiho Mission, mimeograph, 1959, p. 171.

'men who had been in touch with Europeans and picked up some of their skills'.[1] Kagubi's daughter was a schoolgirl in the Catholic mission at Chishawasha. I have myself described elsewhere how in the Makombe rising of 1917 in Portuguese East Africa there was a return to the new opportunities of leadership by men who had gone to seek their fortunes in the colonial economy, producing a 'leadership of paramounts and spirit mediums and returned waiters and ex-policemen'.[2]

Of course these attempts to create a large-scale mass movement failed. Although in a single tribal situation, as with the Nandi or the Kipsigis, the charismatic leadership of the prophets continued to provide coherence even after defeat, where attempts at unity had been made over much larger areas, involving many more disparate peoples, defeat brought the new forms of co-operation to an abrupt end. In some cases, indeed, defeat led to a sudden abandonment by many of the ex-rebels of their commitment to African religious leadership and a turning instead to mission Christianity. The new religion was felt to have proved itself the more effective.

It has often been said that the collapse of African resistance and rebellion was followed by a hiatus of leadership. 'Tribal risings ceased', wrote Norman Leys in 1924,

...because they were always hopeless failures. Naked spearmen fall in swathes before machine guns, without inflicting a single casualty in return. Meanwhile the troops burn all the huts and collect all the livestock within reach. Resistance once at an end, the leaders of the rebellion are surrendered for imprisonment and of the rest of the tribe some return to build their homes again, while others go to work for the conqueror in order to find the money to pay tax on these homes. Risings that followed such a course could hardly be repeated. A period of calm followed. And when unrest again appeared it was with other leaders...and other motives.[3]

The future belonged, it seemed, to the representatives of the 'defter nationalisms' which operated 'in the idiom of the Westernisers'. Leadership passed into the hands of the educated élite, often drawn from co-operating groups with access to modern ideas and skills.

[1] Gann, *Southern Rhodesia*, p. 136.
[2] T. O. Ranger, 'Revolt in Portuguese East Africa: the Makombe rising of 1917', in *African affairs*, no. 2 (Oxford University, St Antony's College, *St Antony's papers*, no. 15), Kenneth Kirkwood, ed. (Carbondale, Southern Illinois University Press, 1963), p. 68.　　　[3] *Kenya* (London, 1924).

So runs the standard argument. But this argument needs to be probed. Students of African nationalism are coming to pay increasing attention to the current of mass political emotion and to the continuity of rural radicalism, as well as to the development of élite leadership. Therefore we must ask if there is any continuity between expressions of mass political emotion in the twentieth century and the risings we have discussed.

I have pursued this inquiry at greater length elsewhere and here will summarize the main points of the argument only. The first point to be made is that there were many mass movements of a millenarian character in the decades after the suppression of primary resistance and rebellion. Some of these took the form of African independent Christianity; others have been labelled as 'nativistic' or 'syncretic'. Many of them have been studied in detail by scholars. There are undoubtedly connexions between these later mass movements and the large-scale resistances described above. The type of leadership and its strategies were often essentially the same. Often there is also a more direct connexion. Thus there are examples of African independent churches which regard those killed in rebellions against the whites as their saints and martyrs. This is true of Shembe's Nazarite Church in Zululand, which glorifies 'the people who were killed in Bambata's rebellion'. It is also true of the Church of the White Bird in Rhodesia, which regarded those killed during the 1896–7 rebellion as its proto-martyrs.

A particularly interesting example of this continuity is the Mumbo cult in the Nyanza Province of Kenya. Mumbo is a 'pan-tribal' sect, promising eventual triumph to the true believers who are merely being tested by the ordeals of the colonial period. It has direct links with the period of the resistance. 'Mumboism turned to the past for inspiration', Audrey Wipper writes;

Fresh meaning was imbued into tribal ways, old dreams infused with new reality...The Gusii's most venerated warriors and prophets, noted for their militant anti-British stance, were claimed by the movement. Zakawa, the great prophet, Bogonko, the mighty chief, and Maraa, the *laibon* responsible for the 1908 rebellion, became its symbols, infusing into the living the courage and strength of past heroes...Leaders bolstered their own legitimacy by claiming to be the mouth-piece of these deceased prophets. Especially successful in effecting such claims were their descendants...Thus with the progeny of the Gusii heroes supporting the sect, a physical as well as a

317

symbolic link with the past was established. Here was a powerful symbolic group whose prestige and authority could well be used to arouse, strengthen and weld the various disunited cults into solid anti-British opposition.[1]

Miss Wipper shows that the cult 'looks to the past for inspiration and to the future for living'. 'Its goals are Utopian and innovative rather than traditional and regressive'. It attacks small-scale traditional customs as well as European values.

There are other striking examples in the recent political past. The Dini Ya Msambwa cult of Elija Masinde, for example, still poses problems to the Kenyan authorities. Masinde focused opposition to the colonial administration in the 1940s by appeals back to the memory of primary resistance. In September 1947 he held a mass meeting at the site of a battle between whites and blacks fought in 1895; as J. D. Welime tells us:

He wanted his followers to remember the dead in their prayers. One interesting thing about this meeting is that they were dressed as in readiness for the 1895 war. At this meeting it is alleged that he unearthed a skull in which a bullet was found buried in the mouth...The crowd became very emotional and destructive.[2]

The second point to be made concerns the relationship of these later millenarian cults and modern nationalism. Clearly the cults are not nationalist in the sense that they do not possess a clear concept of territorial nationality. Nor do they have any practical notions of how to modernize society. Moreover such millenarian movements have often clashed with nationalist parties as the Lenshina church clashed with U.N.I.P. in Zambia. But they do have common elements. They both try to renovate society and they both try to achieve mass commitment to this renovation. The hostility between them sometimes arises not from their essential differences but from the fact that they are competing for exclusive mass loyalty on the basis of promises to transform society.

It is worth while bearing in mind what John Lonsdale has written of modern mass nationalism in the Nyanza Province of Kenya. He shows

[1] Audrey Wipper, 'The cult of Mumbo', East African Institute of Social Research, *Proceedings of the EAISR Conference, January 1966*, pt. D. Kampala, Makerere College, 1966.

[2] 'Dini ya Msambwa', research paper, University College, Dar es Salaam, 1965.

how Nyanza independent churches have their roots in pre-colonial religious movements. He shows how the first and second generations of the new modernizing élite could not come to terms with this tradition of mass protest. 'Only after the start of popular, mass nationalism did the politicians court the independents.' But then they did so and in a wider sense, he suggests, the values of the independents triumphed over the values of the early élite.

The independent's selective approach to Western culture has triumphed over the early politician's desire to be accepted by, and participate in, the colonial world. It is symbolic of the victory of the mass party over the intellectual and occupational élite of the inter-war years.[1]

I myself have seen how in Southern Rhodesia the themes and memories of the rebellions have flowed back into nationalism as soon as it became a mass movement with support in the villages. 'In rural areas', writes Nathan Shamuyarira,

meetings became political gatherings and more...the past heritage was revived through prayers and traditional singing, ancestral spirits were invoked to guide and lead the new nation. Christianity and civilisation took a back seat and new forms of worship and new attitudes were thrust forward dramatically...the spirit pervading the meetings was African and the desire was to put the twentieth century in an African context.[2]

So George Nyandoro, grandson of a rebel leader killed in 1897, and nephew of a chief deposed in the 1930s for opposition to rural regulations, appealed in his speeches to the memory of the great prophet Chaminuka, around whom the Shona had rallied in the nineteenth century; so Joshua Nkomo, returning home in 1962, was met at the airport by a survivor of the rebellions who presented him with a spirit axe as a symbol of the apostolic succession of resistance.

In these ways it can be suggested that the resistance tradition runs into modern mass nationalism just as does the tradition of the 'Christian Revolution'. But I do not wish to suggest an essential conflict between the élite solutions of the co-operating societies and the mass solutions of the resisters. The 'resisters' and 'collaborators' were not fundamentally distinct. There has always been a complex interplay, also, between

[1] J. M. Lonsdale, 'A political history of Nyanza, 1883–1945' (Ph.D. thesis, Cambridge University, 1964), chs. 11 and 12.
[2] Nathan M. Shamuyarira, *Crisis in Rhodesia* (London, 1965), pp. 68–9.

mass and élite expressions of opposition. The establishment of colonial rule took a long time. 'Primary resistance' to the whites still continued in some areas of East, Central and Southern Africa, while 'secondary' oppositions had already developed elsewhere. Independent churches, trade unions and welfare associations overlapped and co-existed with tribal or pan-tribal resistance. There was a fascinating interaction between them.

In 1897, for example, Tengo Jabavu, the great South African political leader, visited Matabeleland to see the consequences of company rule; he found 'such friction as to compel the poor, ignorant people without enlightened advisers, to surrender to despair and even wish to be exterminated';[1] he returned to South Africa to warn readers of *Imvo* that this was what Rhodes's native policies meant. Jabavu's ideas in turn influenced African politics north of the Limpopo. Later on, in 1904, during the Rhodesian hut-tax crisis, the Chief Native Commissioner sent copies of *Imvo* to the Administrator's secretary. These contained attacks by Jabavu on Jameson with reference especially to the hut-tax increase. 'The information gathered therefrom', the C.N.C. alleged: 'is passed along by the educated native to his less advanced brother and in the course of transmission from one to another becomes twisted and exaggerated beyond recognition'; hence, he naïvely suggested, 'the native's anxiety as regards his future'.[2]

Another example derives from Shepperson and Price's account of the contacts between Nyasaland and Zululand. In 1896 Joseph Booth, the radical missionary, travelled from Nyasaland, taking with him one Gordon Mathaka, because the Yao wished 'to send a messenger to the other tribes in the south who had known the white man a long time to find out what they thought.' Mathaka heard the opinion of the Zulu Christian élite. 'No matter what the Yao thought', they told him, 'no living white man, whether carrying guns or not, would in the end, when war came, be friends of the black men.' And when Booth himself gathered together 120 African intellectuals to discuss his projected African Christian Union,

after a twenty six and a half hour session they rejected his scheme...on the simple grounds that no white man was fit to be trusted, not even Booth himself...No trust or reliance at all could be placed in any representative

[1] Report on Jabavu's visit to Rhodesia, *Cape Times*, 22 Nov. 1897.
[2] Chief Native Commissioner, Bulawayo, to Private Secretary, Salisbury, 12 Feb. 1904, A11/2/13/11, National Archives, Salisbury, Southern Rhodesia.

of 'the blood-stained white men, who had slain scores of thousands of Zulus and their Matabele relations'.[1]

These Zulu intellectuals did not perceive as sharply as modern historians the alleged gulf between primary and secondary resistance.

This sort of interplay continued into the 1920s and 1930s. African trade unionists in Bulawayo in 1929 looked to the resistant Somali as an example of successful unity; on the other hand, surviving leaders of the Ndebele rebels looked with envy at the successful collaborators, Lewanika and Khama, who had retained their land. The resistant Kikuyu looked with admiration at the institutions of the accommodating Ganda and sought at first to achieve them through a Kikuyu Paramount Chief movement. The ancestry of modern African politics, in short, is a complicated one. What we *can* say with certainty is that its patterns do not derive merely from decisions conceived in the capitals of the colonial powers and put into effect in East and Central Africa. In so far as they derive from the period of the 'Pacification' and of the establishment of the colonial administrations, they owe their origin to the participation of African societies in those processes; through both accommodation and resistance; through eager demands for modernization and stubborn defences of a way of life.

BIBLIOGRAPHY

Austen, Ralph. 'Political generations in Bukoba, 1890–1939', in East African Institute of Social Research, *Proceedings of the EAISR Conference held at the Institute*, June 1963, pt. D. Kampala, Makerere College, 1963.

Braginskiĭ, Mosei I., and Y. Lukonin. *Aperçu d'histoire du mouvement de libération nationale dans les pays d'Afrique orientale*. Moscow, 196–.

Cairns, H. Alan C. *Prelude to imperialism: British reactions to Central African society, 1840–1890*. London, 1965.

Davidson, A. B. 'African resistance and rebellion against the imposition of colonial rule', in *Emerging themes of African history*, T.O. Ranger, ed. Nairobi, 1968.

Davidson, Basil. *Guide to African history*. London, 1963.

Doutreloux, M. A. 'Prophétisme et culture', in International African Seminar, 3rd, Salisbury, Southern Rhodesia, 1960, *African systems of*

[1] George Shepperson and Thomas Price, *Independent African: John Chilembwe and the origins, setting, and significance of the Nyasaland native rising of 1915* (Edinburgh University Press, 1958), pp. 70, 71, 76.

thought: studies presented and discussed...at the Seminar... London, Oxford University Press, 1965.

Ebner, Elzear. 'History of the Wangoni.' Peramiho Mission, 1959. Mimeograph.

Gann, Lewis H. *A history of Southern Rhodesia: early days to 1934.* London, 1965.

Gifford, Prosser, and William Roger Louis, eds. *Britain and Germany in Africa: imperial rivalry and colonial rule.* New Haven and London, Yale University Press, 1967.

Halpern, Jack. *South Africa's hostages: Basutoland, Bechuanaland and Swaziland.* Harmondsworth, Middlesex and Baltimore, 1965.

Harlow, Vincent, and E. M. Chilvers, eds., assisted by Alison Smith. *History of East Africa*, vol. II. Oxford, Clarendon Press, 1965.

Hemphill, Marie de Kiewiet. 'The British sphere, 1884–94', in *History of East Africa*, vol. I, Roland Oliver and Gervase Mathew, eds. Oxford, Clarendon Press, 1963.

Iliffe, John. 'The effects of the Maji Maji rebellion of 1905–1906 on German occupation policy in East Africa', in *Britain and Germany in Africa: imperial rivalry and colonial rule*, Prosser Gifford and William Roger Louis, eds. New Haven and London, Yale University Press, 1967.

'The German administration in Tanganyika, 1906–1911: the governorship of Freiherr von Rechenberg.' Ph.D. thesis, Cambridge University, 1965.

International African Seminar, 3rd, Salisbury, Southern Rhodesia, 1960. *African systems of thought: studies presented and discussed at the Third International African Seminar in Salisbury, December 1960.* London, Oxford University Press, 1965.

Keltie, J. S. *The partition of Africa.* London, 1893.

Leverhulme Inter-collegiate History Conference, University College of Rhodesia and Nyasaland, Salisbury, Southern Rhodesia, 1960. *Historians in tropical Africa: proceedings of the Leverhulme Inter-collegiate History Conference held at the University College of Rhodesia and Nyasaland, September, 1960.* Salisbury, University College of Rhodesia and Nyasaland, 1962.

Leys, Norman. *Kenya.* London, 1924.

Lonsdale, J. M. 'A political history of Nyanza, 1883–1945.' Ph.D. thesis, Cambridge University, 1964.

Low, D. Anthony. 'British East Africa: the establishment of British rule, 1895–1912', in *History of East Africa*, vol. II, Vincent Harlow and E. M. Chilver, eds., assisted by Alison Smith. Oxford, Clarendon Press, 1965.

Low, D. Anthony, and R. Cranford Pratt. *Buganda and British overrule, 1900–1955: two studies.* London, Oxford University Press, 1960.

Matson, A. T. 'The pacification of Kenya', *Kenya Weekly News*, 14 Sept. 1962.

Meinertzhagen, Richard. *Kenya diary, 1902–1906*. Edinburgh, 1957.

Oliver, Roland, and John D. Fage. *A short history of Africa*. Harmondsworth, Middlesex and Baltimore, 1962.

Oliver, Roland, and Gervase Mathew, eds. *History of East Africa*, vol. I. Oxford, Clarendon Press, 1963.

Ranger, T. O. 'Revolt in Portuguese East Africa: the Makombe rising of 1917', in *African affairs*, no. 2 (Oxford University, St Antony's College, *St Antony's papers*, no. 15), Kenneth Kirkwood, ed. Carbondale, Southern Illinois University Press, 1963.

    Revolt in Southern Rhodesia, 1896–7: a study in African resistance. Evanston, Northwestern University Press, 1967.

    'Connexions between "primary resistance" movements and modern mass nationalism in East and Central Africa', *Journal of African History*, 1968, **9**, nos. 3 and 4.

Rea, W. F. 'The Bemba's white chief.' Historical Association of Rhodesia and Nyasaland, local series 13. Salisbury, Southern Rhodesia, 1964.

Redmayne, Alison H. 'The Wahehe people of Tanganyika.' Ph.D. thesis, Oxford University, 1964

Rennie, J. K. 'The Ngoni states and European intrusion', in *The Zambesian past: studies in Central African history*, Eric Stokes and Richard Brown, eds. Manchester University Press, 1966.

Robinson, Ronald E., and John Gallagher. 'The partition of Africa', in *The new Cambridge modern history*, vol. XI: *Material progress and world-wide problems, 1870–1898*, F. H. Hinsley, ed. Cambridge University Press, 1962.

Shamuyarira, Nathan M. *Crisis in Rhodesia*. London, 1965.

Shepperson, George, and Thomas Price. *Independent African: John Chilembwe and the origins, setting, and significance of the Nyasaland native rising of 1915*. Edinburgh University Press, 1958.

Stahl, Kathleen Mary. *History of the Chagga people of Kilimanjaro*. London, 1964.

Stenning, Derrick. 'Salvation in Ankole', in International African Seminar, 3rd, Salisbury, Southern Rhodesia, 1960, *African systems of thought: studies presented and discussed at the…Seminar…* London, Oxford University Press, 1965.

Stokes, Eric. 'European administration and African political systems, 1891–1897', in Rhodes–Livingstone Institute, Conference, 17th, Lusaka, Northern Rhodesia, 1963, *Conference of the history of the Central African peoples: papers presented at the…conference…May 28th–June 1st 1963*. Lusaka, 1963.

    'Malawi political systems and the introduction of colonial rule, 1891–1896', in *The Zambesian past: studies in Central African history*, Eric Stokes and Richard Brown, eds. Manchester University Press, 1966.

Stokes, Eric, and Richard Brown, eds. *The Zambesian past: studies in Central African history.* Manchester University Press, 1966.

Sundkler, B. G. M. Bantu prophets in South Africa. 2nd ed. London, Oxford University Press, 1961.

Van Velsen, J. 'The establishment of the administration in Tongaland', in Leverhulme Inter-Collegiate History Conference, University College of Rhodesia and Nyasaland, Salisbury, Southern Rhodesia, 1960, *Historians in tropical Africa: proceedings of the...Conference...* Salisbury, University College of Rhodesia and Nyasaland, 1962.

'The missionary factor among the Lakeside Tonga of Nyasaland', *Rhodes–Livingstone Journal*, 1960, no. 26.

Welime, J. D. 'Dini ya Msambwa', research paper, University College, Dar es Salaam, 1965.

Wipper, Audrey. 'The cult of Mumbo', in East African Institute of Social Research, *Proceedings of the EAISR Conference, January 1966*, pt. D. Kampala, Makerere College, 1966. (Contents page gives title as 'Religious sects in Nyanza'.)

Wright, Marcia. 'Chief Merere and the Germans', seminar paper, University of London School of Oriental and African Studies, Jan. 1965.

CHAPTER 10

THE BRITISH IMPERIAL FACTOR
IN SOUTH AFRICA FROM 1870 TO 1910

by D. W. KRÜGER

When the Netherlands and England successively occupied the Cape of Good Hope, both were motivated primarily by strategical considerations. But contrary to their original intentions each found itself becoming more and more involved with the interior. And as a result, southern Africa gradually developed into a white settlement in the midst of a large non-white population. The Cape was founded by the Dutch East India Company in 1652 chiefly as a supply station for ships plying between Holland and its trading stations in the Far East. At this time there was no intention of colonizing; but during the course of the eighteenth century the sparsely inhabited interior gradually came to be occupied by white farmers. This movement forced the hands of the company. In 1779 its officials proclaimed the Fish river as the eastern boundary of the colony, thus creating a geographical and political border between the white settlement and the Xosa tribes to the east. Before the end of the century the frontier farmers had thrown off the yoke of the company, whilst still claiming allegiance to the Dutch States General. By this time the Dutch East India Company was politically and financially at the end of its tether.

In 1795, during the French Revolutionary wars, Britain forcibly occupied the Cape to safeguard British interests in the East. As the result of the peace of Amiens the Cape Colony was handed back to Holland, but taken once more in 1806. The second occupation was legalized by the Congress of Vienna in 1814, at which time the Cape became a British crown colony.

Contrary to Britain's original intention, her commitments in South Africa increased steadily. The main problem was to safeguard the Fish river border area, which was in a chronic state of unrest. Population pressure from the Xosa tribes led to a number of expensive wars between the tribes and British imperial forces during which the white farmers in the frontier districts suffered severe losses. In 1836–7 a mass emigration of Dutch (Boer) farmers began. Dissatisfied with British rule, they crossed the Orange river into the sparsely habited northern plateau. Here they attempted to form an independent republic in Natal, which had been largely depopulated a decade before as a result of raids by the Zulu chief Shaka. London, however, refused to acknowledge the independence of another white settlement in the coastal area which might in future endanger Britain's strategical position. Hence the British forcibly annexed the short-lived republic in 1842. The Boers had no option but, recrossing the mountains to the interior, to establish independent settlements in the areas beyond the Orange and the Vaal rivers, which later became known as the South African Republic and the Orange Free State. The independence of the two states was recognized by Britain through formal conventions in 1852 and 1854.

During the middle years of the nineteenth century British statesmen would not consider any extension of British rule toward the far interior, and the Colonial Office was satisfied to limit British control to the Cape Colony and Natal, leaving the Bantu tribes in the coastal area between these two colonies and in the interior completely independent. Towards the late sixties, however, there was a revival of imperial interest. Ever since the Great Trek by the Boers, the position on the eastern border, where many British immigrants had settled since 1820, had remained unchanged. Constant border raids led to a further series of wars and the annexation of tribal territory in an attempt to create order. Thus, in 1866, the Ciskei, the area between the Fish and Kei rivers, had been annexed to the Cape Colony; and for the first time a white settlement area had acquired a considerable black population.

Events beyond the Orange compelled Britain to interfere in that direction as well. The Orange Free State had practically no black population, but there was constant friction with the independent Basuto nation in the mountainous area to the east that led to two wars between the republic and the Basutos in 1858 and in 1865–6. The Basutos were defeated at last and their chief, Moshesh, claimed British protection against the Boers. In March 1868 Basutoland was formally annexed by Sir Philip Wodehouse, Governor of the Cape, as a crown colony. The Secretary of State for the Colonies, the Duke of Buckingham, consented only reluctantly, and for administrative and security reasons the territory was formally taken over by the Cape colonial government in 1871. The Cape, however, had little direct interest in the country and was unable to deal with questions such as land settlement and the disarmament of tribesmen. It was glad to get rid of the burden when Downing Street took over control in 1884. Basutoland then became a crown colony where the chief with his council was allowed to govern under a system of indirect rule. No white settlement was allowed. The territory remained under the supervision of the British High Commissioner for South Africa, locally represented by a Resident. British control was little more than nominal and advisory.

During the late sixties, under humanitarian pressure, Britain's imperial interest in the interior revived, but philanthropical motives did not play the largest part. Although the desire to protect the native tribes living within or near the borders of the Boer republics was not a negligible impulse, this factor was overshadowed by economic interests. In 1867 white frontiersmen discovered the world's richest diamond fields near Kimberley, in the south-west of the Orange Free State. The area acquired a sudden and unexpected economic key position at a time when the whole of South Africa was in a state of severe depression. A petty Griqua chieftain, incited by a white adventurer, laid claim to the territory which had always been recognized by Britain as part of the Orange Free State. In spite of evidence to the contrary, Britain supported the Griqua claim; the British accepted the sovereignty over the diamond fields offered to them by the Griqua chief under the influence of Cape officials.

The Free State government protested in vain. In 1871 the imperial government formally annexed the whole area on both sides of the Vaal river at its confluence with the Orange as British territory. The event caused much bitterness in the adjoining republic, which was powerless to interfere. In June 1872 the Cape Parliament refused to accept responsibility for the territory, which remained a British crown colony with its own lieutenant-governor at the new diamond metropolis, Kimberley. Britain's sole motive in this sordid affair was to deny the neighbouring Republic possession of the country's enormous diamond resources. At the time, the Cape Governor, Sir Henry Barkly, admitted that he could not maintain the fiction that he was acting in the name of the Griqua chief. Four years later a Cape Land Court, after careful weighing of the evidence, rejected the Griqua claim to the territory; but by that time it was too late for the Free State.

The annexation of the diamond fields was the first of a series of British attempts to extend its influence toward the interior. The Portuguese harbour of Delagoa Bay on the east coast also quickened

British interest. In 1867 the German explorer Carl Mauch had discovered signs of gold-bearing quartz in the territory north of the Limpopo river. Diamonds had already been found on the southwestern border of the Transvaal, and in 1868 President M. W. Pretorius of that republic issued a proclamation extending the boundaries of the republic far to the west and eastwards along the lower course of the Maputo river to Delagoa Bay. This action both Britain and Portugal immediately protested; and Britain furthermore laid claim to the harbour itself. Both parties agreed to arbitration, and in 1875 the French President, Marshal MacMahon, decided in favour of Portugal. Although Britain acquiesced, the Colonial Office was determined at least to keep the Boers away from the east coast.

Meanwhile Britain had strengthened her position in the Cape Colony by granting that territory a new constitution, leaving it free to conduct its own internal affairs with an elected bicameral parliament and a ministry responsible to the legislature. The constitution was liberal, with equal voting rights for all citizens, irrespective of race, subject to low property and educational qualifications. For the first time Dutch colonists were in a position to make their influence felt in the legislature, particularly after 1881 when the use of the Dutch language was permitted in Parliament.

The advent in Britain in 1874 of the Conservative government under Disraeli inaugurated a period of active imperial interest in the affairs of South Africa. The new Secretary of State for the Colonies was Lord Carnarvon, who had successfully brought about the federation of Canada in 1867. He had similar aims in regard to South Africa. His objective was a federation of the British coastal colonies, Griqualand West and the two Boer republics. The Cape Governor, Sir Henry Barkly, served as his representative until 1876. Carnarvon's policy was opposed by the Transvaal Boers, who under their President, Thomas François Burgers, were determined both to maintain their independence and to safeguard it in the economic sphere through a railroad connexion with the Portuguese harbour of Delagoa Bay. The Free State Boers likewise showed little enthusiasm for Carnarvon's scheme, especially after the loss of their diamond fields. The people of the Cape also resented attempts from Downing Street to force federation down their throats. They could not forget that theirs was a self-governing colony, and they felt that any constitutional change should come from within.

Set on his course, Lord Carnarvon in September 1874 sent James

Anthony Froude, the well-known British historian, to South Africa to explore the whole situation. He travelled extensively, spoke to the leading politicians in the different territories, and made a provisional report. Local British officials supported him. They assured the Secretary that his proposals would be favourably received by the majority of the white population, that federation would permit of a common native policy and save the British taxpayers a considerable amount of money.

Carnarvon in 1875 proposed a conference of representatives from the different territories, and even went so far as to suggest some specific names. The Secretary's tactics were not at all to the liking of Cape Premier Molteno, who was supported by his Parliament. Carnarvon's representative, Froude, added to the discord by openly supporting a separation movement in the eastern province of the colony. When Carnarvon next suggested London as the venue of the conference, the Cape government refused to co-operate. Only the crown colonies of Griqualand West and Natal would attend. The governments of the two republics stood aloof and were only willing to discuss common problems. Froude, on his return to England in November 1875, reported that the Cape and the two republics were unwilling to discuss federation and that the movement had to develop spontaneously in South Africa. But Carnarvon determined to go ahead. The conference, held in August 1876, was a failure.

A new opportunity came for Carnarvon when the Transvaal became embroiled with a Bantu tribe, the Bapedi, whose chief, Sekhukuni, had refused to acknowledge the overlordship of the Republic. In May 1876 war had been declared, but the campaign had been a failure. Just after the conference the news reached Carnarvon that the Republic was too weak to maintain order and even to withstand the Zulus, who were adopting a threatening attitude in the south-east. Financially the Transvaal was in a bad state, unable to raise sufficient funds to construct the railway to Delagoa Bay. A vociferous minority of British gold-diggers were adding their voices and clamouring for a British take-over of the country. Carnarvon thought this too good an opportunity to waste. Accordingly, in October 1876 he empowered Theophilus Shepstone, a trusted Natal official, to go to Pretoria and to annex the Republic to the British empire providing he found sufficient support. At the same time, he appointed a new Cape Governor and High Commissioner for South Africa, Sir Bartle Frere, who had special instructions to carry out his federation policy.

Shepstone arrived in the capital of the Transvaal Republic in January of the following year and embarked at once on a series of discussions with the Boer government concerning the internal state of the Republic, its relations with the Bantu within its borders and with the independent Zulu nation. The president attempted financial and constitutional reforms; but these came too late, for after protracted negotiation, Shepstone in April 1877 summarily proclaimed the annexation of the Transvaal as a British colony. The republican government protested in vain. But it was powerless to act decisively in view of Shepstone's diplomatic use of the Zulu threat. The whole episode was a dramatic attempt by Carnarvon to force the Republic to accept federation. The Transvaal was occupied by British troops who had stood ready in Natal.

Too weak to fight back, the Transvaal Boers were nevertheless not prepared to accept British rule. A deputation led by Paul Kruger, the Vice-President of the defunct Republic, was sent to London. The delegates explained to the Secretary for the Colonies that the majority of the people were not satisfied. Carnarvon, misled by Shepstone's optimistic reports to the contrary, refused to undo the high-handed annexation. Kruger returned to the Transvaal only to find a growing feeling of unrest. Public meetings were held, and a plebiscite clearly showed that British rule was rejected by an overwhelming majority of the Boers. A second deputation to London in 1878 proved fruitless; and a personal visit by the High Commissioner, Sir Bartle Frere, failed to persuade the people to accept the situation. Opposition continued to build up, and there was talk of a military revolt even though the odds were heavily against the badly armed and numerically weak Boers.

The British at the same time were having more than the Transvaal to reckon with. In 1878 there was serious trouble on the eastern border of the Cape Colony where the independent chief of the Galekas, living in the Transkei, had refused to obey an order of Frere to meet him for a discussion concerning the problem of the Fingo tribe within his territory. Tembus and Gaikas had joined the Galekas in an inroad into the colony. The invaders were defeated and placed under colonial control, although the country was not annexed outright. The tribes of the Transkei would not remain independent much longer. In 1879 Tembuland and Griqualand East were joined to the Cape Colony. By 1894 the whole of the Transkei were incorporated with that colony after Britain had acquired the coastline of Pondoland. Meanwhile in the Transvaal the new British administration had had to put down a rising of the Bapedi in 1878. Sekhukuni's tribe was completely subjugated, but shortly afterwards Britain had become embroiled with the Zulus under Cetewayo. After several pitched battles and a severe British military disaster at Isandhlwana in January 1879, the military power of the Zulus was broken. Zululand came under white control and was formally annexed by Britain in 1887.

Frere's difficulties with both the black population and the Transvaal Boers were not yet at an end when the Cape Parliament rejected a Federation Bill introduced by the governor in 1880. A majority of the Cape colonists clearly sympathized with the Transvaal Boers in their political campaign against British rule. When Gladstone and his Liberal Party came to power in England shortly afterwards, Kruger fully expected the new government to revoke the annexation policy. Gladstone, however, though prepared to grant the Transvaal a liberal measure of self-government, would not undo the work of his predecessor. This was the last straw. Kruger, up to that time, had maintained the fiction that the republican government was still functioning, though acknowledging the *de facto* British administration. Now he was forced by public opinion to act at last. Accordingly, in December 1880 he raised the standard of revolt. The British garrisons were besieged in the principal towns of the Transvaal and a force posted on the Natal border, the only direction from which the Transvaal could be reconquered. In a series of sharp clashes the British were defeated. The Boers crowned their achievement by the battle of Majuba on 27 February 1881, when a British regular force of veteran troops was utterly routed by a few Boer sharpshooters.

Kruger was keenly aware through all this that in the long run his forces would be no match for the overwhelming forces of Britain. Even before the battle of Majuba he had been willing to negotiate on the basis of the restoration of the independence of the Republic, subject to British suzerainty. This offer was now accepted by Britain, where there was considerable sympathy for the Boers, and where the Liberal government was glad to get out of a difficult situation in view of a possible general rising in South Africa against Britain. Morally, the British were in a bad position. The vast majority of the white population was opposed to British imperial methods, and during the period 1878–9 British policy had estranged the Bantu also. The political and military reputation of Britain was nowhere highly rated, and the Transvaal

Boers profited by the general situation. A large portion of Boers and blacks, alike, rejected imperialism. British liberal opinion in England stood firm on one point—the safeguarding of the position of the African population.

Peace negotiations led to the appointment of a royal commission headed by the new High Commissioner, Sir Hercules Robinson. Its findings resulted in the Pretoria Convention between Britain and the Transvaal in August 1881. The independence of the Republic was recognized, but Britain retained a suzerainty over the country, including the right of supervising its external and native affairs. A new western boundary was delimited so as to exclude from republican rule many of the Tswana people in that area. In addition, the Transvaal was held responsible for a comparatively large debt that the colonists considered to be an unjust burden on the small white community.

The Transvaal government was not satisfied with these terms, and between 1883 and 1884 sent a deputation to London, led by Paul Kruger, the newly elected President of the Republic and the recognized leader of his people. The Transvaal emissaries persuaded Lord Derby, the Secretary of State for the Colonies, to remove the suzerainty clause, to lessen the debt to Britain and to modify the western border slightly in favour of the Republic. Out of this came a new agreement, the Convention of London, signed on 27 February 1884. By this instrument Britain retained only a partial supervision over the external affairs of the Transvaal; British consent still had to be obtained by the Republic for treaties with foreign nations, including the black tribes to the east or west, excepting its neighbour, the Orange Free State.

The Transvaal deputation, before returning, visited the principal capitals of Western Europe. They concluded some commercial treaties, especially with Portugal, and granted a concession to a Dutch group to build a railway connecting Pretoria with Delagoa Bay. The Republic was too impoverished to undertake this task itself and the Dutch concessionaries were at first not able to raise the necessary capital.

In the meantime, Transvaal affairs on the western or Bechuanaland border had also been in a state of confusion. The boundary proclaimed in 1881 had cut several Tswana tribes in two, sometimes leaving a chief independent whilst a number of his subjects were living within the borders of the Republic. There were quarrels between various chiefs; and white adventurers from the Transvaal and the diamond fields in Griqualand West took part on opposing sides, tempted by lavish promises of farms in conquered country. The Cape colonial government as well as the Transvaal took a keen interest in the intertribal struggle. Both hoped for territorial advantages.

Just prior to these events a new man had arisen in Cape politics—Cecil John Rhodes, a Cape politician who had made a fortune on the diamond fields. As a member of the Cape Parliament, he had consistently advocated the right of the Cape Colony to expand to the north, carrying with it the British flag and the Pax Britannica. But Rhodes also wished to exclude what he called the 'imperial factor' from South African affairs. He was an idealistic and ardent imperialist, but he regarded direct imperial interference as injurious. In his view the Cape was able to manage its own affairs. He dreamed of a commercial and political road from the Cape to the north, eventually joining the Cape to Cairo. He regarded Bechuanaland as the bottleneck between the Transvaal and German South West Africa, the 'Suez Canal' to the north that should be kept open in the interests of the Cape and of the British empire. Hence he meant to prevent any western expansion of the Transvaal that might create a link between that country and the German protectorate on the west coast. The interests of the Tswana tribes, which were mostly located near the Transvaal border, were not taken into account. The Cape colonial government was induced by Rhodes to take part in the affair.

Thus when Kruger in October 1884 impulsively attempted to extend the authority of his Republic over part of Bechuanaland, he was forced to reckon with both the Cape Colony and Great Britain. He hastily withdrew, but Britain, after the humiliation of Majuba, was determined to teach the Republic a lesson. An armed force, commanded by Sir Charles Warren, was sent to Bechuanaland. Two tiny Boer republics that had been established during the troubles were frightened into submission. British agents induced several Tswana chiefs to sign treaties establishing a British protectorate over the whole of Bechuanaland from the Zambezi in the north to the Cape colonial border in the south, including the whole Kalahari from the western borders of the Transvaal to the German territory of South West Africa. The southern part of this huge territory, south of the Malopo river, was directly annexed as British Bechuanaland; the remaining portion was proclaimed a protectorate. British Bechuanaland in 1895 became part of the Cape Colony after a resolution, proposed by Rhodes, had been adopted by the Cape Parliament. Bechuanaland in its turn served as a jumping-board for Rhodes's next adventure. He was already looking at the territory north of the Limpopo. He had succeeded in preventing Boer westward expansion and he was determined further to isolate the South African Republic by blocking the way to the north.

In 1886 an event occurred that exerted a profound influence on the destinies of South Africa. This was the discovery of the fabulous gold reef along the Witwatersrand (the Ridge of the White Waters) barely forty miles from Pretoria, the capital of the Transvaal. The economic result was immediate; and its political, sociological and cultural consequences, although somewhat slower in appearing, were no less momentous. Almost overnight the Transvaal, heretofore the poorest of the white settlements, became the most prosperous. Thousands of diggers from many parts of the world, but mostly British subjects, swarmed into the area. A host of new companies were formed; and as mining shafts were sunk ever deeper below the surface, capitalist exploitation took over. A new metropolis arose in the heart of the Republic with an alien population out to make its fortune, but not for long content with Boer or Afrikaner control. The gold mines, like the diamond diggings before, attracted thousands of tribesmen from the reserves, thus complicating the racial problem.

The way was paved for industrial development, although the Transvaal for the most part remained a pastoral country with the majority of the Bantu people still living in tribal reserves. The presence of thousands of British subjects in an alien Boer republic provided a suitable pretext for fresh British interference, with the result that the Republic was drawn even farther into the orbit of South African and imperial politics. It would take all the astuteness of Paul Kruger to maintain his country's independence in the face of overwhelming odds during a period when Britain had entered the phase of militant imperialism, and when the Empire stood at the zenith of its power. The Transvaal had suddenly become a glittering prize, ready to be grasped by any means, fair or foul.

Paul Kruger understood the situation completely and did everything possible to strengthen his country. The railway to the east coast, when completed, would provide him with an independent outlet to the sea. It would enable the Republic to claim its proper share of customs duties on imported goods, which up to that time had filled the coffers of the British coastal colonies controlling the commerce with the interior. Because Kruger considered the railway to be the lifeline of the

Republic, he refused to enter a customs union proposed by the Cape government, now keenly conscious of the prospective economic advantages. The discovery of gold enriched the state treasury of the Transvaal and brought prosperity to the whole country; but it also started a race to extend the railway lines from the harbours of the Cape Colony and Natal to distant Johannesburg.

Kruger did his utmost to promote his own railway scheme and to retard the construction of competing lines from the south. The Dutch concessionaries in 1887 found the necessary capital and formed the Netherlands–South African Railway Company where the Republic had the controlling interest. By 1888 lines from Delagoa Bay, Durban and Cape Town, all government-controlled, were being built simultaneously, each eager to be first in Johannesburg and to carry the major share of the traffic. The winner would get the lion's share of traffic dues, as well as customs duties levied at the ports of entry. Kruger was never more determined to maintain the independence of his country, because there was also at stake the larger issue of the future of the Afrikaner people.

Ever since the British occupation of the Cape of Good Hope, the British authorities had been trying systematically to anglicize the Dutch colonists. They succeeded only to a limited extent in the area adjacent to Cape Town, but the majority of the colonists clung tenaciously to the Dutch cultural heritage. During the seventies latent Boer national sentiment had been awakening. At first this took the form of a movement in the Cape in favour of spoken Afrikaans (the Cape form of Dutch) as a literary language.

During the Transvaal war of 1880–1 Afrikaners in the Cape and the Free State sympathized with their kinsmen in the north. Shortly after the war two Cape Afrikaner leaders, S. J. du Toit and J. H. Hofmeyr, began to organize their followers. The movement started as a Farmers Protection Association, but the economic motive soon took second place to politics. It was an important sign of a group feeling existing amongst Afrikaners. The first Transvaal war against the British was a major factor in changing the character of the movement. In 1879 the Reverend S. J. du Toit, leader of the movement in favour of Afrikaans, advocated the forming of an 'Afrikaner Bond' to serve Afrikaner political interests throughout South Africa. Its proposed aim was a united South Africa as a national home for all white South Africans. In 1882–3 the Farmers Protection Association was absorbed by the new organization, which took an active part in politics, and even had branches in the republics in the north.

A new feeling of Afrikaner nationality was fostered by this amalgamation. But Cecil Rhodes, recognizing the value of the movement, decided to use it to further his schemes of territorial expansion. While Paul Kruger, suspicious of the Cape Colony as an instrument of British politics, tried to maintain his country's political and economic independence, Rhodes exploited colonial sentiment in the south. Between 1885 and 1895 he succeeded in estranging Afrikaners in the south from their brethren in the Transvaal. Already the most powerful man in financial circles with vast diamond and gold interests, he rapidly became the strongest political leader in the Cape. With the support of the Bond he assumed office as Prime Minister of the Cape in 1890. Even before then the Bond had stood by his schemes of expansion to the north, had supported him in Bechuanaland, and had even backed his policy in the territory farther north. Many Afrikaners in the Cape Colony shared the objection of Rhodes to the imperial factor because he fostered a sort of colonial patriotism which favoured them. It remained to be seen whether this alliance of interests would be able to withstand a sudden national crisis unleashing deeper, emotional forces.

The closer the co-operation between Rhodes and the Afrikaners of the south, the more suspicious Paul Kruger became, and the more determined to go his own way. He began to distrust even his kinsmen in the Cape Colony. Cape Afrikaners for their part accused him of favouring imported Hollander officials. They also censored his reliance on the Netherlands Railway Company to the detriment of the Cape government railways, which were steadily pushing north towards Johannesburg. Here Kruger was in a strong position, for his own line, when completed, would run for most of its length through republican territory. This enabled him to regulate railway tariffs in such a way as to discourage traffic over the Cape and Natal railways over which he had little control. Railway competition was ultimately to cause a serious clash with both Britain and the Cape Colony.

Meanwhile Kruger had to face new difficulties concerning the alien population on the gold-fields. He was not prepared to grant equal voting rights to people who were regarded by his conservative followers as Outlanders, interested only in making their fortunes and then departing. The new immigrants were certainly not easily assimilable, and their very numbers seemed to threaten to destroy the homogeneous character of the Boer people. In an effort to meet this threat, the Transvaal Volksraad or Legislative Assembly in 1890 adopted a new franchise law. A second legislative chamber was created to deal particularly with mining affairs, but the first Volksraad could still veto its acts. Newcomers could vote for this body two years after registration as citizens, but for presidential and ordinary Volksraad elections the residential qualification was raised to fourteen years. The law was designed to prevent the Outlanders from outvoting the older established population.

The Outlanders naturally were unhappy with this situation, although many of them were little concerned with politics. Their leaders and English-language newspapers started to agitate against the Kruger regime, and mounted a campaign that continued for many years. The President, though personally vilified on many occasions, stuck to his guns. He was concerned both with the internal situation in the Transvaal and with the larger South African position, particularly in view of steady outside pressure for a general customs union, which Kruger regarded as the beginning of the end for his republic.

Rhodes saw in Kruger the major stumbling-block to his policy of expanding the Cape and unifying the whole of South Africa under Cape leadership. He therefore steadily opposed Kruger's policy and encouraged the Outlanders of Johannesburg, where he himself had vast gold-mining interests, to oppose the Kruger régime. The British government through its High Commissioner, Sir Henry Loch, likewise strove to isolate the Republic. Both directly and indirectly Loch supported Rhodes in preventing the expansion of the Transvaal to the north and in denying the Republic an independent outlet to the east coast through Swaziland.

For several years Rhodes had had his eye on the country north of the Limpopo where Lobengula, the king of the Matabele, held sway. Rumours of golden riches in the Far North had been circulating ever since Mauch had discovered gold in the interior. Rhodes thought that the region north of the Limpopo might prove to be a second Witwatersrand. Economic and political motives were clearly entwined in his policy of expansion in this direction. Accordingly, in 1888 he sent agents to obtain a concession from Lobengula to prospect for minerals and to exploit any discoveries. The Matabele king, fearing the coming of the white man, for a long time refused to listen to the blandishments of these agents. Again and again he was assured that the Europeans were not interested in his country and that they only sought economic

337

advantages. At last Lobengula was persuaded to grant the concession in return for a monthly salary, rifles and cartridges as well as a steamboat on the Zambezi. Rhodes thereupon formed the British South Africa Company (1889), which obtained a charter by the British Parliament with extensive governmental powers. The occupation of Matabeleland followed soon afterwards.

Lobengula realized too late that the new settlers were not only trying to find gold, but also wanted Mashonaland, his traditional raiding sphere. His war parties clashed with the settlers and in 1893 hostilities broke out. In due course, Lobengula's power was destroyed, and he himself perished in flight. The British South Africa Company now took over the whole region, which became known as Southern Rhodesia.

Rhodes had gained his object of making Rhodesia British. But he was faced also with the task of keeping out Kruger's Transvaalers, and in this he availed himself of the High Commissioner's assistance. He was supported also by the Afrikaner Bond, since he had assured the Afrikaners that he wanted only to further the interests of the Cape Colony, and to work for a federation in South Africa. His Chartered Company was precisely meant to exclude the 'imperial factor'. Just at that time (1890) Sir Henry Loch was conducting negotiations with the Kruger government regarding the Swaziland question. Before the British annexation of the Transvaal in 1877, Swaziland had been an autonomous country under the nominal suzerainty of the Republic. When the Republic regained its independence in 1881, Swaziland recovered complete freedom; but the Boers considered the country to lie within their own sphere of interests. The British were not interested in Swaziland as such, but realized its value in their bargaining with the Boers. Kruger thought that Swaziland might provide an alternative outlet to the sea, since his Republic was surrounded on three sides by British territory. The matter became urgent after the Chartered Company had entered Rhodesia.

Both Sir Henry Loch and Cecil Rhodes saw a new opportunity to force the Republic into a customs union with the British colonies, and to exert pressure on Kruger to allow the colonial railways to be extended to the borders of the Transvaal. In addition, they wanted Kruger to prevent Transvaal subjects from advancing beyond the Limpopo in armed trekking groups. In March 1890 Kruger met Loch and, with Rhodes present, discussed the whole question. He was willing to leave Rhodes a free hand in Rhodesia, and provisionally undertook to join a customs union and allow extension of the southern railways as soon as his own road had sufficiently advanced. In return he was promised a three-mile-wide corridor through Swaziland to Kosi Bay on the east coast. On this basis a Convention between Britain and the Republic (the first Swaziland Convention) was signed in 1890. The Republic, however, was unwilling to enter a customs union unless it had acquired its own outlet to the sea. On this condition the Republican government was persuaded to ratify the Convention, which it regarded as a temporary measure.

Swaziland, where order was maintained jointly by British and Transvaal representatives, again became a subject of discussion when the Republic gave notice that it would terminate the Convention in August 1893. This time Kruger demanded that the territory be incorporated into the Republic and be subject to its laws. The High Commissioner was willing to agree to a Transvaal protectorate over the Swazis, who were otherwise to remain independent. Kruger, for his part, agreed with a British demand that a railway between Swaziland and the sea could only be built with the consent of Britain. The terms of this agreement were embodied in a second Swaziland Convention (November 1893). But this instrument never became effective because the Swazis would not comply with its main condition, which was to accept the protection of the Republic. In a Third Convention Britain then allowed the Republic to establish a protectorate even without the consent of the Swazis.

In February 1895 the Transvaal at last realized its aim, but the triumph was short-lived; for a few months later Britain annexed the native territories of Zambane, Mbegisa, and Tongaland, between Swaziland and the sea, thus finally cutting the Republic off from any outlet to the sea, except through Portuguese territory. The Republic was hemmed in. But in the meantime the railway to Delagoa Bay had been opened, and the Transvaal became more than ever unwilling to enter into any form of federation or even a customs union. Rhodes was now forced to resort to different tactics; and this time he saw a new way of gaining his objective in the grievances of the Rand's alien population.

Paul Kruger's republic had during the past few years acquired great economic and political importance. The inauguration of the railway to Delagoa Bay in which Germany, amongst others, had taken part, reminded British statesmen of a possible German threat to British hegemony in southern Africa. The interests of Cecil Rhodes and British statesmen in the Transvaal became identical, particularly since July 1895, when Joseph Chamberlain became Secretary of State for the Colonies in Lord Salisbury's Conservative government. Paul Kruger at this time publicly stressed the importance of German–Transvaal friendship, thereby strengthening British suspicions that Germany was secretly seeking advantages for herself to the detriment of British paramountcy, even to the extent of obtaining a protectorate over the Transvaal. Germany, too, had financial interests in the Netherlands Railway Company and a considerable stake in the gold-mines.

Downing Street was determined not to allow the Transvaal to achieve international status. When Chamberlain during the second half of 1895 was approached by agents of Rhodes regarding the possibility of bringing about the fall of the Kruger régime, he was not unsympathetic. Rhodes hoped to use the grievances of the Outlanders as a lever against the Transvaal government. In June 1895 he sounded out Lionel Phillips, the chairman of the Transvaal Chamber of Mines, and Charles Leonard, President of the National Union, a pro-British organization that voiced the grievances of the Outlanders. When Rhodes became assured that these leaders favoured the idea of an armed revolt in Johannesburg, supported by outside intervention, he proceeded to make sure that he could rely on Chamberlain, who was in favour of a South African federation and of British rule in Pretoria. And in the course of the plans that followed, Chamberlain actively connived with the plotters.[1]

Shortly afterwards an event occurred that drew Rhodes and Chamberlain closer together. After the completion of the railway to Delagoa Bay, there was keen competition between the different lines which by that time had all reached the terminus, Johannesburg. In order to attract overseas traffic to his own line, Kruger in October 1895 increased the freight rate on the fifty-mile stretch of the Cape line under his control. Rhodes countered by reducing the rate over the rest of the line from the Cape to the Transvaal border and by boycotting the Transvaal section. He had the goods off-loaded just before the border and conveyed by ox-wagon for the rest of the way. Kruger promptly closed the fords through the Vaal river. There then arose a very serious situation

[1] The complicity of Chamberlain, also believed in by the Boers but not supported by direct documentary evidence, has recently been proved conclusively by Johannes Stephanus Marais, *The fall of Kruger's Republic* (Oxford, Clarendon Press, 1961), pp. 70 ff. and particularly pp. 94 ff.

(known as the Drifts crisis), for Kruger now faced the Cape Colony as well as the British Colonial Office, which backed the Cape and threatened to take military action. Kruger, wisely, gave in and reopened the fords. The episode, however, estranged him both from the Cape Colony and from Great Britain. It helped also to push Chamberlain into supporting Rhodes in his anti-Transvaal conspiracy.

Strangely enough, matters had come to the point where the very man who had always rejected the imperial factor came to invoke that factor to gain his ends. In this policy he had another ally in the new High Commissioner, the aged and ailing Sir Hercules Robinson.

The last remnants of his conscience went overboard. The Prime Minister of the Cape Colony, one of Her Majesty's Privy Councillors bound by several holy oaths, instigated and took an active part in the smuggling of arms from the Cape into the Transvaal, arms which were destined to help conspirators against the lawful government of a friendly state ! It was the end of Rhodes as a responsible politician. He had turned a political adventurer.[1]

Rhodes arranged with some leaders of the mining industry that, with arms smuggled into the Republic, a rising would be staged before the end of December 1895. As a pretext for outside intervention a spurious letter, undated, was drawn up calling upon Leander Starr Jameson, Rhodes's lieutenant in charge of his private army in British Bechuanaland, just across the border, to come to the aid of British women and children whose lives were supposedly threatened by the Boers. After the revolt had started, Jameson was to march in with 600 mounted troopers and some quick-firing guns. At the request of the High Commissioner in the Cape, Britain would then intervene to maintain order. Kruger would be driven from power, but the conspirators were not very clear about what was to happen subsequently.

Rhodes's calculations, however, were thrown out of gear by the impatience of Jameson, who would not wait for the signal to start. He jumped the gun; but before his force had reached Johannesburg he was forced to surrender to the rapidly mobilized Boer forces. The Outlander revolt was put down without bloodshed before it could properly develop. Kruger was left completely master of the situation and more firmly in the saddle than ever. He wisely handed over Jameson and his men to be punished by Britain. They were subsequently found guilty by a British court but let off with light sentences. The

---

[1] Felix Gross, *Rhodes of Africa* (London, 1956), pp. 269–70.

ringleaders of the revolt in Johannesburg were tried in Pretoria, found guilty of high treason and condemned to death. The sentence was commuted by Kruger to heavy fines; but as a consequence of the raid the Republic began to import arms from Europe.

After the Jameson Raid had forced Rhodes to resign as Prime Minister of the Cape Colony, he was finished as a political leader in South Africa. His perfidy brought about a complete break with the Afrikaner Bond, which turned to Kruger instead. The raid caused a wave of anti-British feeling throughout South Africa and tended to consolidate Afrikanerdom. The Free State was driven into the arms of its northern neighbour. A House of Commons Committee of Enquiry found Rhodes guilty, but Chamberlain got off scot-free through lack of written evidence. Rhodes, allowed to remain head of the Chartered Company, in return refused to implicate the astute Colonial Minister.

The Jameson Raid had international repercussions too. On 2 January 1896 the German Emperor sent a congratulatory telegram to Kruger, implying that if Britain intervened in the Transvaal, Germany would come to the assistance of the Republic. The Kaiser's telegram caused a wave of resentment in England and seemed to remove the stain of infamy from the raiders and their British accomplices. Britain was more determined than ever to maintain British paramountcy in South Africa. At the same time anti-German sentiment was awakened and British suspicion as to Germany's intention was never afterwards properly assuaged. The British found themselves diplomatically isolated and for the time being had to proceed warily.

But in the long run, the alliance between imperialism and a major section of the mining capitalists on the Rand proved to be too strong for Kruger. The Jameson Raid had clarified the struggle between the two white elements in South Africa as one between British imperialism and Afrikaner nationalism, of which Kruger was the champion. Chamberlain, who was rapidly becoming known as the arch-priest of imperialism, at first tried to induce Kruger to come to England in order to revise the Convention of London that Kruger had demanded. At the same time, however, Chamberlain determined not only to demand constitutional reform in the Republic, an unwarranted interference in the Republic's internal affairs rejected by Kruger, but also to supervise the Republic's external relations. The Transvaal President thereupon refused the invitation.

The appointment of Sir Alfred Milner as Governor of the Cape

Colony and British High Commissioner for South Africa in 1897 marked a distinct change in imperial policy, with the British steadily becoming more aggressive. Milner became the agent of Chamberlain's policy for uniting the whole of South Africa under the Union Jack. The indigenous tribes had lost their independence during the two previous decades; and the sole remaining stumbling-block was Kruger, backed by the Free State and Afrikaner national sentiment in the rest of South Africa. Milner's task was to overcome all the obstacles. Educated in Germany and a trusted and zealous official with an excellent reputation in the administration of Egypt, he was considered to be the right man to carry out the policy of Chamberlain, with whom he shared the idea of British superiority. He firmly believed in the high destiny of the empire, called upon to rule South Africa. During his first few months in South Africa he carefully studied the situation, but from 1898 onwards he gradually began to apply harsher pressure.

In February 1898 Kruger was re-elected president with an overwhelming majority. He strengthened the position of his government by appointing the state secretary, Dr W. J. Leyds, a brilliant young Dutch lawyer, as special envoy in Europe in order to plead the Republic's cause overseas. His new state secretary was Francis W. Reitz, formerly President of the Orange Free State. Kruger brought in also Jan C. Smuts, an outstanding Cape barrister trained at Cambridge, as state attorney and chief legal adviser. The new appointments implied that Kruger was prepared to work with his Afrikaner compatriots in the Cape. The *rapprochement* between the Transvaal, the Orange Free State and the Afrikaners of the Cape was interpreted by Milner as preparation for a vast Afrikaner conspiracy against British influence in South Africa, instead of a natural reaction against British imperialist designs.

With Kruger's re-election, Milner's last hope to achieve his aims by peaceful methods vanished. He began to press the Kruger régime for the removal of 'substantial wrongs and injustice', as he called it.[1] When in a public speech he accused Afrikaners in the Cape Colony of disloyalty to England, Chamberlain had to warn him to be careful. He was not sure as to the attitude of foreign powers if it came to a military showdown. In the course of the year, however, the international situation had changed in Britain's favour. The Fashoda crisis with France was surmounted and relations with the United States improved with strict British neutrality during the war with Spain. In addition,

[1] Cecil Headlam, ed., *The Milner papers* (London, 1931–3), I, 221–3.

Britain gained an important diplomatic victory as the result of an understanding with Germany in August 1898. An Anglo-German agreement to assist Portugal financially was guaranteed by a lien on the Portuguese territories in Africa and Timor. In the event of Portugal's inability to repay, the two great powers were to divide her possessions between them with Delagoa Bay going to Britain. In effect, the British–German treaty meant that Germany was withdrawing her support from the Transvaal. Consequently, by the end of 1898 British statesmen were assured of a free hand in their dealings with the Transvaal and Milner could safely proceed. He became all the more determined by the elections in the Cape Colony, which in 1898 brought to power the Afrikaner Bond, with W. P. Schreiner as prime minister. The new government was in complete sympathy with the Transvaal Republic, and in 1898 the two republics concluded a defensive and offensive alliance and so set the stage for the final act.

Milner needed the full support of the Outlanders, amongst whom a new movement against the existing régime was started. The capitalist leaders of the movement agitated for a government amenable to mining interests. They were after larger profits in the first place, and their press continuously attacked the Republic's policy in regard to railway traffic, customs dues, state monopolies and labour. They stirred up the mass of the alien population on the gold-fields, who did not realize that they were being used by the capitalists. The purpose of the press campaign was also to create the impression in England that the Outlanders were being oppressed as a class and that only British intervention could save them. Their grievances, real and imagined, were wildly exaggerated. In March 1899 they drew up a petition, signed by more than 21,000 persons, that was sent to Milner, who, in turn, forwarded it to Chamberlain. A counter-petition, signed by even more people, had no effect. Milner in May 1899 assured the Colonial Office that the Outlanders, mostly British, were being treated as 'helots' and that there was every reason for interference.

In the meantime Chamberlain had begun to exceed Britain's legal powers by claiming British suzerainty over the Transvaal. In an unguarded moment State Secretary Reitz, not content with refuting the claim, insisted that the Republic was a sovereign independent state, notwithstanding the London Convention that provided for British supervision of the Republic's treaty-making right. Reitz thereby provided Chamberlain with new grounds for attacking the Republic.

Events were rapidly building up to a crisis when President Steyn, at the request of the Cape politicians, invited Kruger and Milner to a conference at the Free State capital, Bloemfontein, in order to discuss the points at issue. Kruger was already aware through reports of Dr Leyds from Europe that he could not rely on any assistance from European powers. During the conference, which lasted from 31 May to 6 June 1899, Milner forced Kruger to limit the discussions to the franchise question. He proposed a residential qualification of five years for all Outlanders as a requirement for full political equality. Kruger offered to reduce the period from fourteen to seven years, but Milner was adamant. At last, in despair, the old president exclaimed that what Milner really wanted was not the vote but the country. The conference ended in failure, but Kruger nevertheless resolved that he would carry out his own proposals.

The situation now deteriorated rapidly. British troops in South Africa were reinforced and all efforts of Free State and Cape politicians to mediate were in vain. Throughout August and September correspondence between the Republic and the Colonial Office continued, but Milner was set on war. In a candid moment he told a Cape politician that he was determined to end the 'dominion of Afrikanerdom'.[1] It was no longer a struggle to achieve political equality of British and Boers, but to make South Africa British.[2] With the British imperial troops beginning to mass near the republican border in Natal, and in the face of the British government's decision to issue an ultimatum to the Transvaal, Kruger suddenly forced Britain to show her hand. On 9 October 1899, with the consent of the Free State government, he dispatched an ultimatum to Britain. Britain was to remove her troops within forty-eight hours and to submit the outstanding questions to arbitration. A refusal would be considered as a declaration of war. As expected, there was no answer; and on 11 October 1899 Britain and the two republics were at war.

The disparity of the opposing parties was manifest. Britain, a world empire, had unlimited manpower and endless resources. She ruled the waves, and from the very beginning was able to impose a complete blockade on the republics. The two Boer states together could not

[1] Sir James Tennant Molteno, *The dominion of Afrikanerdom: recollections pleasant and otherwise* (London, 1923), pp. 184–5.
[2] That Milner was bent on war has recently been proved by Godfrey H. L. Le May, *British supremacy in South Africa, 1899–1907* (Oxford, Clarendon Press, 1965), pp. 19–26.

mobilize more than 50,000 men, mostly untrained farmers, but all mounted, highly mobile and armed with modern German Mausers. They were aided by a few thousand foreign volunteers and later by some 5,000 Cape rebels. The Republican artillery consisted of a few modern batteries and a dozen vintage field pieces. Although efficient and well-drilled, it could not stand up to British overwhelming superiority. The only hope of the republics lay in taking the offensive as soon as possible and before Britain had time to bring in the full weight of her resources. At first the Boer strategy of conducting the war on enemy territory succeeded. British garrisons were isolated and beleaguered at Ladysmith in Natal, Kimberley, and Mafeking in the western Cape. During December British relieving forces were thrown back with heavy loss, but in February 1900 the tide turned. A new commander-in-chief, Lord Roberts, with Lord Kitchener as chief of staff, was sent out from England with numerous reinforcements. The British applied new tactics of outflanking the weak defending Boer forces and forcing them to retire or to be captured. The defences crumbled; Kimberley and Ladysmith were relieved after heavy fighting, and early in March Roberts occupied the Free State capital.

In May 1900 the British crossed into the Transvaal and occupied Johannesburg. On 4 June Pretoria, undefended, fell, and the Boer forces retreated to the east astride the railway to Delagoa Bay. President Kruger with his government had quitted the capital shortly before and had set up a new capital on the railway line, far to the east. At the end of August the Boers lost the last pitched battle. In a conference of leaders it was decided to continue the war by guerrilla tactics. Kruger, by then too old to accompany his men in the field, was sent to Europe to plead the cause of the republics with foreign governments. Accordingly, he crossed the border in September and was conveyed by a Dutch cruiser to Marseille. Although he received an enthusiastic welcome on the continent, neither France nor Germany was willing to intervene. Kruger thereupon took up residence in Holland and later moved to the south of France. He died in exile at Clarens near Montreux in Switzerland on 14 July 1904. His remains were brought to South Africa and interred at Pretoria. He was remembered ever afterwards by his people as a patriot and national hero.

Meanwhile, Roberts, thinking that the resistance of the Boers was practically at an end, had annexed both republics as British colonies. Before the end of 1900 he returned to England, where he received a hero's welcome, leaving Kitchener as his successor to conduct mopping-up operations. The British high command, however, had seriously underrated the capacity of the Boers to resist; and the war continued for another eighteen months. Steyn proved to be an inspiring political leader who accompanied his men in the field. The Boers produced brilliant tacticians in C. R. de Wet of the Free State and J. H. de la Rey in the Transvaal, whilst Louis Botha remained in the field as Comman-dant-General of the Transvaal forces. British communications were continually attacked, and isolated garrisons were immobilized. Early in 1901 the British controlled no more than the towns and the few railways in the new colonies. The Republican forces even took the offensive by invading the Cape Colony.

Kitchener, seeing that the war was by no means won, decided on a drastic new scorched-earth strategy. Unable to beat the Boers in the field, he thought to deny them the means of subsistence. Farmhouses were systematically burnt, crops destroyed and all livestock captured. These measures forced him to provide for the Boer civilian population in concentrations camps, established at numerous centres during the first half of 1901. Malnutrition and contagious diseases caused a high rate of mortality, particularly amongst children. In July 1901 the death-rate stood at 116 per thousand per annum; by October it had risen to the appalling figure of 346 per thousand. Amongst children below five years of age it was much higher; and towards the end of the war, out of a total camp population of 118,000, no fewer than 26,000 Boer women and children had died.

The policy of farm-burning and concentration camps, aimed primarily at the civilian population, caused a tremendous outcry throughout the world. A part of the liberal press in England and of the Liberal Party, led by Sir Henry Campbell-Bannerman, protested publicly against what Sir Henry labelled 'methods of barbarism', until at last the government was forced to take action. Towards the end of 1901 conditions improved; but for thousands of camp inmates reform had come too late.

Meanwhile Boer resistance did not slacken, and in August 1901 Kitchener threatened the Boer leaders with banishment and their men with confiscation of property if they did not surrender before a given date. The Boers laughed Kitchener's 'paper bomb' to scorn and intensi-fied their efforts. By this time, however, they had hardly 20,000 men in the field as against twenty times that number of British soldiers.

During the second half of 1901 and in 1902 Kitchener employed new tactics. He constructed lines of blockhouses connected with barbed wire which divided the whole country into sections whilst large mobile forces conducted systematic drives against the Boer commandos. It seemed to a weary and disillusioned England as if the war would never end. Britain had hardly any friends left in Europe, and a large segment of the continental press was jeering at Britain and holding up her leaders to scorn. But the strength of the Boers was slowly being whittled down. Already thousands of them were prisoners of war in St Helena, India, Ceylon and the Bermuda Islands. They could expect no outside assistance and there was no general revolt of their kinsmen in the Cape Colony.

In January 1902 the Dutch government of Dr A. Kuyper offered to mediate. This offer was rejected by the British, who held that negotiations could only be carried on by Kitchener and the Boer leaders in South Africa. Finally representatives from both parties did meet at a conference at Vereeniging on the Vaal river. The Boers, remembering particularly their women and children in the camps, decided to end the struggle and to accept the British terms. Accordingly, peace was signed on 31 May 1902. The Boers agreed to lay down their arms and to recognize King Edward as their lawful sovereign. The British, on their part, undertook to make a contribution towards the repair of war damage as well as a loan to the new colonies. They promised also that self-government would be introduced as soon as possible, and that the matter of voting rights for Bantu people would not be raised before that time.

The new administration's main task was to rebuild the devastated country and to resettle the civilian population. When Milner set out to anglicize the schools, the Afrikaners, now led by their one-time generals as politicians, reacted by establishing private schools. Before the end of 1904 a political revival of the Afrikaners took place, led by Generals Botha and Smuts in the Transvaal and Abraham Fischer, seconded by Generals J. B. M. Hertzog and C. R. de Wet in the Free State. Milnerism was fought tooth and nail on the political platform. When the High Commissioner returned to England in 1905, the Afrikaners were glad to see the last of a man they considered to be their deadly enemy. A significant cultural revival also commenced with a new movement in favour of Afrikaans, which was now proving to be an effective medium for the noblest literary expression. The lost war served as an inspiration, and a new generation grew up, as anti-British as their forebears.

The victory of the Liberal Party at the polls in England in 1905 brought Sir Henry Campbell-Bannerman to power as Prime Minister. In consequence the former republics were granted self-government much sooner than expected. The Transvaal in 1906 and the Free State in 1907 obtained constitutions which made provision for full local self-government and ministerial responsibility. General Botha, the last Commandant-General of the old Republic, became the first Prime Minister of the Transvaal, with Smuts as one of his ministers. In the Free State, Fischer became Premier with Hertzog as his chief adviser and power behind the throne.

The achievement of constitutional equality between the northern and the coastal colonies was a necessary preliminary step towards a South African federation or union. Railway tariff and customs competition between the colonies had not lessened after the war, and there was a general feeling in favour of closer political ties. War had strengthened the Afrikaners' sense of national solidarity, and there was a unanimous desire for closer union. In May 1908, therefore, representatives from the four colonies assembled at a Customs Conference at Pretoria. They decided that the customs and tariff problems could only be solved by uniting the country. With this purpose a National Convention met in Durban before the end of the year. This body, representing all shades of white opinion, drew up a constitution for the Union of South Africa. The three High Commission territories of Basutoland, Bechuanaland and Swaziland were not included because the majority of the members of the Convention would not grant equal voting rights to the inhabitants. Rhodesia, which had not yet attained the status of a self-governing colony, was likewise excluded from the Union for the time being.

The Convention further decided that each colony, now to be a province of the Union, would retain its own laws concerning Bantu and other non-white political rights. The Cape franchise was entrenched in the constitution. In practice the Bantu and coloured people would accordingly acquire the suffrage on the same terms as white people in the Cape, and theoretically also in Natal. In the two northern provinces, where non-whites had always been excluded, their position remained unchanged. In regard to the Union itself there would be no further attempt at direct intervention from Downing Street.

The Union of South Africa was established formally on 31 May

1910, with General Louis Botha as its first Prime Minister. With its mixed population, with deeply rooted differences between the two white elements on the one hand and between white and non-white on the other, the young state had accepted a fearful legacy of the past.

BIBLIOGRAPHY

Butler, Jeffrey. 'Sir Alfred Milner on British policy in South Africa in 1897', in *Boston University papers in African history*, vol. I, Jeffrey Butler, ed. Boston University Press, 1964.

Butler, Sir William. *Autobiography*, London. 1913.

The Cambridge history of the British Empire, vol. VIII: *South Africa*. Cambridge University Press, 1936.

Colvin, Ian Duncan. *The life of Jameson*. London, 1922.

Davenport, Thomas Rodney Hope. *The Afrikaner bond: the history of a South African political party, 1880–1911*. Oxford University Press, 1966.

De Kiewiet, C. W. *The imperial factor in South Africa: a study in politics and economics*. Cambridge University Press, 1937.

Gross, Felix. *Rhodes of Africa*. London, 1956.

Hancock, Sir William Keith. *Smuts*, vol. I: *The sanguine years, 1870–1919*. Cambridge University Press, 1962.

Headlam, Cecil, ed. *The Milner papers*. 2 vols. London, 1931–3.

Hofmeyr, Jan H. *The life of Jan Hendrik Hofmeyr*. Cape Town, 1913.

Jaarsveld, Floris Albertus van. *The awakening of Afrikaner nationalism, 1868–1881*, trans. by F. R. Metrowich. Cape Town, 1961.

Krüger, Daniel Wilhelmus. *Paul Kruger*. 2 vols., in Afrikaans. Johannesburg, 1961–3.

Le May, Godfrey H. L. *British supremacy in South Africa, 1899–1907*. Oxford, Clarendon Press, 1965.

Lockhart, J. G., and C. M. Woodhouse. *Cecil Rhodes: the colossus of Southern Africa*. New York, 1963.

Marais, Johannes Stephanus. *The fall of Kruger's Republic*. Oxford, Clarendon Press, 1961.

Miller, E. B. I. *Lord Milner and South Africa*. London, 1902.

Molteno, Sir James Tennant. *The dominion of Afrikanderdom: recollections pleasant and otherwise*. London, 1923.

Newton, Arthur Percival, ed. *Select documents relating to the unification of South Africa*. 2 vols. London, 1924.

Pakenham, Elizabeth, Lady Pakenham. *Jameson's raid*. London, 1960.

Preller, Gustav. *Lobengula: the tragedy of a Matabele king*. Johannesburg, 1963.

Thompson, Leonard M. *The unification of South Africa, 1902–1910.* Oxford, Clarendon Press, 1960.

Vindex (pseud. of F. Verschoyle). *Cecil Rhodes: his political life and speeches, 1881–1900.* London, 1900.

Vulliamy, Colwyn E. *Outlanders: a study of imperial expansion in South Africa, 1877–1902.* London, 1938.

Williams, Basil. *Cecil Rhodes.* New ed. London, 1938.

Worsfold, W. Basil. *Lord Milner's work in South Africa from its commencement in 1897 to the Peace of Vereeniging in 1902.* London, 1906.

Wrench, Sir Evelyn. *Alfred Lord Milner, the man of no illusions, 1854–1925.* London, 1958.

CHAPTER II

UNECONOMIC IMPERIALISM: PORTUGAL IN AFRICA BEFORE 1910

by RICHARD J. HAMMOND

'Poor Portugal!' wrote the British Prime Minister, Salisbury, on the occasion of the treaty of 1891 that ended the Portuguese dream of coast-to-coast dominion in Central Africa.[1] 'Poor Portugal!' echoed Miguel de Unamuno in December 1908, at the end of an essay entitled 'A Suicidal Nation' (*Un Pueblo Suicida*) that commented on the ingrained pessimism of Portuguese leaders, not infrequently carried to the point of self-destruction. The writers Antero de Quental, Camilo Castelo Branco and Trindade Coelho, the sculptor Soares dos Reis, the sometime colonial governors Cabral Moncada and Mousinho de Albuquerque—all men tolerably successful, or more, by mundane standards—had one and all taken their own lives within the previous twenty years.

The same spirit of pessimism runs through the work of the great historian Oliveira Martins; not for nothing was he, along with the great novelist Eça de Queiroz, a member of a group styling itself *Vencidos da Vida* ('Those defeated by Life'). The feeling was shared by the King, Carlos I—mainly German by blood and dilettante by temperament—who (Unamuno says) styled Portugal 'a lousy hole' (*uma piolheira*). Unamuno adds that the assassination of the king in February 1908, which virtually ended the dynasty, was also a suicide, morally speaking.[2] To despair of the commonwealth, at any rate in private, was almost (one might think) a requirement for Portuguese public men; to despair of the overseas territories, even more so. '...the annals of our colonial administration', wrote Oliveira Martins in 1880, 'are a web of misery and disgrace'; he went on to urge that the colonies, with the possible exception of Angola, be leased to those 'who can do what we most decidedly cannot'. 'Our colonies', declared

[1] Lady Gwendolen Cecil, *Life of Robert, Marquis of Salisbury* (London, 1932), IV, 275.
[2] Reprinted in Unamuno, *Por Tierras de Portugal y de España*, 2nd ed. (Buenos Aires, 1944), pp. 82–90.

A. F. Nogueira, a senior official of the Banco National Ultramarino, some years later,

oblige us to incur expenses we cannot afford: for us to demand more sacrifices from the home taxpayer so as to conserve, out of mere ostentation, mere display, mere prejudice (as is the case), colonies that serve no useful purpose and will always bring us into discredit, is the height of absurdity and barbarity besides.[1]

That was in 1893, at a time when the Portuguese state, after incurring debts for forty years on the sort of terms habitually extended to borrowers with poor credit, had at length justified its low credit rating by a declaration of national bankruptcy. In 1895 the very Minister of Marine and Colonies, the naval officer Ferreira de Almeida, was a man who had twice introduced parliamentary motions in favour of selling some of the colonies and using the proceeds to develop the remainder. In 1909 another minister, Augusto de Castilho, told the Lower House that his department was the Cinderella of cabinet discussions. Even in 1890, at the height of the controversy with England over Nyasaland, a government spokesman admitted not knowing where one of the key places at issue was situated.

Outside political circles indifference toward, and ignorance of, colonial questions was even more marked. Emigrants from the over-populated northern provinces went not to the African territories but to Brazil; wealthy investors, such as there were, mostly fought shy of colonial enterprises; of middle-class colonists, such as Great Britain sent to countries like Rhodesia, there were none. 'The *Montepio Geral*', wrote a colonial governor-general indignantly in 1907, 'is replete with Portuguese funds, yet of all the *contos* of *réis* deposited therein, not one is drawn out to be invested in Moçambique.'[2]

In the light of these sentiments the historical phenomenon that actually occurred, and that left the infant Portuguese republic of 1910 effectively controlling a greater area of African territory than the kings of Portugal had ever controlled, is something calling for explanation. The Hobson–Lenin theory of economic imperialism seems evidently ruled out, in this instance even more than in the others where its most

[1] J. P. Oliveira Martins, *O Brasil e as colónias Portuguesas*, 5th ed. (Lisbon, 1920), p. 223; A. F. Nogueira, *A ilha de S. Thomé, a questão bancaria no ultramar e o nosso problema colonial* (Lisbon, 1893), p. 154.
[2] A. Freire de Andrade, *Relatórios de Moçambique* (Lourenço Marques, Imprensa Nacional, 1908), III, 5.

obvious weakness was its failure to explain the *modus operandi* by which the capitalist seeking new fields to exploit was able to manipulate the machinery of the imperialist state. Oddly enough, a Portuguese Minister of Foreign Affairs, Barbosa de Bocage, anticipated Hobson in part by nearly a generation when he wrote in 1885:

At this time the attention of Europe is directed avidly toward the Black Continent, and the most powerful nations are making ardent efforts to find markets there for the over-abundant products of their industries, and to secure raw materials the known supplies of which are threatened with exhaustion.[1]

This reference to the economic imperialism of *others*, however, took for granted something that certainly required to be explained—namely, why Africa should appear to be a promising field for capitalist exploitation. '...the negroes of Senegal and the Congo', remarked the French economist Yves Guyot in that selfsame year 1885, '...have no need of our products, or, having need, have not the purchasing power with which to buy them.' 'Our colonies', he declared, 'are an outlet not for our industry and commerce, but for the taxpayers' money.'[2] Goschen, the British Chancellor of the Exchequer whose name was a synonym for financial conservatism, evinced the same views when he refused Harry Johnston a paltry two thousand pounds for treaty-making with Central African chiefs. One wonders whether the alleged economic advantages of imperial conquests, as set out by such men as Joseph Chamberlain and Jules Ferry, were not in part at least a cover for the innate predatoriness of national states—using capitalists as a stalking-horse, rather than being used by them. Such a view is more plausible than the other in that it admits the possibility that governments constitute in themselves an autonomous political force, and asserts no imperative need to look for the puppet-master manipulating the strings of the professional politician.

At any rate, one will look in vain at nineteenth-century Portugal for signs of imperialist motives extraneous to her small and socially homogeneous governing group. When Eça de Queiroz wrote sardonically that the Portuguese wanted colonies simply for the pleasure of contemplating them on the map, he neither strayed beyond, nor fell

[1] Quoted in F. M. da Costa Lobo, *O Conselheiro José Luciano de Castro e o segundo período constitucional monarquico* (Coimbra, 1941), p. 141.
[2] *Lettres sur la politique coloniale* (Paris, 1885), pp. 99, 101.

far short of, the simple truth. Along with the pleasure of contemplation went not only a consciousness of past national glory, but a belief—which still persists and for which no rational explanation suffices—that the possession of territory overseas constituted some kind of justification, and hence some guarantee, for the continued existence of Portugal as an independent national state. (The real guarantee is constituted by the great natural strength of the country's land frontiers, coupled with its ability to summon help overseas in case of attack from or through Spain.)

Such motives would have been insufficient to set Portugal on an empire-building path *de novo*, in competition with the great powers to which much of its former imperial inheritance had fallen. But, even after the Peninsular War, the loss of Brazil and a generation of almost incessant civil strife, an exhausted and impoverished kingdom was left with title to a sizeable portion of the seaboard of Africa, both east and west—a patrimony so meagre, it seemed, as to be worth no one's taking—and it was this that by dint of tenacity, the forbearance of others, and a certain amount of good fortune, was transformed into the relatively solid holdings of 1910. The process is at once a vivid illustration of the power of past history to influence events and a testimony to the impossibility of historical prophecy. No one, Portuguese or not, looking at the state of the realm in 1860, would have forecast the actual outcome, for its overseas possessions, of the next fifty years; and half-way and more through that period that outcome would have appeared, if anything, even less probable than before. (Perhaps it is partly because Portuguese colonial rule, by its very persistence, seems to defy the inevitable trends and broad movements to which a certain type of historical exegesis is addicted that it has frequently been so unpopular in circles considering themselves intellectually enlightened: but that is by the way.)

The *disjecta membra* of empire that were left to Portugal in and around Africa by the middle of the nineteenth century consisted, apart from the South Atlantic islands (the Cape Verdes, São Tomé and Príncipe), of a number of scattered settlements on the coast or on off-shore islands, together with their immediate environs. Their possession served as basis for claims to suzerainty over the hinterland, claims sporadically enforced by military incursions and alliances with native rulers, but seldom undisputed by these for any considerable period. Repudiation of Portuguese political control, as with the Dembos of northern

Angola after 1872 or the Cruz family in Zambezia about the same time, was quite consistent with professions of Christianity, with the adoption of quasi-European ways of life, and with the use of Portuguese as a lingua franca. In these ways, as in the use of crops like maize and manioc that originally derived from Brazil, the influence of Portuguese-speaking missionaries and traders far transcended the limits of political authority.

For centuries previously, of course, there had been a mutually advantageous link between the coast settlers and the native authorities in the form of the slave-trade. On the west coast particularly, slaves constituted the staple, almost the sole, export and hence the principal means by which desired imports were secured: as late as 1825 nine-tenths of the exports of Luanda by value consisted of slaves, and the export tax on slaves constituted four-fifths of the total revenues of the province of Angola. (A similar situation prevailed at Benguela, the province of which, together with that of Angola, made up the 'government-general' of Angola.) It is not surprising that when the reforming liberal minister, Sá da Bandeira, decreed (1836) the abolition of the slave-trade everywhere in the Portuguese dominions, the decree should have proved impossible to enforce in the overseas provinces. Not until first a unilateral and typically high-handed Act of the British Parliament, passed in 1839 at the instance of Lord Palmerston, and thereafter an Anglo-Portuguese treaty of 1842, provided for the right of search to be exercised in Portuguese–African waters by the British navy, were powers available to make the law effective. Their exercise contributed, no doubt, to the economic decline which was noted by visitors to Luanda in mid-century and from which some measure of recovery began in the sixties, triggered perhaps by the temporary stimulus to cotton production that arose from the American Civil War.

Just as the Angolan settlements, for the greater part of their history, had been essentially tributary to Brazil, so those on the coast of Moçambique, from Ibo south to Lourenço Marques, had been tributary to Portuguese India; it was not until the mid-eighteenth century that Moçambique became a government-general separate from that at Goa, and the Archbishop of Goa retained spiritual jurisdiction in Moçambique for at least a century more.

The slave-trade here was on a smaller scale, but took longer to suppress; the indented coast was difficult to police and over much of it there was no European control; the slave-ships, Arab dhows for the most part, were small and hence difficult to intercept; the haul, mostly to Indian Ocean islands, was short compared with that across the Atlantic. The Portuguese settlements, by the nineteenth century, were poverty-stricken and isolated from one another, even by sea. When, in 1842, the southern outpost among them, Lourenço Marques, was destroyed and the governor killed in a native raid, the authorities at Moçambique did not hear of the happening until a year later, by way of Rio de Janeiro.

If to dislodge the Portuguese from such natural strong-points as the islands of Moçambique and Ibo was beyond the capacity of the neighbouring chiefs, advance into the interior was equally beyond that of the forces at their governors' command. Only in and near Zambezia, where the private armies of the great prazo-holders might on occasion be put at the disposal of constituted authority, was there some prospect of strengthening Portuguese hold on the dominion to which they laid nominal claim. It was with the aid of such forces that Angoche was occupied in 1861 (and, for that matter, the Barué district subdued as late as 1902); but no fewer than four similar expeditions mounted against the 'rebel' prazo-holder of Massangano on the Zambezi, António Vicente da Cruz ('O Bonga') in the late sixties were complete failures, and a fifth was abandoned after two years of preparation before it could set out. Such expeditions were undertaken on grounds of prestige alone, for there is no evidence that the Bonga interfered seriously with the trade route to the upper Zambezi. Even had they been successful, they could nowise have been justified economically—not because they were excessively expensive in blood and treasure, even in terms of Portuguese resources, but because the net return must have been, mundanely speaking, negligible.

These strivings, feeble though they were, bear witness to the vitality of the Portuguese imperial idea and to their ability to prevent themselves from being wholly swallowed up in what Winwood Reade, with Victorian bluntness, called 'Savage Africa'. In common with other visitors, he noted the 'European' character of the city of Luanda. A Portuguese writer in the mid-seventies, describing the streets and squares of the city of Moçambique, remarked that the principal square contained 'an elegant bandstand...where the band of the 1st battalion of chasseurs plays on Thursdays and Saturdays, attracting a numerous attendance'.[1] He might have been writing of any small provincial town

[1] Manuel Ferreira Ribeiro, *A Província de S. Thomé e Príncipe* (Lisbon, Imprensa Nacional, 1877), p. 257.

in Portugal itself. A generation earlier the persistence of the Portuguese tradition had been exemplified in the lonely and successful effort of Honório Pereira Barreto, the black African Governor of Portuguese Guinea, to prevent the French from taking over the whole littoral of Senegambia. It would have been easy for Barreto to make himself into an independent ruler; he simply preferred to regard his country as 'a tiny and unfortunate, but integral part' of the Portuguese nation, and he was hurt when the prime minister of the day referred to him as 'a coloured man'.[1]

The ability of the home government either to help or to control these outposts was, of course, extremely limited, the more so since it was for a time unable to compel its own armed forces to serve overseas. Conditions in most of the African settlements did not permit Europeans to settle and multiply, and the population there was maintained only by the shipment of convicts and by miscegenation. Contrary to the speculations of Gilberto Freyre and the statements of some modern Portuguese authorities, racial mixture has always been a matter of necessity rather than policy; willingness to cohabit with black or mulatto women being, come to think of it, perfectly compatible with keeping black men in a state of servitude or social inferiority. Portuguese imperialists like António Enes (Ennes) or, in the present century, Vincente Ferreira, regarded the practice with as much abhorrence as any British proconsul of the old school:

Going native [wrote Enes in 1893] is a species of reversion of civilized man to savagery, and its main agent is the negress. Africa charged the negress with avenging her [conquest] on the European, and it is she, the hideous one—for there is no negress that is not hideous!—who causes the proud conquerors of the Black Continent to fall victim to the sensuality of the monkey, to the base and inhuman practices of the slavemonger, to the delirium of alcoholism, to all the brutalizations of an inferior race, and even to the teeth of the hyenas scavenging in the graveyards.[2]

Half a century later, Ferreira was to recommend segregation as a means of preserving the racial purity of Portuguese agrarian settlers in Angola who, he thought, should not be allowed to employ black labour. Both these influential men were, in effect, repudiating as a 'necessary mistake' the historical basis of Portuguese dominion in Brazil and Africa alike.

[1] Barreto observed bitterly many years afterwards that the offending phrase had been printed in italics (Jaime Walter, *Honório Pereira Barreto* (Bissau, 1947), pp. 79, 166).
[2] *Moçambique; relatório apresentado ao govêrno*, 3rd ed. (Lisbon, 1946), p. 193.

Dominion in Africa could scarcely have survived into the twentieth century were it not for that very process of opening-up which at one time bid fair to be fatal to it. In the last quarter of the nineteenth century, first the Moçambique coast and then the hinterland ceased to be backwaters remote from the mainstreams of international trade and communication. The Suez Canal was opened in 1869; in 1879 the Eastern Telegraph Company's cable, en route to Cape Town, established 'anchor points' at Moçambique town and Lourenço Marques; in 1867 gold and diamonds had been discovered in southern Africa. In 1886 the telegraph line reached Luanda, likewise en route to the Cape. For the first time in history there were reliable and swift communications between Portugal and the overseas capitals—the importance of which for effective government can hardly be overestimated. Moreover, the prospect, if no more, of economic development presented itself, for it was hardly conceivable that some of the progress being charted elsewhere in Africa should not rub off, so to speak, on Angola and Moçambique. On her own, Portugal could expect to accomplish little in Africa; but if others should set things moving, she might, given luck and skill, be able to extract some advantage at least from her historic claims.

The Portuguese statesman who saw most clearly what had to be done was João de Andrade Corvo, in some ways a disciple of Sá da Bandeira but possessed of a more powerful analytical mind. Sá da Bandeira's liberalism, which led him almost single-handed to undertake the outlawry of the slave-trade and the abolition by stages of slavery in the overseas provinces, was a matter of moral conviction; it was an article of faith with him that such a course could not but lead to better things for Portugal's African subjects. Corvo shared these beliefs, but, living as he did in the age of the Franco-Prussian War and the re-emergence of a frank militarism in Europe, was less inclined to suppose that liberalism would triumph by reason of its innate merits. For him, the war of 1870 constituted a latent threat to the existence of the smaller European nations; and the way of safety for Portugal lay in strengthening the bonds of the alliance with Great Britain, whose interests were likewise threatened by the appearance of strong military powers on the continent.

Unfortunately the alliance was regarded by the majority of Portuguese politicians, who were usually French in cultural, if not political, sympathies, as at best a necessary evil; the frequent exhibitions of high-handedness by the British in their dealings with their ally, coupled with the Philistine arrogance of many British residents in Portugal and the attacks of Livingstone and his followers on alleged Portuguese mis-government overseas, were not calculated to make the connexion popular. For the British government, the relationship was that between a wealthy patron and a client of such long standing and such dependence that his dignity and self-respect were of little account. 'It is far better', ran a Foreign Office minute of 1876, 'to have to deal with the worst savages than with the best-intentioned Portuguese':[1] and it was on this principle (supplemented latterly by traders' objections to the Portuguese tariff) that the British had, for thirty years previously, refused to admit the long-standing Portuguese claim, embodied in the Consti-tutional Charter of 1826, to the coast on either side of the Congo mouth.

When one party to a prospective deal is indifferent and the other touchy, only the strongest sense of mutual interest is likely to bring them to terms; and such a sense was only intermittently present during the Anglo-Portuguese negotiations concerning Africa, which were all but continuous for the better part of a decade after 1875. They had begun propitiously enough, with the settlement by French arbitration of a dispute of half-a-century's standing, one of several that had embittered relations between the allies. In an award of July 1875, President Mac-Mahon confirmed the Portuguese claim to the whole of Delagoa Bay and rejected that of the British to the coast immediately south of the settlement of Lourenço Marques, which thus became the undisputed outport for the Boer republic of the Transvaal. (In view of later misunderstandings it is important to emphasize that the possession of Lourenço Marques itself was not an issue in the arbitration.)[2] Portugal and the Transvaal thereupon concluded a revised version of their existing territorial treaty of 1869, in which they made specific provision for the building of a railroad from Lourenço Marques to Pretoria. This treaty would have needed to be ratified by the British as suzerain power over the Transvaal; eventually it was so ratified, in 1882, but only after a bizarre episode that did harm to Anglo-Portuguese relations and was thought by some to have endangered the stability of the Portuguese monarchy.

[1] Quoted in R. T. Anstey, *Britain and the Congo in the nineteenth century* (Oxford, 1962), p. 54.

[2] An official British publication of 1907 (the so-called Selborne Memorandum on the future of South Africa, actually drafted by Lionel Curtis) fell into this error. See p. 53 of the reprint edited by Basil Williams (London, 1925).

This episode, the first of many in which Portugal was involved willynilly in the complex and turbulent course of Anglo-Boer relations, arose from no action of her own, but from the British annexation of the Transvaal in 1877 and its subsequent retrocession in 1881. A fresh agreement over the Lourenço Marques railway was necessitated by the annexation; and negotiations for a comprehensive treaty were begun between Corvo and Robert Morier, the forceful British Minister in Lisbon from 1876 to 1881. But the British Colonial Office, at whose instance the negotiations had been started, blew hot and cold over the financial provisions; the Zulus' defeat of the British at Isandhlwana cast temporary doubt on their prospects in South Africa; and the Fontes government, in which Corvo was Foreign Minister, fell on the morrow of the signing of the so-called Lourenço Marques treaty (May 1879). The terms of that treaty were admittedly not obviously favourable to Portugal, and they were so bitterly attacked, particularly by the rising Republican party, that both monarchist parties sought to avoid the odium of ratifying it.

Some modifications were made in the hope of appeasing the opponents of the treaty; but in the meantime the Boers had risen against the British and defeated them at Majuba Hill (February 1881). In face of this Gladstone, the British Prime Minister, reverted to the anti-annexation policy that he had proclaimed before the General Election of 1880 but had thought better of after coming into office: by the Pretoria Convention of August 1881 the Boers once again acquired autonomy and the still unratified Lourenço Marques treaty became otiose, inasmuch as its railway and transit clauses were no longer the direct concern of the British government. Incidental casualties were a provision for freedom of navigation on the Zambezi; an agreement for mutual action against the slave-trade on the east coast of Africa; and the ministerial career of Corvo. (Morier, whom his political chief Granville described as having the dangerous habit of turning small things into great, was transferred first to Madrid and subsequently to St Petersburg, where he was credited with the peaceful solution of the Penjdeh incident.)

The intense anti-British feeling that had been aroused in Portugal by the time the treaty was dropped was to some extent synthetic, the work of the Republicans who were anxious for any stick to beat the monarchy with, along with the habitual factiousness of Portuguese politics—what Morier in his trenchant way called 'morbid pseudo-patriotism'. But behind the shouting and exaggeration there lay a genuine sense of the national dignity which was anything but mercenary and which Morier and his compatriots persistently underrated. Most Portuguese political leaders were intensely sensitive to any charge of sacrificing this dignity for the sake of material advantage, even when that advantage was more obvious than in the case of the Lourenço Marques treaty; and they generally preferred to yield to *force majeure* rather than incur the odium of willingly sacrificing a national interest or a slice of territory howsoever insignificant.

Corvo, disinterested and magnanimous, was indeed prepared to admit that the natural northern frontier of Angola was the 'Zaire' (Congo) and that the Portuguese 'fort' at Ouidah was 'a mere source of expense and vexation'. But even he acknowledged that any proposal to alienate territory included in the Constitutional Charter was fraught with political difficulty. Corvo, indeed, might be said to be a believer in the 'imperialism of free trade', though not in the sense in which recent writers have employed that phrase, to mean the use of free trade as a weapon of expansion. Admitting (as who could not?) the improbability that Portugal would ever become able to develop her overseas possessions from her metropolitan resources, he was prepared to open them to foreign trade and investment and let the question of sovereignty take care of itself. Hence the new liberal tariff introduced in Moçambique in 1879, in which transit duties were reduced to a mere three per cent.

One of the criticisms levelled at Corvo over the Lourenço Marques treaty had been based on his failure to demand as a *quid pro quo* for the concessions to the British—such as a separate customs-house for the transit trade in Lourenço Marques—that they recognize the old claim to the Congo coast between latitudes 8° and 5° 12′ S. This had, in fact, been no more than a tactical omission, agreed upon between Morier and Corvo with the intention of making a separate treaty creating a condominium of all the interested powers to administer the territory north of the Congo mouth. Whether the Côrtes would have ratified such a scheme, which was embodied by Morier in a sketch for a treaty drawn up in 1881, is more than doubtful; but it would have had the enormous tactical advantage of inviting the concurrence of other interested countries from the outset, and it would have disarmed the opposition of trading interests that professed to fear the traditional exclusiveness of Portuguese tariff policy. The result of the long wrangle over the Lourenço Marques treaty was to delay the Congo negotiations, and to place them in the hands of men—less far-seeing than Corvo and Morier—who anticipated neither the objections of other European powers nor the opposition from British trading-cum-philanthropic interests, egged on by King Leopold of Belgium.

It was partly, perhaps mainly, in an effort to placate these interests that the British stiffened their terms during the course of negotiations, and so delayed their conclusion. The Portuguese, for their part, made the tactical error—in which the British concurred—of proposing an Anglo-Portuguese commission to control navigation on the Congo in lieu of the international commission that had originally been suggested. The effect was to make the treaty as signed look like an attempt to settle the Congo question by a private deal between two powers, of which the greater had not even the *locus standi* conferred by a territorial claim. Such obtuse high-handedness received its deserts when Bismarck, in agreement with the French, announced in June 1884 that he could not accept the treaty and proposed that the question be settled by mutual agreement of all the interested powers.

The ensuing Berlin West African conference and the territorial settlement that accompanied it were galling to the Portuguese, the more so since the territories in the Congo hinterland they were obliged to renounce went, not to a great power, but to King Leopold's Congo Association—'a private company, of uncertain nationality and no known articles of association', as the Portuguese Foreign Minister, Bocage, indignantly described it. They felt that the British ally had been indecently ready to throw them over, and that the propaganda of the humanitarians had deprived them of their historic rights.

In terms of 'effective occupation'—the new principle laid down by the Conference for adjudging claims to the African coastline—they had not, however, done at all badly. They were given title to the Angolan coastline as far as the Congo mouth, and to its left bank up to and including Noki. The Cabinda enclave, north of the Congo, embodied at any rate part of their old claims. Moreover, they had secured these without the concessions on which the British had insisted as a *quid pro quo*: freedom of navigation on the Zambezi, and the fixing of the western boundary of Moçambique at the junction of the Shire and the Ruo. Though their new acquisitions were to form part of the low-tariff 'conventional basin' of the Congo, an attempt to neutralize them in time of war had been, with French help, beaten off. No one other than a Portuguese would say that they had been hard done by, or that due respect had not been afforded to history, or that they did not retain title to far more of Africa than they could hope to exploit. Corvo was almost alone among Portuguese in being *willing* to compromise on such points: as a member of the British Foreign Office remarked a few years later, the Portuguese would accept a *fait accompli*, 'but will never abandon the dogma that Africa belongs to Portugal'.[1]

Certainly the disappointments of the Berlin conference did not diminish the Portuguese resolve to hold on in Africa, more particularly to the hinterland between Angola and Moçambique—what one writer, in 1880, called 'our Angolo-Moçambiquan province'—that had long fascinated Portuguese travellers and had most recently been traversed by Serpa Pinto. They had at that time no notion of administering the area directly, but rather, as an article added to the boundary conventions signed with France and Germany in 1886 put it, that the 'King of Portugal' should 'exercise his sovereign and civilizing influence in the territories'— that the king should be, in practice, a kind of paramount White Chief.

At no time were Portuguese military resources equal, without the aid of numerous African auxiliaries, to the task of occupying large areas of the continent. The total establishment of first-line troops in Angola in 1886, for instance, was less than 3,000 officers and men, who were badly housed and armed; and any attempt to raise native levies in inland areas like Bailundo and Bihé was apt to bring about a complete paralysis of the bush trade on which the exports, and hence the income, of the province depended. There was nothing in Angola, of course, that corresponded in a military sense to the *prazo* system in Zambezia. (The *prazos* were great semi-feudal estates, initially granted by the Portuguese for the purpose of encouraging European settlement and assuring Portuguese control in the far interior. As time went on, the *prazos* came to be held mainly by estate owners of Goan and mulatto origin.) The Portuguese penetrated deeper into the inland regions of Moçambique than into those of Angola; military expeditions, dispatched usually from Quelimane, extended Portugal's 'sovereign and civilizing influence' into some of the remoter areas of Portuguese East Africa. The Portuguese thus encountered British opposition rather earlier, perhaps, than they might otherwise have done.

[1] Villiers Lister, quoted in Richard J. Hammond, *Portugal and Africa, 1815–1910: a study in uneconomic imperialism* (Stanford University Press, 1966), pp. 77–8.

After the fiasco of the Congo treaty, the Portuguese abandoned Corvo's policy of co-operation with the 'faithful ally'—a phrase frequently used in sarcasm by the Lisbon press—and strove rather to win the support of France and more especially of Germany. The figure commonly identified with this policy is the *progressista* Foreign Minister, Barros Gomes, but it had actually been initiated by his *regenerador* predecessor Bocage. (*Regeneradores* and *progressistas* were members of opposing political parties which succeeded one another in office under a system scathingly referred to as *rotativismo*.) It seems to have been based on pique and an excessive respect for Bismarck's prowess at the Berlin conference rather than on a close calculation of diplomatic forces; for while it was true that the Congo treaty had come to grief through ignoring French and German interests there, this did not constitute a case for making the same error in reverse and ignoring British interests around Lake Nyasa. The acquiescence of France and Germany in Portuguese ambitions was indeed obtained in principle (though in the latter case only by the surrender of a strip of Angolan territory south of the Cunene River); but, significantly, subject to the rights of other powers and without definition of the territory affected. Only a naïve politician would have read the provisos of the 1886 agreements (by which France and Germany acknowledged Portuguese sovereign rights to an extensive territorial belt linking Angola and Moçambique) as a licence to Portugal from France and Germany to go ahead; as events were to prove, they were a warning to her that those powers would do nothing to help if she embroiled herself with Great Britain.

If Barros Gomes and his colleagues had played their cards more skilfully they might, even so, have achieved their object; for the British long seemed reluctant to show their hand and declare a protectorate over the missionary settlements in the Nyasa region. Indeed, as late as 1888–9 Foreign Office minutes were describing this as 'impracticable', and such apostles of empire as Harry Johnston and John Kirk were recommending that the area be ceded to the Portuguese as not being worth quarrelling over. The only access to it from the outside world lay through territory acknowledged as Portuguese; even though the British claimed—contrary to the opinion of their own leading international lawyer, Sir Travers Twiss—that the Zambezi was an international, and not a Portuguese, river. The portage overland from the channel above Quelimane was over territory unquestionably Portuguese; hence the capital importance of Daniel Rankin's discovery, or rather rediscovery, of the Chinde mouth of the Zambezi, which became known in London in late April 1889. ('The free passage along the Zambezi', Salisbury at once noted, 'we can take for ourselves whenever the Zambezi becomes physically accessible from the sea.'[1])

The discovery came at a time when the British government and public were becoming increasingly exasperated with Portugal both for obstructing the passage of arms and ammunition wanted by the Nyasa settlers for defence against Arab slave-raiders from the north, and on account of a variety of other provocations. These varied from such trivia as the arrest of a vice-consul on a charge not so much trumped-up as unintelligible, and a decree enforcing the wearing of trousers on British Indian traders whose religion forbade it, to the furtive sending of treaty-making expeditions into precisely those areas of the hinterland in which the British were known to have an actual or prospective interest, and the revocation of the Delagoa Bay railway concession (June 1889). Some of these actions were due, not to Lisbon, but to over-zealous officials on the spot; for most of them a case in law could be made out. But they were one and all not calculated to promote a peaceable settlement between British and Portuguese—a settlement that was only possible if the chauvinists and the religious zealots could be kept in check.

The last occasion on which such a settlement might have been possible was that of the unofficial Johnston mission to Lisbon in the spring of 1889; the stumbling-block was the proposed cession to Portugal of Blantyre, which aroused strong opposition from the Church of Scotland. But it is arguable that Salisbury virtually organized that opposition, against the advice of his permanent officials, in order to have an excuse to drop the negotiations now that the existence of the Chinde mouth was known;[2] it is also arguable that Barros Gomes, by giving up the trans-African sphere of influence, had made concessions that his government would never have been able to carry in the Côrtes. Upon the very tail of the Johnston mission, moreover, Cecil Rhodes arrived in London to promote his Mashonaland venture and offered to meet the expenses—denied by H.M. Treasury—of a treaty-making trip in the Nyasa region that Johnston had proposed to make in his capacity as Consul at Moçambique. Thereafter, both sides rapidly moved in the direction of a

[1] Minute by Lord Salisbury, 26 April 1889, F.O. Conf. Print No. 5970, Doc. 107.
[2] This is the view taken by Roland Oliver, *Sir Harry Johnston and the scramble for Africa* (London, 1957), pp. 150–1.

showdown; the occasion for it came when the Portuguese, in face of a local and as yet unconfirmed declaration of a British protectorate over the Makololo, crossed the river Ruo in force and annexed the disputed territory. The British had apparently already resolved on a demonstration in force against some Portuguese possession, and now were able to represent the Portuguese as aggressors. In January 1890 Salisbury forced them to withdraw by a public threat to break off diplomatic relations, in which no effort was made to spare the feelings of an ally. That ultimatum is a source of resentment in Portugal to this day.

Patriotic indignation at the time was so great that the Côrtes repudiated the Convention that had been signed with Britain in August 1890, embodying a territorial settlement in Africa. This gave Rhodes's Chartered Company the chance of making further annexations at Portuguese expense, notably on the Manica plateau, supposed to be a second Rand gold-field. This area Salisbury insisted on retaining in the eventual settlement; but he refused to allow the company to retain Macequece (Massi Kessi), or establish suzerainty over Gungunhana, chief of Gaza, which would have brought its territory to the Indian Ocean. The Portuguese dream of a link between Angola and Moçambique was to be ended. Nevertheless, the settlement ultimately imposed on the Portuguese by a treaty of June 1891 was, like that of 1885, moderate, having regard to their actual possessions as distinct from their aspirations. Rhodes, who had wanted to take over virtually everything south of the Zambezi, was hardly less indignant about it than Lisbon. Both France and Germany—less from sympathy with Portugal than from fear of republicanism in the Iberian Peninsula—had urged moderation on the British, and doubtless would have demanded an equivalent for any extensive annexations on their part. Moreover, there was no evident need to hasten a process of disintegration that—to most European and perhaps to most Portuguese politicians—must have seemed inevitable anyway.

The disappearance of Portugal from the African scene seemed to be brought a stage nearer when, in June 1892, she defaulted on two-thirds of the interest on her foreign debt: being already in peril—it was hopefully believed—of having to pay a swingeing indemnity for expropriating the London company that was building the railway from Lourenço Marques to the Transvaal border. Smiling vultures of various nationalities looked forward, first to the mortgaging of the colonies for fresh loans, and thereafter to the day of foreclosure. Successive Portuguese governments hung on in a kind of despairing tenacity, hardly hoping, for a time, to do more than retain a nominal suzerainty, in Moçambique especially, over the administration of chartered companies whose capital was largely if not wholly foreign. Two of these—the Moçambique and Nyassa companies—were actually brought into being; and a third, for the district of Inhambane, failed to materialize because its promoters were unable to raise the capital. Had it done so, only the immediate environs of the city of Moçambique, the lower Zambezi, and the district of Lourenço Marques would have been subject to direct Portuguese administration.

For a time even Lourenço Marques, which had become something of a boom town since the discovery of gold on the Rand and the building of the Transvaal railway—opened to through traffic in November 1894—seemed likely to escape from Portuguese control. It had, of course, long been coveted both by Great Britain and the Transvaal republic; and in the last quarter of 1894 the town appeared to be threatened by a native insurrection, and hence by foreign occupation on the pretext of maintaining order. Behind the insurrection, perhaps correctly, the Portuguese saw the hand of Gungunhana, paramount chief of Gazaland: behind Gungunhana, 'Sir' Cecil Rhodes and his Chartered Company, to them the root of all evil. The Chartered Company had indeed endeavoured in 1890–1 to induce Gungunhana to place himself under their protection rather than that of the Portuguese, but had been forced to desist by the British government, once the treaty of 1891 had been ratified. António Enes, who as Royal Commissioner in Moçambique had been charged with putting the provisions of the treaty into effect, was sent out once again to restore order in the district, and determined, if he could, to deal with Gungunhana once and for all. The general belief was that this was beyond Portuguese capacity, for the impis of Gungunhana were feared as far north as the Zambezi. But after a scratch force of Portuguese and Angolan troops, thanks to a combination of resolution and superior armament, had decisively beaten off an attack from five or six times their number at Marracuene, a few miles from Lourenço Marque—leaving the task of mopping up the defeated enemy to their native allies—Enes appears to have made up his mind that Gungunhana was neither militarily nor politically invincible.

To mount an offensive against him was impossible, however, with the resources to hand in the province. Some troops were sent from Portugal (and from Angola); horses, mules and the indispensable draft oxen and wagons were procured in Natal. Two columns, one based on Lourenço Marques and the other on Inhambane, slowly converged upon the chief's kraal, at Manjacaze just north of the Limpopo, during the third quarter of 1895, while parleys for the surrender of the original 'rebel' chiefs went on between Gungunhana and Enes' emissaries. Although the chief appears not to have realized until later that he might no longer turn to the British for support, he had shown a disposition to submit; and it was Enes' desire to put things to the test of force while his fever-ridden armies were still in being, rather than a genuine impasse in the negotiations, that caused them to be broken off. The occasion was another victory at Magul, in September, when the experience of Marracuene was repeated. Even so, it was with the greatest difficulty that the northern column was eventually prevailed upon to leave its advance base and begin the twenty-five-mile march to the kraal. At Coolela, on 7 November, it was attacked by Gungunhana's army of upwards of 8,000 men; and yet again superior fire-power and discipline sufficed to put the enemy to flight. Gungunhana fled from his kraal shortly before the victors approached it; less than two months later he was captured, unresisting, in a bold stroke by the dashing officer Mousinho de Albuquerque. The news of the exploit of Chaimite reached Portugal hard on the heels of the news of Jameson's fiasco; in a single week the two great opponents of Portugal in Africa had been humbled.

The downfall of Gungunhana came at a comparatively early stage of the effective occupation of Moçambique, which was not completed until the eve of the First World War. The occupation of Angola was accomplished only after the Germans of South West Africa, who invaded the colony in September 1914 without the formality of a declaration of war, had been defeated by a South African force under General Botha. The length of the process was due not so much to the amount of resistance to be overcome as to the inability of the Portuguese to afford any but small-scale military expeditions. None the less, the victories of 1895 were decisive, for they restored the national self-respect that had been hurt by the British ultimatum and by a pervading sense of impotence.

After Chaimite there could be no more talk of selling Moçambique. But the financial problem remained. In the first period of shock after the partial repudiation of June 1892, some attempts had been made at budgetary retrenchment; but these had fizzled out at the end of 1893 with the removal of the last of a series of would-be reformers at the Ministry of Finance, Augusto Fuschini; and the successful exploits of 1895, though remarkably inexpensive as colonial wars go, were still a burden on the exchequer. Moreover, large sums needed to be spent on harbour works at Lourenço Marques if it were to retain its paramount position as the port of the Transvaal. By early 1897 the Portuguese government—shut out from the money markets of Europe pending a settlement with its foreign creditors, of whom the majority were French and German—was trying to get a fresh loan through the good offices of the British government, in consideration for effective control of the port and railway of Lourenço Marques. The tense relations between the British and the Transvaal Boers had made such control all but a *sine qua non* of British imperial policy: a Colonial Office memorandum of October 1895 had spoken of the absolute necessity of acquiring Delagoa Bay 'at any cost'.[1]

It was known, however, that other powers would object to such a move: the Germans had made the point brutally clear by sending two warships to Lourenço Marques at the time of the 1894 insurrection, and by the notorious telegram to Kruger on the failure of the Jameson Raid. Some months before that event, Edward Fairfield, the most knowledgeable in African matters of any among the Colonial Office staff, had suggested an arrangement over Delagoa Bay 'confined to the Germans and ourselves'; and German Colonial Office officials had talked earlier of an Anglo-German agreement to settle the inheritance of the Portuguese possessions in Africa. Between such a deal and an open quarrel no third course was open, other than that on which both powers professed to be agreed—the maintenance of full Portuguese control at Lourenço Marques. When, therefore, in the spring of 1898, the Portuguese renewed their request for a loan, which—perhaps at British suggestion—was now to be guaranteed by a charge on the Moçambique customs, it should have been no cause for surprise that the Germans should at once have taken the opportunity to demand an equivalent. The result was the secret treaties of August 1898, providing for a contingent partition between Great Britain and Germany that would include not only Moçambique, but Angola and Portuguese Timor.

[1] *Memorandum* [by G. V. Fiddes] *on the Question of the Delagoa Bay Railway*, Oct. 1895, C.O., Conf. Print, Africa [South] no. 508, 38.

(Portuguese Guinea was not mentioned; it may have been overlooked, or perhaps tacitly left to France by way of compensation.)

For the Germans, the treaties made sense only if one read between the lines a British undertaking to expedite the process of mortgage and foreclosure, in return for a free hand in dealing with the Boers and a united front against the French in south-east Africa; and they considered themselves as having been swindled when the British insisted on the strict letter of the terms. Yet this—as the Germans should have made it their business to verify in advance—was as far as the British could go without an overt breach of long-standing engagements to Portugal. Their obligations under this head were merely reiterated with fresh corollaries in the Anglo-Portuguese Secret Declaration of 1899, concluded after the Boer War had already broken out.

The only substantial effect of the treaties, in fact, was something that had not apparently been intended, namely the discouragement of fresh foreign investment in the Portuguese colonies. Great Britain and Germany had agreed that neither would seek concessions in territory earmarked for the other, and that any substantial concession not in breach of this undertaking should entitle the other power to an equivalent. This agreement in restraint of trade was calculated to discourage the Portuguese from offering concessions to either side, and it discouraged the British, as having the largest existing stake in Moçambique, from trying to increase it. Much of the concession-hunting that had gone on in Lisbon during the nineties was in any case more political than economic, predicated on the continuing rivalry of the powers and the Transvaal. Such a speculation was the Eiffe or Katembe concession at Lourenço Marques, which was actually mentioned in the secret treaties and which was rendered worthless, because politically null, by the Boer War.

By a pleasing irony it was French financial interests that probably gained most influence in Portugal as a result of treaties that were directed against them. The Portuguese government naturally abandoned all intent of raising any loan on the strength of the colonial customs, and instead made arrangements to borrow in France; eventually, with the good offices of the British, it achieved a long-term settlement with its foreign creditors. The British element in the Moçambique Company, which for some years had been planning to oust the French and Belgian elements in order to complete a virtual British take-over in the province of Manica e Sofala, was discouraged by the Foreign Office, so that by

1914 French influence in the company's counsels, though not in its local administration, had become paramount. British interests in the Nyassa Company, whose territory was in the German inheritance, had actually sold out to German banks when the Great War broke out and prevented the deal from being consummated. An attempt by an Anglo-German group to take over the mainly French-owned Mossamedes company was abruptly abandoned on account of the 1898 treaties, which placed the territory in the German inheritance. Most important of all, the British Foreign Office gave the builder of the Benguela Railway, Robert Williams, no assistance in securing his concession, and when he required extra capital advised him to seek it in Germany; while a proposal to establish a chartered company with British capital to develop Portuguese Timor was discouraged on the ostensible ground that the Dutch had been granted the reversion in a reciprocal treaty of 1904 with Portugal.

In these circumstances it was not altogether fitting for the British Foreign Secretary, Grey, and the avowedly pro-German Colonial Secretary, 'Lulu' Harcourt, to complain of the undeveloped state of the Portuguese colonies, or to encourage a revision, which inevitably implied a revival, of the 1898 treaties in the supposed interests of Portugal. The original treaties had had at least an intelligible purpose, and had been made on an appropriate occasion; but with the Boers inside the British Empire, the French attached to the British by the *Entente cordiale*, and the Portuguese not actively seeking a loan secured on the colonial customs, the revised agreements could have no point, other than appeasing Germany, except the greater convenience of some of their details. (Germany was to be entitled to the whole of Angola, together with São Tomé and Príncipe, which were not in the original agreement; Timor was to be excluded and the British were to be compensated by a larger prospective slice of Moçambique.)

If there is one thing more baffling than the willingness of Grey and Harcourt to enter into a deal of this kind, without the evident motive, whether one approve it or not, that inspired their predecessors Chamberlain and Balfour, it is Grey's belief—nay, insistence—that the agreements both with Germany and with Portugal were fit for publication. The German objection to this course, which alone prevented the revised agreements from being ratified, had at any rate logic, and even a kind of propriety, on its side.

Grey's frank dislike of the alliance with Portugal, contrasting with the indifference of most British public men, appears to have been rooted in humanitarian disapproval of her colonial administration. The two aspects of it that he objected to most were the alleged oppression of native workers that took place on the Zambezia *prazos*, and the recruitment of contract labour in Angola for work in the cocoa islands of São Tomé and Príncipe. It is by no means clear whether the acts of individual brutality on the *prazos*, such as the use of the *palmatória* on the hands of offenders, which had been practised from time immemorial, were on a scale that would justify Grey's description of the whole institution as 'abominable', and a limit to economic exploitation, here as elsewhere in Portuguese Africa, was set by the impossibility of preventing the *prazo* inhabitants from leaving. (They were said, for instance, to escape forced labour on the left bank of the Zambezi by crossing to the Moçambique Company's territory on the right bank.) The case of the cocoa labourers, on the other hand, did call in question the very system of administration, and incidentally provided a splendid weapon with which interested parties could attack the continued possession of colonies by Portugal.

In effect, the system of recruitment constituted essentially a survival of slavery in substance though not in legal form. The labourers and their families were technically free, having indeed been freed from slavery by the very process by which they were recruited. But they were seldom if ever in a position to understand the terms of their contracts, and no case was known of any contracted labourer ever having returned from the islands to the mainland.

The device of a contract appears to have been invented by the French for the benefit of their plantation islands in the Indian Ocean and had originally been frowned upon by Portuguese liberal legislators. Indeed, it had occasioned an international *cause célèbre*—the seizure of the French barque *Charles et Georges* in Moçambique waters in 1857—in which the Portuguese, for want of adequate support from their British ally, had had to pay an indemnity to the government of Napoleon III. It had nevertheless been embodied in a Portuguese decree of 1878 that won the encomiums of Morier, the British Minister in Lisbon. But as early as 1882 Granville, on the strength of a report by the British Consul in Luanda, described the system in a dispatch as 'simply a form of slave trade', and in view of the eagerness of British commercial and humanitarian interests to attack Portugal at that time, it is perhaps odd that massive agitation about it was delayed until the twentieth century.

What brought matters to a head was the increasing prosperity of the cocoa industry and hence a much greater demand for labour from Angola at a time when the supply was being affected by the spread of sleeping-sickness in the interior. It was no longer a case of a comparatively decorous recruitment of a regular supply of war captives from areas outside Portuguese jurisdiction, but of the payment of inflated prices that encouraged officials to connive at flagrant illegalities and trenched upon the supply of labour available to planters in Angola itself. In 1901 a decree issued by the government in Lisbon sought to put a stop to recruitment by violent means, such as the forcible seizure of members of trading caravans; pamphlets denouncing the traffic appeared in Luanda; the Bailundo revolt of 1902 was attributed to the same cause; and in 1903 fresh regulations were issued which were immediately denounced in Luanda as an elaborate subterfuge. Not that the Portuguese government or its colonial administrators objected to forced labour: on the contrary, the official view, embodied in a law of 1899, was that it was an essential part of the civilizing process—provided it were done decently and in order. In Angola, as elsewhere on the mainland of Portuguese Africa, the arm of the administration did not reach sufficiently far for such a proviso to be capable of fulfilment: but this was difficult to admit in public.

When the great English muck-raking journalist, H. W. Nevinson, began to expose the scandals of the cocoa islands in *Harper's Magazine* (1905), he set off an agitation that culminated, early in 1909, in a reluctant boycott of the cocoa by the leading British and German manufacturers, and in a libel suit by one of them, against the *Standard* newspaper, which amounted to putting the Portuguese administration on trial without benefit of counsel. By the time that suit was tried, the Portuguese government had held an official inquiry and had actually prohibited the recruitment of labour for the islands until more effective regulations could be devised. But many engaged in the humanitarian agitation were reluctant to give the Portuguese government credit even for good faith—as distinct from efficient administration—and the persistence of the campaign aroused suspicion in the British Foreign Office that the agitators were in connivance with, or at any rate cat's-paws of, German designs on the Portuguese colonies. 'Missionary polemics', remarked Eyre Crowe, 'are notorious for their lack of candor.' (One of the leaders, John H. Harris, a former missionary, was shown to have made allegations of widespread cruelty in São Tomé on the basis of a couple of days' stay in the British Vice-Consul's house.)

The Foreign Office itself, however, might have kept the agitation from reaching such extravagant lengths if it had published, in 1906, its own Consul Nightingale's report, based on a detailed investigation on the spot. This had clearly brought out that the evil lay, not in conditions on the islands (except that sleeping-sickness had become endemic on Príncipe) but in the means of recruitment on the mainland and the want of repatriation. In an attempt to avoid stirring up ill-feeling, the report had been given to the humanitarian organizations in a bowdlerized form and therefore could not be published without exposing the fact. It is, of course, open to question whether the needed reforms might have been brought about by diplomatic pressure alone; but certainly the way in which they were brought about generated the maximum of ill-feeling between the allies.[1]

What incensed many Portuguese was the contrast between the attacks to which they were subject over the contract labourers from Angola and the unwillingness of the British to dispense with the recruitment of Moçambique labourers for the Rand gold-mines, where conditions were just as dysgenic as they were on São Tomé and the numbers involved far greater. Leaving aside the obvious economic motive for this difference (which was one of the reasons for not publishing the Nightingale Report, lest the Portuguese retaliate against the Rand), it could be argued that recruitment for the mines was genuinely voluntary, the workers' welfare a prime concern, and that they did return to Moçambique. In any event, successive Portuguese governments were reluctant to forgo either the invisible exports represented by the repatriated earnings of the workers, or the *quid pro quo* represented by the treaty-guaranteed share of the rail traffics from the Transvaal through Lourenço Marques; for all that the opponents of the export of labour claimed that it was a menace to the health and social stability of the native population and a hindrance to economic development within Moçambique itself.

The export of labour from Angola and Moçambique was not so

[1] James Duffy, *Portuguese Africa* (Cambridge, Mass., Harvard University Press, 1959), pp. 158–65, has not used the Nightingale Report, which remains unpublished; it is F.O. Conf. Print No. 8806. Eyre Crowe's remark is in a minute dated 3 Dec. 1912 commenting on a letter from J. H. Harris to *The Spectator*, F.O. Archives, vol. 367/287, file 52779 of 1912.

much a reason for their lack of economic development as a symptom of it; just as it was in Portugal itself, where emigration reached record heights in the period immediately before World War I. The Portuguese territories were not the only parts of Africa to disappoint investors; had not Rhodes declared that the gold-reefs of Mashonaland were richer than the great Rand itself, and was not his Chartered Company at one with the Moçambique, Nyassa, and Mossamedes companies in being unable to pay a dividend, year in, year out? Perhaps Yves Guyot was not so far out when he wrote of 'la folie coloniale', and recalled Peter the Hermit and the seventeenth-century Darien scheme (which, oddly enough, was promoted by the same man, Paterson, who founded the Bank of England).

What had become clear by 1914 was that a great deal had to be invested in Africa without hope of return, before much could be invested with any such hope; the function of what economists nowadays call the infrastructure of an economy was beginning to be made plain— along with, incidentally, the looseness of much talk about private enterprise as the source of all wealth. Railroads, for instance, were at once more than usually indispensable to economic growth, in a country lacking navigable rivers and infested by the tse-tse fly, and more than usually expensive to construct, given the climate and the terrain, and the need to import not only materials but labour. (Even in temperate South Africa before 1914, the extent of railroad construction was by no means justified by the traffics in immediate prospect; hence the part played by the rival routes from the Transvaal to seaboard in the nego- tiations leading to the creation of the Union of 1909.)

The failure to estimate traffics with any degree of realism accounts for the great chimera of the Cape-to-Cairo route, as it does for the so-called Trans-African route from Luanda, which stopped abruptly some two hundred-odd miles inland, and whose principal effect appears to have been the diversion of traffic from the steamers on the Cuanza river. As was pointed out at the time, it would have made a great deal more economic sense if the line had been begun at Dondo, the head of navigation on the Cuanza; this, however, would have deprived the capital of Angola of the glory of a railroad and a passenger terminus, and so was not to be heard of. But this error of judgement, though it must have greatly increased the subsidy to the line—which in any case was so calculated as to encourage the proprietors to carry as little traffic as they dared, so as to keep down running expenses—is unlikely to have made much difference to the level of economic activity in the Luanda hinterland.

The hopes that had been expressed at the time the line was inaugurated, like the hopes implicit in the unrealized plans for a railroad to be built inland from Porto Amelia in the Nyassa Company's territory, rested on the belief that the mere creation of means of communication would generate economic activity in proportion to its cost. What had been overlooked, as in so many other cases, such as the Zambezi *prazos*, was the utter dependence of all such schemes on an export market whose prices and requirements were beyond the control of the promoters. Even after 1892, when Corvo's low-tariff policy was abandoned, the ability of Portugal to provide a market for colonial produce was limited by her own poverty and small size.

It was thus reasonable, economically speaking, that exports from Angola and Moçambique, excluding the latter's transit trade through Beira and Lourenço Marques, should continue to consist almost entirely of wild products gathered in the interior, whose production did not tie up capital in quantity or for a long period. It was also reasonable that such European activity as there was in Angola should consist largely in the production of rum from sugar-cane for use in barter with the natives; or rather would have been, had not the forces of European humanitarianism, in successive conferences at Brussels from 1889–90 onwards, decided that the liquor traffic between Europeans and Africans (north of the twenty-second parallel of S. latitude) was to be discouraged by progressive increases in import duty. To these measures Portugal was an adherent, and it was decidedly inconsistent with the intent, though not with the specific wording, of the Brussels Act of 1890, for her to promote a new protected distilling industry in Angola under cover of its provisions. The mistake boomeranged, for eventually the industry had to be forcibly converted, with compensation for the owners, into one producing sugar for export in competition with the small but established industry of Moçambique. The result, a generation later, was an overall colonial sugar surplus of embarrassing proportions.

Even more important than the elements of an economic infrastructure, such as communications, was a settled administration; and this, outside a few areas of long settlement, the Portuguese had barely begun to provide before 1914. Some of their colonial experts, notably Eduardo Costa, had begun to think seriously about the requirements of a widespread civilian administration, as distinct from military occupation;

but, aside from a few professional judges, the characteristic colonial administrator was a soldier, and a sergeant turned colonial officer at that. Until the founding of the Escola Colonial in the first decade of the twentieth century there was no regular cadre of trained civilian recruits on which to draw. The result was an almost complete absence of the routine competence that is indispensable to good administration anywhere and that minimizes the effect of inevitable variations in the calibre of political appointees to the highest positions. Portugal was able, in the last decades of the monarchy, to command the services of some colonial governors of high ability; men who compared favourably in sophistication, breadth of view, and practical good sense with the best the British could show. But such men were caught between the upper millstone of an unstable administration in Lisbon, with its attendant bureaucracy, and the nether millstone of inadequate subordinates. The reports of Paiva Couceiro in Angola, of Enes and Freire de Andrade in Moçambique, reflect this state of frustration in varying degrees, while Mousinho de Albuquerque tried, with the best of intentions, to take the law into his own hands and was broken by the Lisbon establishment. Another reflection of the same feeling was the demand in Angola for autonomy for the few thousand white settlers.

The Portuguese could not but be aware that administrative reforms were likely to be a condition of continued imperial dominion, if only because administrative incompetence played into the hands of covetous great powers upon whose continued mutual jealousy it would be unwise to count. They could not foresee that the murder of an Austrian Archduke would rule out the philanthropic partition envisaged in the Anglo-German agreements and give their threatened rule a further respite. But, in the years when the House of Bragança was finally sinking in a slough of political confusion and financial scandal, no less than those in which the victorious republicans seemed bent on proving that all that had united them was a negation—opposition to the monarchy—it was even easier than usual to write brilliant memoranda about colonial reform, and even harder than usual to accomplish it. The defects of the colonial régime were indeed so patent that there was a tendency to hold them, rather than economic circumstances beyond the control of any régime, responsible primarily for the backward state of the colonies and to overrate the likely effects of administrative reforms.

That such problems should face Portugal in 1914 was, however, an index of what had been achieved in a quarter of a century. Nothing, of course, could have saved her dominions overseas if the powers had been determined on partition and had been willing to incur the political consequences in Europe. Overt action might not have been necessary; if the British had been unhelpful on several occasions, from the time of the campaign against Gungunhana onwards, the task of consolidation in Moçambique might have been beyond Portuguese capacity. The Germans likewise might have hampered the occupation of southern Angola more than they actually did.

Given these favourable chances, a handful of Portuguese colonial leaders, with a minimum of material assistance from Lisbon, had exceeded all expectations, including perhaps their own. Theirs was not the triumph of a governmental system, nor even of a class, but of a tradition reincarnate in a few determined individuals: the civilian António Enes, the soldiers Caldas Xavier, Mousinho de Albuquerque, Freire de Andrade, Aires de Ornelas, Paiva Couceiro; the sailor Azevedo Coutinho, and a handful of comrades and disciples. It was a tradition that some had thought dead and others anachronistic: significantly, it more often than not went along with strong royalist sentiments that saw in the dilettante Coburg scion, Carlos I, a rein-carnation of the patriot kings of earlier centuries. It contained, too, a strong tinge of quixotry—not for nothing did Oliveira Martins refer to Portugal as the kingdom of Barataria—that would have been absurd but for its effectiveness.

One cannot but ask why, at a time when most would have thought Portuguese imperialism a doomed survival, the tradition should have reasserted itself. It seems that the challenge—and the insult—represented by the British ultimatum of 1890 produced an effect different from what Lord Salisbury intended. His disdainful and impatient move underrated the tenacity of Portuguese leadership and the solidity of Portuguese patriotic sentiment, just as today the attacks of African nationalism and the disapproval of world opinion provoke Portugal to devote ever more resources to the defence and development of her overseas provinces.

BIBLIOGRAPHY

Anstey, Roger. *Britain and the Congo in the nineteenth century.* Oxford, Clarendon Press, 1962.

Bell, Herbert Clifford Francis. *Lord Palmerston.* 2 vols. London, 1936.

Boxer, Charles R. *Race relations in the Portuguese colonial empire, 1415–1825.* Oxford, Clarendon Press, 1963.

[Capello, Guilherme Augusto de Brito]. *Relatório do governador-geral da província de Angola.* Lisbon, 1889.

Cecil, Lady Gwendolen. *Life of Robert, Marquis of Salisbury.* 4 vols. London, 1921–32.

Corvo, João de Andrade. *Perigos.* Lisbon, 1870.

Costa Lobo, F. M. da. *O Conselheiro José Luciano de Castro e o segundo periodo constitucional monarquico.* Coimbra, 1941.

Couceiro, Henrique de Paiva. *Angola: dois anos de govêrno, junho 1907–junho 1909.* 2nd ed. Lisbon, 1948.

Coutinho, João de Azevedo. *A campanha do Barué em 1902.* Lisbon, 1904.

Duffy, James. *Portuguese Africa.* Cambridge, Mass., Harvard University Press, 1959.

Eça de Queiroz, António. *Cartas da Inglaterra.* Oporto, 1905.

Ennes, António. *A guerra de Africa em 1895.* Lisbon, 1898; reprinted with additional contemporary material, Lisbon, 1945.

Moçambique: relatório apresentado ao govêrno. 3rd ed. Lisbon, 1946.

Ferreira, Vicente. 'Colonização étnica da Africa Portuguesa', *Estudos ultramarinos,* vol. IV: *Colonização e diversos.* Lisbon, 1955.

Ferreira Ribeiro, Manuel. *As conferencias e o itinerário do viajante Serpa Pinto atravez das terras da Africa austral nos limites das províncias de Angola e Moçambique, Biè a Shoshong, junho a dezembro de 1878: estudo crítico e documentado.* Lisbon, 1879.

A província de S. Thomé e Príncipe e suas dependencias. Lisbon, 1877.

[Fiddes, G. V.] *Memorandum on the question of the Delagoa Bay Railway.* Colonial Office Confidential Print, Africa [South], no. 508, Oct. 1895.

Freire de Andrade, Alfredo. *Relatórios de Moçambique.* 6 vols. Lourenço Marques, 1906–10.

Great Britain. Foreign Office. 'Great Britain, Germany and Portugal,1898–9', *British documents on the origin of the war, 1898–1914,* vol. I: *The end of British isolation,* G. P. Gooch and Harold Temperley, eds. London, 1927,

Great Britain. Foreign Office. 'The Portuguese colonies, December 1911–July 1914', *British documents on the origin of the war, 1898–1914,* vol. X, part II: *The last years of peace,* G. P. Gooch and Harold Temperley, eds., with the assistance of Lillian M. Penson. London, 1938.

Guyot, Yves. *Lettres sur la politique coloniale.* Paris, 1885.

Hammond, Richard J. *Portugal and Africa, 1815–1910: a study in uneconomic imperialism.* Stanford University Press, 1966.

Johnston, Sir Harry H. *The story of my life.* London and Indianapolis, 1923.

Lavradio, Marquês de. *Portugal em Africa depois de 1851.* Lisbon, 1936.

Lovell, Reginald Ivan. *The struggle for South Africa, 1875–1899: a study in economic imperialism.* New York, 1934.

Lyne, Robert Nunez. *Mozambique: its agricultural development.* London, 1913.

Macedo, José de. *Autonomia de Angola.* Lisbon, 1910.

Maugham, Reginald Charles Fulke. *Zambezia: a general description of the valley of the Zambezi River, from its delta to the River Aroangwa, with its history…and ethnography.* London, 1910.

Nogueira, A. F. *A ilha de S. Thomé, a questão bancaria no ultramar e o nosso problema colonial.* Lisbon, 1893.

Oliveira Martins, Joaquim Pedro. *O Brasil e as colónias portuguezas.* 5th ed. Lisbon, 1920.

Oliver, Roland. *Sir Harry Johnston and the scramble for Africa.* London, 1957.

Palmer, William Waldegrave, Earl of Selborne. *The Selborne Memorandum: a review of the mutual relations of the British South African colonies in 1907.* Introduction by Basil Williams. London, 1925.

Pinheiro Chagas, Manuel. *As negociações com a Inglaterra, 1887–1890.* Lisbon, 1890.

Ramm, Agatha, ed. *The political correspondence of Mr. Gladstone and Lord Granville, 1876–1886.* 2 vols. Oxford, Clarendon Press, 1962.

Reade, Winwood. *Savage Africa: being the narrative of a tour in equatorial, south-western, and north-western Africa; with notes on the habits of the gorilla; on the existence of unicorns and tailed men; on the slave trade; on the origin, character, and capabilities of the negro and on the future civilization of Western Africa.* London, 1863.

Rita-Ferreira, António. *O movimento migratório de trabalhadores entre Moçambique e a Africa du Sul.* Lisbon, 1963.

Sá da Bandeira, Bernardo de Sá Nogueira de Figueiredo, Marquêz de. *O trafico da escravatura, e o bill de Lord Palmerston.* Lisbon, 1840.

Stanislawski, Dan. *The individuality of Portugal: a study in historical-political geography.* Austin, University of Texas Press, 1959.

Teixeira Botelho, José Justino. *História militar e política dos portugueses em Moçambique de 1833 aos nossos dias.* 2nd ed. Lisbon, 1936.

Unamuno y Jugo, Miguel de. *Por tierras de Portugal y de España.* 2nd ed. Buenos Aires, 1944.

Vieira de Castro, Luís. *D. Carlos I.* Lisbon, 1936.

Vilhena, Ernesto de. *Questões coloniaes: discursos e artigos.* 2 vols. Lisbon, 1910.

Vogel, Charles. *Le Portugal e ses colonies: tableau politique et commercial de la monarchie portugaise dans son état actuel.* Paris, 1860.

Walter, Jaime. *Honório Pereira Barreto.* Bissau, 1947.

Warhurst, Philip R. *Anglo-Portuguese relations in South-Central Africa, 1890–1900.* London, 1962.

Webster, Charles Kingsley. *The foreign policy of Palmerston, 1830–1841: Britain, the liberal movement and the Eastern Question.* 2 vols. London, 1951.

CHAPTER 12

THE GERMANS IN AFRICA BEFORE 1918

by ROBERT CORNEVIN

The bibliography on German Africa published in 1965 by the Hoover Institution lists 493 general works and 303 others concerning specifically one or another of the four former German territories. The general works may be divided into two main categories according to their date of publication. Those published before 1914 are almost all by German authors and have essentially a documentary and didactic character. They aim at instructing the metropolitan country about the economic importance of these colonies, so rapidly acquired during the course of 1884 and 1885. Those published after 1918 are written by Germans, English, French, Americans and Belgians who are all more or less biased and pass moral judgements on German colonization in Africa. From 1945 onward the communist writers of East Germany come to confirm, in works written from the archives in Potsdam, the charges against German colonialism published between the two wars by English and French authors, and to utter a cry of alarm against the neo-colonialism of West Germany.

All these books, even the most impartial ones such as Henri Brunschwig's *L'expansion allemande outre-mer du XVe siècle à nos jours*, present colonial history in its classical concept. They treat Africans as either the objects of German goodwill or the victims of cruelty, all initiative on the black man's part being by definition ruled out. This kind of history appears particularly easy to write, now that fifty years have passed since the end of the German colonial empire. In the four former German colonies two generations have been exposed to other influences and have learned to speak a language other than German. It is these generations who hold the levers of command in three of the territories now formed into five independent states: Cameroun on 1 January 1960; Togo on 27 April 1960; Tanganyika on 9 December 1961; Ruanda and Burundi, on 1 July 1962. It is striking to read encomiums on German colonization by Cameroun authors of the first rank such as R. P. Engelbert Mveng or Jean Ikellé-Matiba; they barely mention the accusations of cruelty against the celebrated Governor von Puttkammer and his associates. On the other hand, Judith Listowel reports the opinions of numerous Tanzanians on Germans: 'They were severe but just', and she insists on the great role played by resistance to the Germans in the formation of a national Tanganyikan consciousness. We ourselves, at the end of the colonial period, often noted germanophilism in Togo, expressed not only by certain old men who still spoke a few words of German and evoked with emotion their youthful memories, but also by intellectuals in the prime of life whose families had taught them to respect the German colonial achievement.

The fourth former German territory, South West Africa, occupies a peculiar position because it is the only one in which a large German community remained after World War I. (Out of 14,830 Europeans in 1913, about 6,000 Germans were expelled in 1920.) Windhoek is the only town in Africa where in 1966 there were both primary and secondary German schools, where newspapers were printed in German and where the pastors preached their sermons in German. With few exceptions these Germans considered the natives of South West Africa as an inferior race, and it would be exceptional to find today a single African from that country who was willing to defend the good deeds of German colonization. However, as in the remaining five independent states that have emerged from the three other former German colonies, the history of German colonization could very well be rewritten essentially from the African point of view. This is what we shall now attempt to do, studying successively each of the four German colonies and leaving aside such general questions as: the causes of German expansion, the policy of Bismarck, the scramble, the delimitation of frontiers and the value of the German colonies to the metropolitan economy, all problems on which numerous detailed studies have appeared.

South West Africa

On 24 April 1884 Chancellor Bismarck telegraphed to the German Consul at Cape Town that 'the establishments founded by Herr Lüderitz to the north of the Orange river are placed under the protection of the Empire'. To this date, marking the first manifestation of German imperialism overseas, the German historians of colonialism have given the name of *Geburtstag*.

In fact, this 'birth' was not so unforeseen as some authors have suggested. By two successive treaties, on 1 May and 25 August 1883, signed, respectively, by M. H. Vogelsang, the agent of the Bremen merchant Adolph Lüderitz, and Joseph Fredericks, the Hottentot chief of Bethanie, Lüderitzland had been defined as extending over the whole coast from the Orange river to 26° S., that is to say, over about 300 kilometres to the south and 100 kilometres to the north of the Bay of Angra Pequena (Lüderitz Bay). On 21 November 1883 the government in London had replied to an official inquiry from Berlin that it had no rights except on the islands facing Angra Pequena and on Walvis Bay (400 kilometres to the north of Angra Pequena) annexed in 1880.

Walvis Bay and Lüderitz Bay are respectively the maritime outlets of Damaraland and Namaland, where for more than forty years German missionaries had been established. South West Africa is, along with South Africa, the oldest Protestant mission field in Africa. In 1814 the German missionary Heinrich Schmelen in the service of the L.M.S. set up a station at Bethanie. Returning towards the north, he penetrated into Damaraland, the country of the Herero. (The Herero are cattle-raisers like the Hottentots, but they speak a Bantu tongue. According to Heinrich Vedder, a leading authority, they arrived in South West Africa during the eighteenth century, having come from the Lake Tanganyika region. They drove the Damara (Bergdama) to the mountains and occupied the best lands.)

Around 1834 the Germans set up the stations of Windhoek and Okahandja. About 1865, the Rhenish Missionary Society (founded in 1819), which since 1824 had preached the Gospel among the Hottentots of Stellenbosch, took over all the stations previously held by the L.M.S. and the Methodists to the north of the Orange river. (For example, stations at Warmbad and as far north as Rehoboth and Gobabies were absorbed.)

In both the Nama country and the Herero country, the missionaries found themselves face-to-face with a society of nomadic stock-raisers, whose chief preoccupation was to search out pasture for their herds, around which centred the whole of their material and spiritual life. The missionaries believed that the only means of 'civilizing' these people was to settle them on the land and to introduce them by degrees into a trading economy. The first requirement for such a programme was peace between the Hottentots and the Herero. Conflicts over the possession of grazing grounds had been constant between these two peoples. Until the arrival in Namaland of the Orlam Hottentots, who possessed fire-arms and who had come from the Cape province at the beginning of the nineteenth century, they had been more or less equal in strength. In 1842 the great Orlam chief, Jonker Afrikaner, subdued the Hereros and confiscated their cattle. But in 1863 Maherero, who had become chief of the Hereros two years earlier, took up arms once again. His mentor was the German missionary Hugo Hahn, who in 1864 had raised the Prussian flag over Otjimbingwe.

The Herero army was directed by two English traders, Green and Haybittel, and by the famous Swedish traveller, K. J. Andersson, who had become the richest trader north of the Orange river and who was named 'general in chief for life' by the Herero. Jan Jonker Afrikaner, grandson of Jonker Afrikaner, was defeated near Rehoboth (100 kilometres south of Windhoek). But in 1868, the Nama, furious at the European intervention in favour of the Hereros, sacked the buildings of the Rhenish Mission and Andersson's store at Otjimbingwe. In consequence of this raid the missionaries sought protection simultaneously from both Berlin and Cape Town. For sixteen years their appeals to Berlin went unheeded.

On the other hand, the Governor of Cape Colony, Sir Henry Barkly, replied to a request for protection from Maherero, who was naturally anxious about the progress of Boer trekkers towards the north. The governor sent an envoy, W. C. Palgrave, who in 1876 negotiated a protectorate over Damaraland. This protectorate, however, was not accepted by the parliament of Cape Colony or by the European traders settled to the north of the Orange river. Walvis Bay alone was occupied in 1880, as we have remarked earlier.

However, in that same year 1880, ten years after peace had been concluded between the Herero and the Nama, hostilities broke out again. As the 'protection' offered by the Cape government appeared to be ineffective, Maherero readily agreed, on 21 October 1885, to sign a treaty with the German government, represented by Dr Heinrich Ernst Goering (the father of the Nazi Reichsmarschall Hermann Goering). On the other hand, the Nama chief, Hendrik Witbooi, formally refused to sign. It was largely because of the long-standing hostility between the Herero and the Nama, which had existed for more than a hundred years, that the Germans succeeded in establishing themselves in South West Africa. (In 1903 the total African population of South West Africa was estimated at about 300,000. The European population amounted to 4,682, that is to say one white man to sixty-four Africans.)

Governor Theodor Leutwein, who headed the administration in South West Africa from 1895 to 1904, calmly explained in his memoirs (*Elf Jahre Gouverneur in Deutsch-Südwestafrika*) that he was not averse to playing off one tribe against another, but maintained that the policy of gradually reconciling the racial differences between white and black was sometimes opposed and finally rendered impossible by the local Europeans. Nevertheless, on 9 March 1900 Leutwein officially informed the missionaries in the Herero country that 'the infantile affection' felt by their late president, Viehe, for 'his Herero' was ridiculous, for the Herero were clearly 'the most useless of natives whether as soldiers or workers'.[1] These lines were written four years before the great Herero revolt.

South West Africa was the only German colony in which the suppression of the natives was envisaged officially, for in this country, which was nine-tenths desert, the only regions suitable for European settlement were already inhabited for the most part by Africans. The exploitation of the new colony was at first entrusted to concessionary companies, beginning with the Deutsche Kolonialgesellschaft für Süd West Afrika, founded in April 1885 by A. Lüderitz with a capital of 800,000 marks and authorized to exercise local rights of sovereignty. André Chéradame refers to four German companies existing in 1903, each with a capital of more than a million marks, and three British companies (South African Territories Limited, South West Africa Company Ltd., Damara Guano Gesellschaft) with a capital of more than 10 millions each (20 millions each in the case of the last two).

The exploitation of the subsoil—essentially copper mining before 1907—had relatively few disadvantages for the native population; but European cultivation of the soil took place directly at the black man's expense. As a result of the country's general aridity, each concession granted to a single European colonist—there were 813 in 1903—deprived numerous African stock raisers of the means of feeding their cattle. In 1903 more than half the Herero herds had passed into German hands. Furthermore, the European traders (of whom there were 277 in 1903) sold on credit, and Africans had to pay in cattle appraised at much below their real value.

[1] Document 67 in Germany, Colonial Office, *Kolonien unter der Peitsche*, Fritz Ferdinand Müller, ed. ((East) Berlin, 1962), p. 148.

These foreseeable consequences of the German protectorate had not escaped Hendrik Witbooi, the Nama chief, who, having unified the Hottentots in 1889 after his victory over Jan Jonker Afrikaner, had refused until 1890 to sign any treaty giving away his independence. Between 1891 and 1893 he carried on intensive guerrilla warfare against the Germans, but was finally beaten at the Nan defile, and in 1894 signed a treaty establishing a protectorate.

Between 1894 and 1904 the economic plight of the indigenous people grew steadily worse. An epidemic of cattle plague in 1897 killed off two-thirds of the cattle. The same year the natives were herded into reserves so as to leave the Europeans in possession of the better lands. At length, on 12 January 1904, Samuel Maherero, son of the great Maherero who had died in 1890, mounted a formidable insurrection that began with a massacre of 123 European colonists. This action met with immediate and terrible repression. Reinforcements were sent out under the orders of General Lothar von Trotha. Five thousand Herero were finally encircled on the Waterberg (1,900 metres high). They fought desperately at Hamakari and were forced to flee into the Omahehe Desert, where almost all died of thirst. Samuel Maherero himself succeeded in finding refuge in Bechuanaland.

Then occurred the most shameful atrocity of the war in South West Africa. Von Trotha, refusing to negotiate with a people whose leaders were either dead or in exile, issued his famous proclamation of extermination (*Vernichtungsbefehl*):

Within the German frontiers every Herero with or without a rifle, with or without cattle, shall be shot. I will not accept any woman or child; I will send them back to their people or have them shot. Such are my words to the people of Herero.   The great general of the most powerful Emperor
Von Trotha.

By the time von Trotha was recalled to Berlin at the end of 1905, because of the agitation caused in the Reichstag by the revelations of his proceedings in South West Africa, it was already too late. Too many Herero had suffered either a violent death or had died of starvation for the tribe to recover. Out of an estimated 80,000 Herero in 1903, no more than 20,000 remained within German territory by 1906. Moreover, the survivors had lost everything: a united tribe of rich cattle-raisers had become a mass of fugitives obliged to live by keeping the herds of others on the land they themselves had once owned.

The massacre of the Hereros was not discussed in Berlin alone. It was watched even more passionately by the Nama, a Hottentot people in the south of the colony, who felt themselves directly concerned. Chief Hendrik Witbooi had in 1894 signed a treaty establishing a protectorate; and he had sent troops to the Germans, who had requested them in order to put down the Herero revolt. But he realized that the next victims of the white men might very well be the Namas; and in 1904, at the age of eighty, he led an insurrection. After a year of guerrilla warfare, the great chief of the Nama was killed in battle near Tses. Another leader of the insurgents was Jacob Morenga, who was not defeated until May 1906. It was only in 1907 that the state of war in South West Africa was declared officially at an end.

During the seven following years, the Germans made efforts to get some revenues from a colony in which they had placed such great hopes and whose conquest had proved so difficult and costly. They were assisted by the fortuitous discovery of diamonds in the Lüderitz region in 1907 and by the exploitation of the copper mines of Tsumeb in the north. In 1910, sixty-three companies were working small concessions; and in 1912 the balance of trade was favourable for the first time.

On the other hand, the recruitment of colonists in Germany encountered great difficulties. On the spot, where many old soldiers had become farmers, the labour problem appeared insoluble. The Herero and the Namas who were in prison could be used for public works; those who remained free, however, refused to toil for white men. There remained the Ovambo cultivators, a Bantu people who lived in the north of the colony on the frontier of Angola, the only non-nomad people in South West Africa. However, the German government in 1906 declared Ovamboland forbidden territory. The Ovambo, who today make up more than half of the African population of South West Africa and provide nine-tenths of the manual labour, were thus not touched by German colonization.

We shall see later how the military campaigns of World War I left their mark upon the historical consciousness of the inhabitants of Tanganyika. Nothing of the kind happened in South West Africa. The war was strictly a white man's affair. When the Bastards of Rehoboth[1] offered their services to the South African General Botha,

---

[1] Eighty families of Bastards of Rehoboth, the children of marriages between the Boers of the Trek and Nama women, had settled south of Windhoek in 1870. They spoke Afrikaans and bore Dutch names.

he replied that 'the coloureds had nothing to do with this war between the Germans and South Africans'. The Bastards of Rehoboth, who had been loyal to the Germans, refused to help them 'because they themselves had come from South Africa and did not want to oppose the troops of that country'. They were rewarded by 'independence' granted to their little republic, an independence which up to the present day remains entirely theoretical. The Nama and the Herero, who had pinned all their hopes on the departure of the Germans, soon came to perceive that, although the methods of government had changed, the respective status of the white masters and the African servants did not improve in the black man's favour, while the proportion of whites began to increase.[1]

Togo

Togo may in some ways be regarded as Germany's first colony. The first treaty of protectorate signed in South West Africa dates only from 8 October 1884, that is to say, three months after the signature of treaties between the chiefs of Baguida, Lomé, Togo, and Dr Gustav Nachtigal representing the German government.

As in South West Africa, the occupation of the coast of the future Schutzgebiet-Togo (Togo protectorate) took place in a region where the Germans had for a long time carried on missionary work and had more recently engaged in commercial activity. With regard to the work of the missionaries, although their political influence was very limited both before and during the colonial period, the members of the Norddeutsche Missionsgesellschaft or Bremen Mission had left behind a vivid imprint. Fifty years after their departure, Protestants are still called Brema in numerous Togo languages. Moreover, the national consciousness of the Ewe springs directly from German Protestant missionary labours.

On 14 November 1847 Pastor Lorenz Wolf of the Norddeutsche Missionsgesellschaft established himself at Peki. Peki, to the east of the Volta (in present-day Ghana), was the westernmost centre of the territory inhabited by the Adja-Ewe peoples, who are spread out between the lower Volta and the lower Mono to a depth of about 140 kilometres from the coast. At that time, the Ewe were unknown to Europeans. They lived in small communities composed of peaceful

[1] In 1960 there were 73,000 whites and 477,000 Africans, or 1 white for 6·5 Africans. Compare the 1903 percentage of 1 white for 64 Africans.

and democratic cultivators who had not formed a warrior kingdom like their neighbours, the Ashanti on the west or the Fon of Dahomey to the east. The Bremen Mission did not want to work in areas already prospected by other missionaries. Thus, to the west of the lower Volta the Basel Mission had worked among the Akwapim since 1827; to the east, the region of Anécho had been visited from the Cape Coast (Ghana) by the Methodist Pastor Thomas Birch Freeman and from Agoué (Dahomey) by the Catholics of the African missions of Lyon, who in 1871 temporarily abandoned Ouidah for Agoué. The excellent reception accorded to Pastor Wolf at Peki encouraged the Bremen Mission to concentrate on the Ewe country.

Despite the death of Pastor Wolf and of the three other missionaries, stations were founded in Keta (July 1855) and Anyako (1857) on the two banks of the Keta Lagoon (now in Ghana). Additional posts were set up at Waya in 1855 and Wegbe-Ho in 1859. Waya and Wegbe-Ho, north-east of Peki, were to belong later to German Togoland and then to British Togoland. (Today, in spite of their vote for temporary continuance of trusteeship in the plebiscite of 9 May 1956, these areas form part of Ghana, along with the station of Amedzofe founded in 1878.) During the forty years before the Germans had established themselves in Togo, the Bremen Mission had sent more than a hundred missionaries to the Ewe country. These emissaries, who, in spite of the name of their mission, generally came from South Germany, had no desire to implant German culture. They evangelized in the Ewe tongue[1] and taught English in their schools. Although they appealed in 1857 to the Bremen trading-house M. Vietor Söhne, they did so because the British had abandoned Keta in 1856 and the mission had need of European supplies. Moreover, the Pastor, Rudolf Vietor, who belonged to the Bremen Mission, was a son of the former head of that trading-house. It was this commercial activity—entirely secondary in the minds of the missionaries—that would later allow the establishment of German political control.

In 1874, Keta—where French and British trade had been established since 1857—was reoccupied by the British. The German traders then sought to establish themselves farther east, on the only portion of the coast not already claimed by a European power, between Lomé (known at this time as Bey Beach) and Anécho (Little Popo). In Anécho

[1] Bernhard Schlegel published in 1857 the first lexicon and grammar of the Ewe tongue. See Hans W. Debrunner, *A church between colonial powers* (London, 1965), p. 89.

they were faced with a strong British influence whose origin went back to the famous Latevi Awoku, mentioned by the Danish surgeon Isert as having studied in England around 1780. Latevi's son, Ezakli Akuete, on his return from England took the name of George Lawson. The Lawson family, all-powerful in Anécho, had consistently favoured the British Methodist Mission and British traders.

The circumstances in which the Germans took control of Togo are well known. Between 4 and 6 July 1884, Dr Nachtigal caused the German flag to be hoisted at Baguida, Lomé and Togo. Treaties with the French (24 December 1885) and the British (28 July 1886) recognized the German protectorate over the 52 kilometres of coast extending between Aflao and Agoué, whose hinterland was to become the Schutzgebiet-Togo.

But this hinterland had first to be explored and conquered. The first aim of the Germans was to extend the Schutzgebiet-Togo between the Volta on the north-west, where they were especially attracted by the important native market for the salt of Salaga, and the Niger to the north-east, in the region of Say. They were interested also in the fact that the Niger's tributary, the Bénoué, would have made a link with Cameroun. Thanks to a series of mishaps, these ambitions could be realized only in part. In rapid succession came, first, the accidental death of the explorer Ludwig Wolf at Ndali (1889); then the defeat of Kling and his death (1892); after that, the conquest of the kingdom of Abomey by the French expeditionary force of General Alfred Dodds (1893), which allowed the French to reach the Niger; and, finally, British claims to Salaga as part of a 'neutral zone', which were ratified in 1899 by the Samoa treaty.

The period that we have elsewhere described as 'from steeple-chase to pacification'[1] lasted practically until 1901. From the African point of view, only the population of the Northern Togo (roughly north of present-day Sokodé) put up serious resistance. The Konkomba insurrection (1897–8) and the open opposition of the Kabre (1898) were put down with vigour, thanks in part to the alliance of the Germans with the small Moslem kingdoms of the Kotokoli (Sokodé) and the Chakossi (Mango). These wars had two important consequences: first, by an ordinance of the Governor, Count Julius von Zech, the circumscriptions of Sokodé-Basari and the Mango-Yendi (Yendi is today in Ghanaian Togo) were declared a forbidden zone, closed to

[1] Robert Cornevin, *Histoire du Togo*, 3rd ed. (Paris, 1969), pp. 136–65.

traders and missionaries; and, secondly, the influence—in reality very restricted—of the Moslem chiefs of the Kotokoli and the Chakossi was enlarged and reinforced by the German military leaders in charge of the northern circumscriptions, for whom Islam was a natural ally of the European authorities in Africa.

It was not until June 1912 that an imperial decree authorized the Protestant missions of Basel to operate in the region of Yendi, and the Catholic missions (Fathers of the Divine Word) in that of Sokodé. Nevertheless, the urban centre of Sokodé, considered as Islamic, was forbidden to the Catholic Fathers, who were forced to establish themselves at Aledjo, 30 miles to the north-east of Sokodé. Fifty years after the German departure, despite the creation of an extensive road network and a French policy that was more favourable to the prolific and hard-working populations of the north, 'the neglect of the north' in economic and social matters during the German period still weighs heavily upon the policy of the independent Togo Republic and gives to the northerners a genuine sense of frustration.

The 'useful Togo' of the Germans thus did not extend beyond the district (*Bezirk*) of Atakpamé. Nevertheless it cannot be denied that German colonization was beneficial. The colony was small in size. There was no easily accessible mineral wealth—the iron of Bassari was too far removed from the coast to be profitably exploited at that time. The mountain ranges were below 1,000 metres in height, and the country was therefore much less attractive to white planters than the highlands of East Africa. Within the Kolonialrat (Imperial Colonial Council) there were moreover strong disagreements on the question of whether the territory should be developed by African peasants or by European planters. The missions and J. K. Vietor, the champion of the small farmers, successfully opposed both the alienation of land to white land concerns and the concept of *Plantagenkultur* (plantation agriculture) as a solution to Togo's problems. Hence Togo attracted neither colonizing companies nor great European plantations. In fact the total area of these plantations in 1914 was not in excess of 12,000 hectares. The country had the further advantage of a well-trained administration, whose members often remained in their posts for long periods and were intent on developing the commerce and agriculture of the little territory. The administration sought to balance the budget by means of customs and tax revenues that were devised in terms of the native community and not of the stock exchange quotations on the shares of colonial companies. Thus, Africans subject to labour services might commute them for money payments, a privilege that was extensively used by the peoples of the south, who had long been accustomed to trade. In 1910 such commutation was on so large a scale that the German administration put into force an additional tax.

The economy of German Togo was marked by a steady development of external trade. The most important export products were palm-oil and palm-kernels, maize and raw cotton. In African eyes, the low value of these products was largely compensated by the fact that they brought the African producer into the money economy and did not merely enrich the European trader, as was the case for minerals or rubber in other European territories.

Moreover, the limited economic possibilities of the Schutzgebiet-Togo led to a much more liberal 'native policy' than in the other three German colonies. The practical realization of this policy was greatly assisted by two factors: the taste for trade manifested by the peoples of the Slave Coast, who had been in contact with Europeans for centuries; and the 'favourable prejudice' towards the white man brought about by the disinterested activities of the Bremen Mission in the Ewe country pursued for more than forty years before the establishment of German political control.

During their administration the Germans carried out a number of important public works. The wharf at Lomé was opened to traffic in 1904; the first railway line from Lomé to Anécho, called 'the coconut line', 44 kilometres long, was inaugurated in 1905; the 'cocoa line' from Lomé to Palimé, 119 kilometres, was inaugurated on 27 January 1907; the 'cotton line' from Lomé to Atakpamé, 173 kilometres, on 2 May 1913. Thanks to a sound organization of trade routes, a money economy developed much more rapidly than in the other German colonies. In 1914, the mark was accepted as currency on the principal markets of the south.

Within Togo there are considerable variations in the density of population. The consequent difficulties of finding labour for the construction of the railroad from Lomé to Atakpamé led the Governor, Count Zech, to institute a form of penal colonization that is noteworthy. By a *Runderlass* (circular) of 23 October 1909 he set up *Besserungssiedlungen* (villages of rehabilitation) for those convicted under common law. The end in view, a ready supply of labour, was naturally not mentioned, but banishment itself was used as a device to give another chance to the criminal. The inmates lived in relative freedom, under the supervision of a chief originally from Timbuktu. The first rehabilitation settlement at Chra was succeeded by another at Djabataure on the road from Atakpamé to Sokodé. These were the forerunners of the thousands of Kabre-Losso colonists who, between the two wars, occupied the vacant land between Sokodé and Nuatja, and achieved one of the most remarkable successes of French policy.

German political control was not welcomed by the missionaries, who waited several years before founding new stations in the heart of the Ewe country, which was now German. For many years, in fact, the missionaries had as a remote objective the setting up of an independent Evangelical (that is to say, Lutheran) Church among the Ewe. Already in 1882 they had ordained the first Ewe pastor, Rudolf Mallet, who had been ransomed by the missionaries in 1860 when he was a twelve-year-old slave. In 1884 three young men were sent to Germany to the house of Pastor Albert Binder in Westheim, Würtemberg. Between 1890 and 1900 Binder undertook the complete education of fifteen other young Togolese, including Andreas Akou, father of Dr Martin Akou, the first Togolese deputy to sit in the French parliament, and Robert Baëta. Both of these men were destined to occupy responsible positions in the future independent Ewe Church. In a public lecture given in Germany in 1890, church inspector F. M. Zahn spoke at length about this independent church.

All this explains the attitude of reserve towards the imperial administration on the part of the German missionaries, who considered themselves in the service of the Ewe Church, and not of German imperialism. The missionaries' desire to remain within the bounds of the Ewe country was reinforced by the fact that the German administration did not establish its headquarters at Lomé until 1897. It had previously been based on Baguida and Sébé close to Anécho, the uncontested fief of the Methodist Mission.

In 1888, Ernst Bürgi, the Swiss missionary in the service of the Bremen Misson, surveyed that part of the Ewe country which nowadays belongs to the Togo Republic; but it was only in 1895 that the catechist Andreas Akou established himself at Lomé, followed in 1896 by a European pastor. Agou-Nyogbo (south of Palimé) became a missionary post in 1895, and in 1900 it became the principal station for an independent district. A period of forty years, nearly two generations, thus separated the foundation of the original missionary stations

at Keta (1853) and at Ho (1859) from those of Lomé (1896) and
Agoua (1900). Keta was in the Gold Coast, Ho in the part of German
Togo that was to become first British and then Ghanaian, Lomé and
Agoua in the future Republic of Togo. Keta remained the head-
quarters of the mission until 1905; Ho and Amedzofé, the centre of the
Bremen Mission until the departure of the Germans. It was from the two
latter places that the seven African pastors ordained before 1914 came.
The training school for catechists was located at Amedzofé, and the
great German pastors (among them Bernhardt Schlegel, Johannes
Knüsli and Jacob Spieth), who, even before Westermann, had studied
the history and linguistics of the Ewe people, were stationed at Ho.

The consequences of German missionary policy were mixed. One
significant consequence relates to the political division of the Ewe
country after 1918 between the Gold Coast, British Togo and French
Togo. The difficulties encountered by the Evangelical Church in Togo
were not due entirely to the competition of the Catholics. They arose
rather from the fact that this church was orphaned in its infancy—
there were only four missionary stations in 1914—while the Church
that sprang from the Bremen Mission, situated in present-day Ghana,
was already full-grown in 1918.

In German Togo, as almost everywhere else in Africa, the schools
were originally established by missions. But in German Togo the
Catholic schools differed from those of the Protestant missions to a
greater degree than elsewhere. Except for the brief efforts of the Lyon
Mission before 1886, Catholic missions began work in Togo at the
same time as the German administration. The fathers belonged to the
Gesellschaft des Göttlichen Wortes in den Heidenländern, which had
been set up at Steyl in Holland following the *Kulturkampf*. These
missionaries of the Divine Word from Steyl were almost all German
by nationality. They thus saw no objection to teaching German in the
schools from 1904, the year when the government gave missions a
premium for each pupil with a sound knowledge of German. In 1912,
the teaching of German was being carried on in 106 out of the 181
Catholic mission schools with a total enrolment of 7,653; elementary
instruction was given in the Ewe tongue.

By contrast, in 1912 Protestants were not teaching German in more
than 65 schools out of 156 (5,654 pupils). The Bremen missionaries, as
mentioned earlier, had from the beginning taught Ewe and also
English (since Ada and Accra, the natural commercial outlets of Ho

and Peki, were in British territory). The missionaries 'in the service of the Ewe people' naturally found it normal to give instruction in the language that would be most useful to their pupils. However, from 1905 onwards it appears that the Protestant leaders, like the Catholics, yielded to the German pride in their 'successful colonial enterprise'.

In the eyes of most German officials, even the educated African belonged to an inferior race. There was a flagrant contradiction between the concept of an 'independent church, the aim of our missionary activity' proclaimed in 1890 by the inspector of the Bremen Mission, F. M. Zahn, and the paternalism, even of an enlightened sort, that characterized German administration in the 'model colony' (*Muster-kolonie*) of Togo.

Cameroun

The names Togo and Cameroun have been so often linked during three-quarters of a century (1885–1960) that a certain confusion is inevitable. It is true that within a ten-day period Dr Nachtigal, the former German Consul in Tunis, signed treaties of protectorate in the two territories: with the chiefs of Baguida, Lomé and Togo on 4, 5 and 6 July 1884; and with the chiefs Bell, Akwa and Deido of Douala on 14 July. Certainly also in these two colonies the Germans limited their efforts at economic and social development to the south and were content in the north with military occupation. Togo, like Cameroun, was divided after the German defeat into two parts, unequal in area, and was first placed under League of Nations mandate and later under United Nations trusteeship. The British zones, relatively very small, were attached administratively to Gold Coast or Nigeria, while the larger French zones were administered separately from the neighbouring colonies of Dahomey and French Equatorial Africa.

The resemblance between the two former German colonies of the Gulf of Guinea, however, ends there. The hinterland of Douala is very different from that of Baguida and Lomé, both from a geographical and a historical point of view. We have seen how important were the activities of the Bremen missionaries in Togo from 1847; we have noted the absence or the rarity in Togo of products like wild rubber or ivory, and the consequent development by the German authorities of native agricultural production, which enriched the African producer directly and only indirectly benefited Germany through the consumption of her manufactured goods and the payment of taxes in money.

At Douala, on 14 July 1884, Nachtigal did no more than confirm on behalf of the German imperial government the treaties by which, on 12 July, King Bell and King Akwa had ceded their rights of sovereignty to Eduard Woermann, J. Jantzen and J. Thormählen, representing the powerful Hamburg firm of C. Woermann. Woermann, who in 1863 had set up a trading establishment at Douala, inaugurated in 1883 a regular line of steamers between Hamburg and West Africa. In October 1883 he urged Bismarck to acquire the Bay of Biafra with a view to combating British pre-eminence in the political and commercial fields. British influence in this area had long been established.

It was an English missionary, Alfred Saker of the Baptist Mission of London, who founded the Protestant Church in Douala in 1845. Between 1862 and 1872 Saker had also translated the Bible into the Douala tongue. He trained numerous Cameroun pastors, of whom the first, Thomas Horton Johnson, was ordained in 1855, and the second, George Nkwe, in 1866. It was Saker who had set up a Christian community that in 1886 numbered 246 members and 1,040 novices and pupils at Douala, 203 members and 368 pupils at Victoria (founded in 1858). It was to Queen Victoria, not to the Emperor of Germany, that King Bell and King Akwa of Douala wrote in 1864, in 1879, and again in 1881, vainly asking for protection. It was the British consuls of the Bay of Biafra, based on Fernando Po, who developed the trade in palm-oil and ivory and presided over the famous Courts of Equity of Douala (1856) and Victoria (1858). It was two English companies, established in this region almost at the same time as Woermann, the John Holt Company (1869) and the Ambas Bay Trading Company,[1] who held their positions solidly in the face of German commercial and political programmes. The Douala treaty of July 1884 was written in English, for King Bell had studied at Bristol in England.

Thus on this short stretch of coast, which was now to become German territory, British preponderance was undeniable. This explains the haste with which the Germans delimited the frontier with Calabar (Nigeria). By the Convention of 29 April 1885 the frontier was fixed at Rio del Rey. The town of Victoria was evacuated shortly afterwards by the British Baptist Mission, who were replaced in 1886 by the Swiss of the Basel Mission. The coastal frontier with Gabon was laid down by the Franco-German Convention of 24 December 1885.

[1] John Holt and Company are still all-powerful in independent Cameroun. The Ambas Bay Trading Company was absorbed in 1920 by the Unilever combine.

It is likewise suspicion of British influence that explains the early establishment of official instruction (*Regierungschulen*) in Cameroun (1886), by contrast with Togo. In 1913 there were 1,194 pupils in official schools in Cameroun, compared with 341 in Togo. On the other hand, the less important place occupied by native tongues in the mission schools, which had 41,500 pupils in 1913, was due to other causes. The Douala tongue, which had been studied by Saker from 1847 onwards, was not spoken by more than 20,000 people at the time the Germans arrived. This was nothing in comparison with the extent of the Ewe tongue. The Anlo dialect of Ewe had been studied and codified by the German missionaries of Bremen in the middle of the nineteenth century; it was spoken by more than 500,000 people. This does not take into account the Adja idioms, which were close to Ewe and which were spoken in the southern parts of Togo and of Dahomey. The variety of tongues used in the Cameroun hinterland was endless; and in a way this helped German penetration, for it allowed the Germans to exploit existing tribal conflicts. But this penetration was much more difficult than in Togo by reason of the great, dense rain forests that existed in Cameroun but not in Togo.

The coast of the present Western Cameroun (formerly Southern Cameroons) is one of the wettest regions in the world. Debundja, south-west of Mount Cameroon (40 kilometres west of Victoria), has twelve times (or 375 inches) the annual rainfall of Lomé. The greater part of Western Cameroun has more than 140 inches annually. These conditions had a strong bearing on the way in which the Schutzgebiet Kamerun was conquered and developed.

We shall not dwell on the details of the conquest. The operation was very difficult because there were no means of crossing the dense forest belt that had to be traversed to reach the desired frontiers: Lake Chad to the north, the Congo Basin to the east. The tropical jungles, of course, meant a sparse population and consequent difficulties in the recruitment of carriers. As in neighbouring French Equatorial Africa, porterage gave rise in German Cameroun to numberless exactions and abuses. Moreover—and this is peculiar to the Cameroun—the European conquest coincided with large movements of African populations, both into the forest zone and into the savannahs to the south of the central plateau of the Adamawa. Thus the Bavoute, who resisted the Germans until 1911, were migrating towards the south, pressed by the Mbum who were themselves pushed by the Fula. So, too, the Maka, who resisted until 1907, were not yet established in the region of Abong-Mbang. Many other examples could be given of these migrations and the conflicts they generated.

When we study the methods by which the Germans colonized the territory, we shall see many additional reasons for the almost permanent hostility of the forest peoples. However, in 1887, the Tappenbeck expedition reached Yaoundé, which is beyond the belt of dense forest, at an altitude of 700 metres. The climate, compared with that of the coast, was ideal, and the Ewondo welcomed the Germans. The celebrated Major Hans Dominik established himself at Yaoundé from 1894 onwards and made it his base for the conquest of the north and the east. While the savannahs offered fewer obstructions to the advance of a European force, the conquest of the Fula lamidates (principalities) of the north was especially arduous. The most northerly of these was Tibati, the strategic key to the whole of the Northern Cameroun. This area resisted first Eugen Zintgraff in 1888 and then Curt Morgen in 1893, and did not fall until 1899, after putting up a fierce resistance. In the following three years all the Fula lamidates fell one after another. In 1902 Major Dominik completed the conquest of the north by taking possession of the Mandara country and fortifying Moro. This territory was to become celebrated through the resistance of von Raven in 1916.

The conquered North Cameroun was not administered in the same way as the south. The Germans admired Islam and were impressed by the power of the Fula horsemen, whom they considered a superior race compared with the pagan Kirdi peasants. They therefore employed a system of indirect rule with three 'residencies' corresponding more or less to the three existing administrative regions of North Cameroun, Bénoué, and Adamawa, the last including the 'residency' of Banyo, which extended into the province of Bamenda in the Southern Cameroons. The Bamum, country discovered in 1901–2, formed a fourth 'residency'. Its sultan, the celebrated Njoya, inventor of an African alphabet, became a firm supporter of the Germans, who allowed him to set up a syncretic religion partaking at once of Islam and Christianity. The most northerly point reached by Christian missions in the German period was Foumban.

The administrative separation of the Northern and Southern Cameroun was now complete. The missions, and hence the schools, had not penetrated among the northern peoples, of whom a small proportion had been converted to Islam, and no effort at economic development was undertaken north of Yaoundé. We have already remarked on the present-day consequences of this neglect of the north by the Germans in Togo. In Cameroun the effects were even more grave because of the enormous differences in the social psychology between the peoples of the forest and those of the savannah, and also because the wealth resulting from colonization steadily grew in the south at the expense of the north, which was too far away from the centres of communication.

The economic exploitation of the Schutzgebiet-Kamerun was thus limited to the south, or more precisely to the 'forest' Cameroun. The economy rested principally on the plantations or concession companies to the north-west of Douala and on the gathering of crops to the south.

The concession companies

Even before the establishment of political control, the German agents of the Woermann Company had taken note of the extraordinary fertility of the volcanic lands to the west of Douala and along the slopes of Mount Cameroon, north of Victoria. The idea of plantations was thus 'in the air' from 1885 onwards. A marked predilection of the Germans for the agricultural sciences and a strong sense of organization seemed to promise miracles in this field. Obviously, however, the lands suitable for plantation were not simply 'idle and without a master'. They had first to be occupied, which was not an easy task. In 1891 an expedition of riflemen recruited in Dahomey and commanded by Freiherr Karl von Gravenreuth, 'the lion of West Africa', was sent to the slopes of Mount Cameroon north of Victoria, where it met disaster. The peoples of Buea were able to resist for another three years; but in 1895 they were finally deprived of their lands, were obliged to pay a heavy indemnity and were condemned to build the town of Buea. This town, situated 900 metres above sea level, was to be the capital of the colony between 1901 and 1909.

In 1895, the year when Governor Jesko von Puttkamer arrived for a stay of twelve years, the Victoria Plantations Company was founded with a capital of 2,500,000 marks. The following year the Bibundi Company—Bibundi is to the west of Mount Cameroon—was incorporated with a capital of 2,100,000 marks. André Chéradame lists twelve more plantation companies formed up to 1902. In 1913 there was a total of 58 plantations with 195 European employees and 17,827 workers.

A few of them were south of Douala, growing chiefly plantation rubber, introduced in 1904 (the plantations of Ngoulemakong east of Kribi and of Sangmelima are still producing today). They also cultivated cocoa, the systematic cultivation of which began in 1905 at Ebolowa and Yaoundé.

But the vast majority of the plantations was situated in the present-day West Cameroun (Southern Cameroons) and in the region of Moungo to the west of Douala. These produced the oil-palm, cocoa and bananas—introduced in 1907. Banana plantations around Tiko, which has remained the great banana-shipping port, covered 2,000 hectares in 1912. Cocoa was also cultivated by Africans from 1905 onwards. The native production in 1912 amounted to 715 metric tons out of a total production of 4,511 metric tons.

The plantations, whether African or European, called for a considerable labour force. The workers were not, however, badly treated during their labour contract. In fact, the plantation system seems on the whole to have been less harmful to the African than that of employing Africans to gather wild products.

The systematic collection of rubber and ivory was the principal activity of the two chartered companies whose record of abuses is still remembered in Cameroun. In fact, the older of the two and the only one that obtained any significant financial advantage, the Süd Kamerun Gesellschaft, had no obligation to fulfil in return for the cession of 9 million hectares in the south-east of the colony, an area which at this time was neither pacified nor indeed known. (In 1898 Von Carnap-Quernheimb reached the junction of the Ngoko and Sangha, the south-east limit of the German colony. The Maka resistance was broken by Dominik in 1907.) Founded by a German–Belgian group in December 1898, linked to Stanley Pool by the Sangha and the Congo rivers, the S.K.G. maintained close relations with the Congo and employed methods of recruitment for labourers and carriers similar to those denounced by E. D. Morel in the Congo Free State. In 1914, it employed 200,000 workers in the rubber-trade. It had 12 'factories' and 10 posts employing 100 Europeans and 700 Africans.

The Nord West Kamerun Gesellschaft, founded on 31 July 1899, received a concession of more than 8,000,000 hectares between Sangmelima on 12° N. latitude and the British frontier, but it was required in return to construct roads and railroads, to share in the costs of exploration towards Chad, and to create plantations and 'factories'. In contrast to the operation of the S.K.G., it did not prosper, no doubt because it had more obligations to fulfil than the S.K.G. Besides, it operated in the richest sector and came up against the interests of planters and the complaints of the missionaries. A Catholic mission was established at Marienberg in 1890, and one at Kribi and one at Edea the following year. An American Presbyterian mission was set up in 1893 at Efoulen south-west of Ebolowa in the Boulou country. This mission founded Ebolowa station in 1895, and it remains today the centre of the mission. Four additional stations in the Boulou country were opened before 1916. The Boulou, who had a monopoly on trade between Kribi and the interior, were upset by the competition of the N.W.K.G., whose centre of activity included the Boulou country. In 1899 they besieged Kribi and sacked the Catholic missionary station. In spite of severe reprisals they continued the war until 1901.

Between the Sanaga and the southern frontier of the territory, the numerous missionaries belonging to the Basel Mission, the Catholic Mission, or the Presbyterian Mission denounced the evils of porterage and forced labour of workers for the plantations. They also drew attention to the ravages of sleeping-sickness. In 1913, 80,000 porters were employed to link Yaoundé to Kribi. A thousand of them passed through Lolodorf daily, loaded with the rubber of the forests of the south-east.

The German Colonial Ministry was set up in 1907 with Dr Bernard Dernburg as minister. Dernburg devoted himself to carrying out a more coherent and more 'social' native policy than heretofore. In Cameroun, as elsewhere, numerous public works of an economic and social character were undertaken. It is from this brief period between 1908 and 1914 that the Camerounians of today date whatever good memories they retain of the German period. The conquest, along with the numerous acts of brutality that marked it, had by then almost ended; and the German local administration had been able to concern itself with the economic and social welfare of the Africans. But the good intentions of Berlin and of the governors often came to nought. Thus in 1908 the Kribi Chamber of Commerce rejected a project presented by Governor Theodor Seitz for the creation of native councils, and for communes and districts directed by a white 'curator'.

This was the period of great public works: of the so-called Northern Railroad, of which the stretch from Douala to N'Kongsamba, 160 kilometres in length, was inaugurated on 11 April 1911; the portion of the central railroad from Douala to Eseka, 174 kilometres long, was opened on 17 June 1914. In 1912 the road from Yaoundé to Kribi was finished; the ports of Tiko, Victoria, Douala and Kribi were fitted out; the cable from Douala to Monrovia was completed in 1913 as well as the Douala radio station.

At the same time the value of exports also began to rise considerably. Furthermore—and more important than anything else for the people of Cameroun—attendance figures for the schools leapt upwards. According to Rudin, the number of students in 1913 included 17,833 in the schools of the Basel Mission; 12,461 in those of the Catholic Mission,[1] whose first school had been opened in Marienberg on the Sanaga in 1891; 9,213 in the schools of the American Presbyterian Mission; 3,151 in the Baptist Mission school; 833 in official schools. In these schools the teaching of German occupied a more important place than it had in Togo. The young people of Cameroun were taught not only the language of Goethe but pride in Germany and disdain for all that was not German. The Germans thus created a Cameroun native élite very different from the Togolese top stratum of the same period.[2]

Whether they agreed or refused to enter the French administration, there is no doubt that a certain number of young Camerounians trained in the German schools became 'African Prussians', who regarded the brutality of German discipline as a necessary evil. One may well wonder what might have been the relations between the white Prussians and these black Prussians in the next generation. They could hardly have failed to become strained. Be that as it may, the Germans had by 1914 given to a small élite a degree of instruction that was remarkable for the period.

[1] Engelbert Mveng, in *Histoire du Cameroun* (Paris, 1963), gives this number on p. 332; on p. 464 he writes that before the declaration of war the Catholic schools had 19,576 pupils (following Hermann Skolaster, *Die Pallottiner in Kamerun*, 1924).

[2] This Camerounian élite's feelings are well described by the Cameroun author Jean Ikellé-Matiba in *Cette Afrique-là* (Paris, 1963). It is striking to hear his hero, the son of a Bassa, speak of 'our Kaiser', or to hear him say, 'We are the Prussian students'. This young African, imbued with German culture from his infancy, saw nothing untoward in the harshness of German discipline because he 'was treated like any other German' (p. 99). The Bassa, who number about 200,000, occupy a vast region situated on one side or the other of the lower Sanga between the ocean and Yaoundé (the Sanga maritime province). The missions had a considerable number of stations in the Bassa country during the German period (Lobetal, Marienberg, Edea, etc.).

German East Africa

In almost every respect, German East Africa was essentially different from the three Atlantic coast colonies. The writers who deal with German colonization as seen from Berlin have emphasized the peculiar way in which this colony was acquired. They have stressed also the personality of Karl Peters, who introduced into 'his' colony the 'energetic' policy called for by the Gesellschaft für deutsche Kolonisation. We shall concern ourselves here with another special characteristic that has been generally misunderstood or little taken into account.

In East Africa, African resistance to colonial control was early (1888), long drawn out (it lasted till 1907) and fierce. Three successive revolts led to heavy German losses, to the dispatch of military reinforcements, and to the voting of special funds by the Reichstag. The Bushiri uprising lasted from August 1888 to November 1890; the Hehe war from 1891 to 1898; and the Maji-Maji insurrection from 1905 to 1906. The last two of these have left a vivid memory in the oral tradition of the peoples of the centre and south of present-day Tanzania.

But the German colonization of East Africa was by no means as unfavourable to the Africans as was that of South West Africa. Conditions varied a great deal in the various parts of German East Africa, and so did the policies carried out by local administrators. There were, so to speak, several 'German East Africas', and even armed resistance to the Germans was limited to certain regions. By developing African cultivation of coffee (in the districts of Bukoba and Mwanza on the side of Lake Victoria, or among the Chagga of the Kilimanjaro), of coconuts (in the coastal area), of sisal and of cotton, the Germans in fact contributed very largely to the economic advancement of the African. Furthermore, by teaching Swahili systematically in schools and missions, they prepared the way for the creation in present-day Tanzania of a national consciousness much more solid than that in other independent African states that are plagued by a multiplicity of languages.

Resistance to German penetration

Scholars must study the pre-colonial history of present-day Tanzania in order to understand the motives and the methods of the African resistance. This history is very different from the past of the three west coast colonies. Two features outrank all others in importance: first, the relative absence on this side of the continent of extensive missionary or commercial European activity before 1884; and second, the existence for some fifty years previously of a trading network solidly organized by the coast Arabs along three great principal routes, of which the two most important were situated entirely on the territory of the German colony, while the third, which came into use somewhat later, was on the territory of present-day Kenya but led to the German East African ports of Tanga and Pangani.

All German works insist on the preponderant position occupied by German traders at Zanzibar after the year 1845, when the firm of O'Swald began a profitable trade in exporting cowries to the west coast of Africa. In 1870 German firms accounted for nearly a third of Zanzibar's commerce. But not one German trader had established himself on the mainland before 1884; nor were there any European merchants of other nationalities.

On the other hand, although no German missionaries worked in the territory of present-day Tanzania, there were several French Catholic missions (the Fathers of the Holy Spirit in Bagamoyo in 1869, the White Fathers at Tabora in 1878) and British Protestant missions (the Universities Mission to Central Africa in 1860 in Usambara and the hinterland of Lindi in 1874, the Church Missionary Society in 1876 in Mpwapwa, the London Missionary Society in 1878 in Ujiji on the edge of Lake Tanganyika). Apart from the Fathers of the Holy Spirit at Bagamoyo, however, none of the missions had by 1884 made much impact on the African societies, which remained essentially free from European influences except as regards trade goods.

Although missionaries had made almost no converts before 1884, they had done considerable work in the study of Swahili. Swahili, which today is spoken or understood by some thirty million people, was at that time confined almost entirely to the coast; but it was one of the few African languages possessed of a written literature—in Arabic characters—going back at least to the seventeenth century and epic poems transmitted by word of mouth since the fourteenth century.

The first Swahili dictionary and the first partial translation of the Bible were undertaken by Johann Krapf, a pioneer of Protestant missionary work in East Africa who was famous for having discovered Mount Kilimanjaro and Mount Kenya. Although he was in the service of the Church Missionary Society, which had a very British and very 'official' character, Krapf himself was German by birth. His work therefore had immediate repercussions in Germany. The scientific study of Swahili was to be pursued by Bishop Edward Steere of the U.M.C.A., who published in 1865 in Zanzibar *A handbook of the Swahili language as spoken at Zanzibar* and, thereafter, *Swahili tales* and a translation of the Bible. During their station at Bagamoyo the Fathers of the Holy Spirit taught their pupils a transcription of Swahili in Latin characters. This preparatory linguistic work of the missionaries was to have major consequences for German colonization.

The only peoples of East Africa who before 1884 had had contact with the outside world were those who lived near one of the great trade routes. The northern route from Mombasa to Lake Victoria (entirely in present-day Kenya) does not concern us except for its outlets at Tanga and Pangani, where in 1888 the Arab revolt at Bushiri broke out. It was the central route that was the most important. This followed roughly the line of the present-day Tanganyika railroad, joining Bagamoyo, on the coast facing Zanzibar, to Tabora in a forty-five days' march. So-called 'Arabs' (usually Mrima Swahili from the coast opposite Zanzibar) had established a colony at Tabora in 1840. From there, one route regularly frequented from 1848 onwards went to Lake Victoria and the kingdom of Buganda; another connected with Ujiji on Lake Tanganyika, which the Arabs crossed around 1856–7 to penetrate into the Ouroua, which is present-day North Katanga.

By 1884 the Arab traffic was sufficiently well established on the Tabora route for the neighbouring people to see nothing but advantage in the passage of caravans. At this time the sources of supply for ivory and slaves were mainly situated in the territories of present-day Uganda and Congo-Kinshasa. The tribal chiefs of what is now Tanganyika exacted from all travellers—European explorers or Arab heads of caravans—a toll or *hongo*. It is understandable that they should have been opposed to German colonization, which threatened to suppress this source of revenues both directly and indirectly (by preventing the setting up of slave caravans).

The southern route from Kilwa (or Lindi) to Lake Nyasa had a very different significance for the people along the way. They were not the beneficiaries of the route but its victims. Slaves were captured within present-day Tanzania as well as in what is now Malawi and Zambia. The Arabs, who arrived on the west bank of Lake Nyasa around 1858, were associated with the Yao. These were a Bantu-speaking people

who had come from Moçambique via the Rovuma river about 1860.
The Yao had been converted to Islam, and had supplied slaves to the
Arab or European slave-traders established at Kilwa, Lindi (in Tangan-
yika) or Ibo (in Moçambique). In addition to being harried by Arab or
Yao slave-traders, the peoples of Tanganyika were the victims of the
war-like Ngoni. The Ngoni, who came from distant Natal, had arrived
in the country between Lake Tanganyika and Lake Rukwa around 1842.
In 1878 and 1882 they had been repulsed by the Hehe of the region of
Iringa. At the time the Germans arrived the Ngoni were centred upon
Songea and took an active part in raids for slaves, who were subsequently sent to the coast.

Around 1890 the balance of African political power in the southern
quarter of the German colony was roughly this: there was one, and
only one, African kingdom, that of the Hehe of the region of Iringa.
It had only recently been formed by Chief Munzigumba, who died in
1879, and his son Mkwawa. Mkwawa was known as 'the warrior': he
had stopped the advance of the Masai towards the south, and in 1882
that of the Ngoni towards the north. He had afterwards attacked the
Nyamwezi, the Gogo and the Sagara and had made himself master
of the section of the 'Tabora route' between Mpwapwa and Kilosa.[1]
He exacted tribute from the Arab trade on the Tabora route and also
from that of the southern route; in addition he was the enemy of the
Ngoni. This explains the range of Hehe reactions to the three great
episodes of East African resistance.

At the time of the Bushiri revolt, Mkwawa was not very much
concerned, for his capital was a good twenty-four days' march from
Dar es Salaam. But when the Germans set up a post at Mpwapwa, he
became apprehensive. Between 1891, the year of the ambush of Lula
Ragaro (16 August), where Emil von Zelewski perished with ten
Europeans, and June 1898, when Mkwawa committed suicide in face of
defeat, Mkwawa waged continuous guerrilla warfare, supported by all
his people.

On the other hand, in 1905 the Hehe abstained from taking part in
the Maji-Maji insurrection, perhaps partly because of the activities of
the soldiers from the military post of Iringa. Apart from the Hehe and
the Ngoni, both of them militarily organized and warlike, the region

[1] Kilosa is in the Usagara. It was with the 'independent sultans' of Usagara that Carl
Peters made his famous treaties of November and December 1884 which were the
origin of the German colony.

of southern Tanganyika, which was to be the scene of the terrible Maji-Maji insurrection, was sparsely populated because of drought and the tsetse fly. The inhabitants consisted of primitive tribes, organized in clans, who lived in perpetual fear of the Arab slave-traders. They could thus be terrorized by the Arab or Swahili officials (*akida*) used by the Germans to enforce the planting of cotton or to recruit labour for the European plantations. These *akida* did not exert anything like the same power over the peoples of the coast nor over those along the Tabora trade route.

To the north of the Tabora route, the Germans had to reckon with only very localized and very slight resistance, for instance, that of the Chagga of Kilimanjaro (in the district of Moshi), who were very brutally treated by Carl Peters in 1891–2. On the Tabora route itself, the Germans encountered Siki, the son and successor of the celebrated Mirambo, the Nyamwezi chief who had set up a kingdom extending from Lake Victoria to Lake Tanganyika and who had died in 1884. But Siki was far from having the personality of his father; at the end of three years of active resistance, rather than surrender he had blown himself up with his powder magazine on 9 January 1893.

The early date of the Bushiri revolt (August 1888) is to be explained by the number and importance of those interested in the movement of caravans. In the coast towns of Tanga, Pangani, Saadani, Bagamoyo, Kilwa-Kivindje, Lindi and Mikindani, practically all the population lived by trade. The Indian bankers invested large sums in the long-term financing of the caravans. Although the tactlessness of von Zelewski in hoisting the flag of the German East Africa Company (instead of the sultan's flag) at Pangani actually set off the revolt, it was none the less clear that the German treaty with Zanzibar of April 1888 would have triggered a sharp reaction by the mere fact that it conceded to Europeans the collecting of taxes in the coastal strip. The revolt, which spread to the whole coast, necessitated reinforcements under Hermann von Wissmann, and an appropriation by the Reichstag of two million marks. In the end, the slave-trader Bushiri was betrayed by the chief of the Usambara and was hanged at Pangani on 15 December 1889.

The year 1890 had great significance for the Germans in East Africa. The Anglo-German treaty of 14 June and 1 July defined the sphere of influence and *ipso facto* rendered obsolete the treaty that Peters had signed the previous 24 February with the Kabaka of Buganda. Emin Pasha, who had entered the service of the German East Africa Company after having been liberated against his will by Stanley, signed a treaty of friendship with the Arabs of Tabora on 1 August. Langheld established the stations of Bukoba and Mwanza, on Lake Victoria. Finally, on 20 November the German East Africa Company handed over its administrative privileges to the Empire, and the Sultan of Zanzibar, in return for an indemnity, renounced his sovereignty over the coast of Tanganyika.

The Germans were defeated at Rugaro by the Hehe in June 1891; and in June 1892 they were repulsed near Moshi by the Chagga. On the other hand, Siki, the chief of the Nyamwezi, killed himself in January 1893, and shortly afterwards Meli, chief of the Chagga, was beaten. The following year was the turn of Bwana Heri, the chief of Saadani, who had supported Bushiri. Furthermore, Governor Freiherr Friedrich von Schele inflicted a serious defeat on Mkwawa in October. In 1896 Captain Tom von Prince established a military post in the centre of the Hehe country at Iringa. Mkwawa committed suicide, as has been noted, on 19 July 1898.

Balance sheet of German activity (1898–1905)

In 1898 the whole of the colony appeared sufficiently quiet for the authorities to demand that Africans pay a head tax. According to some writers, a positive programme of development had already been set in motion. Given the exceptional difficulties arising from the existence of Arab traders in the German colony, this would seem a remarkable achievement. In 1896 there were twenty-three plantations, of which fifteen were in the Usambara and eight on the coast. The hinterland of Tanga and the district of Moshi around Kilimanjaro remained the most favoured area for German plantations, and it was here that all the experiments with new crops were conducted. These crops included coffee, quinine, cotton, tobacco, tea, vanilla, and above all sisal, which was introduced in 1892 from Florida and which became Tanganyika's most important cash crop. The construction of roads and bridges, particularly the road from Tanga to Kilimanjaro, was begun about 1894. However, at this time more than two-fifths of all exports still consisted of ivory exchanged by Arab merchants for fire-arms—a figure that points up the relative unimportance of plantation agriculture at that time.

By 1894 Christian missions had already established a considerable number of stations. Since 1887 the Evangelische Missionsgesellschaft für Deutsch-Ostafrika had founded posts at Dar es Salaam and Tanga, two posts in the Usambara, and one in the Usaramo in the hinterland of Dar es Salaam. The Moravian Brothers (Brüdergemeinde) had shared since 1891 with the Evangelical Mission Society of Berlin the missionary work in the mountainous regions to the north of Lake Nyasa. The Leipzig Lutheran Mission (Evangelisch-Lutherische Missionsgesellschaft zu Leipzig) had laboured among the Chagga of Kilimanjaro since 1893. These missions, in addition to some other German bodies, all began their evangelical work in East Africa after 1884. The Catholic missions established before 1884 had been considerably extended by 1894. The Fathers of the Holy Spirit had besides their old post at Bagamoyo (1869) two stations in the Useguha and the Nguru behind Saadani, two in the Moshi district, and two near Morogoro. The White Fathers, who had arrived in the region of the Great Lakes in 1878, had eight stations between Lake Victoria and Lake Tanganyika. Lastly, the Benedictine Mission of Bavaria had established itself at Dar es Salaam in 1889.

With the exception of the two long-established stations of the U.M.C.A. founded in 1876 in the hinterland of Lindi, there was no missionary activity at all in the southern quarter of the colony that was to be the scene of the Maji-Maji insurrection in 1905. However, before the rebellion the Benedictines had attempted to establish a Catholic mission; they had set up a station in 1898 at Peramiho (near Songea) in the Ngoni country and two others in the Hehe country in 1896 and 1898.

The Christian missions played an important role in the diffusion of Swahili in the interior of the German colony. In 1887 a chair of Swahili was created at the University of Berlin, held by the Lutheran missionary G. C. Büttner. Except in a few government schools, German was hardly taught in East Africa, and there was nothing corresponding to the Prusso-African élite that existed in the Cameroun and Togo. Swahili was used everywhere. It was current from the beginning of German colonization, and was employed as a lingua franca even in countries that had little contact with the coast. Swahili was understood as far as Ruanda and Burundi, remote residencies that the Germans had neither the time nor the means to exploit, but where many missions were established at the beginning of the twentieth century. The spread of Swahili brought with it the diffusion of Islam in the interior of the country where before colonization Islam had reached only the Yao in the south—a result not intended by the Christian missionaries. The German administration of East Africa suffered perhaps more than that of any other colony from a want of men, both in numbers and in quality. In 1903 the colony was divided into twenty-two districts (*Bezirke*), of which ten were civilian and twelve military. With the exception of the circumscription of Langenburg (between Lake Nyasa and Lake Rukwa), all regions more than 200 kilometres from the coast were under military administration, that is to say, under direct administration that used the native chiefs as collectors of taxes or recruiters of labour. In the districts under civil administration, the Germans used very largely the system of *akida*, of Swahili or Arab origin, who shared their powers with certain influential natives (*jumbes*). We have already said how great a mistake it was to employ *akidas* among the peoples of the south, who had been victims of slave-hunters for over a century.

The Maji-Maji insurrection

Beyond the region of Iringa, which had been closely studied since the establishment of a military post there in 1896, the south-east of the colony was practically unexplored by 1903. (This is shown by the maps drawn at this period and by those in the book of Chéradame.) The area where the Maji-Maji insurrection was to break out corresponded to the civil districts of Morogoro, Rufiji, Kilwa and Lindi, and to the military districts of Mahenge and Iringa. The last area was in the Songea in the south and was the fief of the celebrated Ngoni warriors. A number of the leaders belonged to the Pogoro tribe, but members of the Ngoni, Bunga, Mwere, Sagara, Zaramo, Matumbi, Kitchi, Ikemba and Bena all participated in the revolt.

The course of events is well-known. In July 1905, the peoples of Kibata in the Matumbi hills (in the hinterland of Kilwa) refused to undertake forced labour in the government's cotton fields and laid siege to the *akida*'s residence. The rebellion was rapidly put down at Kibata, but it spread to the districts of Mahenge and Kilosa (on the great Tabora route), and then to Liwale, the only German post existing between Kilwa and Songea. All foreigners (Europeans, Swahili and Arabs) were attacked by warriors using magic water (Maji-Maji) that 'turns rifle bullets into water'. At Lindi the missionaries' establishments were destroyed. The town of Kilosa was sacked. The missionary station of Maneromango, 50 kilometres south of Dar es Salaam, was burned. At the end of August the capital itself appeared to be seriously menaced.

In September Bishop Cassian Spiss was murdered with his attendants while on his way to the Benedictine station at Peramiho (Songea). In October two cruisers brought reinforcements recruited in Somaliland and New Guinea. A cruel repression swept the country beginning in November. The rebel villages were systematically burned and their harvests destroyed. By the middle of 1906 the Germans had taken the offensive. By the end of the year they again controlled the more important settlements in the southern part of the country. The Ngoni of Songea, however, continued to resist until 1907. Their chief, Chabruma, was finally forced to flee into Portuguese territory, and all remaining leaders of the rebellion were executed.

It is impossible to calculate exactly the extent of losses in human life in that rebellion. To the 26,000 Africans officially counted as direct victims of the repression must be added some tens of thousands who died of hunger or sickness. Even today the southern province of Tanzania, very sparsely peopled, bears the marks of the insurrection of 1905–6; and it would be difficult to find there any supporters of German colonization.

Nevertheless, it is undeniable that the change of attitude that took place in 1907 in the German colonies after the creation of the Ministry of Colonies was particularly spectacular in East Africa. The first task of the new minister, Dr Dernburg, was to inform himself as to the causes of the Maji-Maji revolt. He then set about instituting many reforms that had already been suggested by various administrators on the spot. He ordered a reduction in corporal punishments, forbade the use of the whip by private persons, instituted health regulations for the benefit of wage-earners, encouraged school attendance, and set in motion a plan for the economic development of the colony that would encourage agricultural production both in European plantations and among native growers.

Governor Freiherr Albrecht von Rechenberg, who held his post from 1906 to 1912, attempted to put these measures into effect. He found at the outset that the labour question posed very difficult problems. The plantation districts (Usambara, Mt Pare, Mt Kilimanjaro), occupied in 1913 by 882 planters, were not themselves sufficiently populated. The tribes capable of furnishing manpower on a large scale were principally the Nyamwezi and the Sukuma, dwelling well away from the coast, south of Lake Victoria. But the central railroad did not reach Tabora until 27 July 1912. Because the delays en route considerably increased the period during which the worker was separated from his family, the villages tended to become depopulated. The consequent ills were aggravated by the spread of venereal diseases brought from the coast by the workers. The administration was called upon to provide not only agricultural workers, but also carriers and labourers for public works. In 1913 there were over 133,000 wage-earners, of whom 91,892 were on the plantations, 3,000 in the mines, 13,000 in railroad construction, 15,000 carriers working for Asiatics, 5,000 working for the whites and 5,000 working for the government.

Missionary work in education developed considerably between 1907 and 1914. According to the somewhat unreliable statistics of the time, there were in 1914 6,100 pupils in government schools and 155,287 in mission schools. Swahili newspapers appeared. A series of religious tracts in Swahili had an edition of 11,000 in 1910. In 1914 persons able to read Swahili were to be found everywhere in the villages, and they gave the chiefs written orders coming from Dar es Salaam. (After the war the British were astonished at the number of people in Tanganyika who could read Swahili.)

The missions took part also in the important medical work undertaken by the administration. It was after a visit to East Africa that Dr Robert Koch in 1907 introduced atoxyl, which for fifty years was to be used against sleeping-sickness. The struggle against smallpox and sleeping-sickness was already taking place on a large scale in 1914.

Between 1907 and 1914 the progress in production was equally spectacular. European efforts in the districts of Tanga and Morogoro were concentrated on plantation rubber and on sisal and cotton. The native farmers in the district of Bukoba produced three-quarters of the total output of coffee, those in the district of Mwanza three-quarters of the ground-nuts. Copra, too, was cultivated by the coast inhabitants.

In February 1912 the extension of the railroad from Usambara to Neû Moshi at the foot of Kilimanjaro was opened. The central railroad reached Kigoma on Lake Tanganyika, 1,252 kilometres from Dar es Salaam, in March 1914. A commemorative exhibition was being prepared just at the time the news of the declaration of war arrived.

The war in East Africa

German East Africa was the sole territory in Africa where military operations lasted more than four years, thanks to the extraordinary personality of General Paul Emil von Lettow-Vorbeck and to his decision to keep the greatest possible number of enemy troops occupied on African soil in order to prevent them from taking part in the war in Europe. He carried out this design to perfection: the Allies arrayed against him 130 generals and 300,000 men; and 967 officers and 17,650 men were killed or wounded. Von Lettow-Vorbeck had only 3,000 Europeans and 12,000 askari.

This war in East Africa has been given the name of 'the last gentleman's war' and has given rise to an abundant literature. Until March 1916 the Germans were masters on their own soil, but General Smuts's offensive caused them to lose first the plantation region in the north of the colony and then the central railroad after Tabora had been taken by the Belgians. From October 1916, although the Germans were no more than fugitives in their colony, they continued to fight. In November 1917 Lettow-Vorbeck crossed the Rovuma with 278 Europeans, 16,000 askari and 4,000 carriers. After a stay of ten months in Portuguese territory, he returned to the north-west in September 1918 only to receive the news of the German capitulation in present-day Zambia, near Abercorn.

The war left unforgettable memories, especially in the southern half of the colony. The blacks recalled not the achievements of the whites but the sufferings and misery consequent upon war: the forced recruitment of thousands of porters, the neglect of European plantations and native crops, the flight of the village people in face of the askaris' exactions. On the other hand, for the askari, who were often recruited among the Hehe and the Ngoni who had fought the Germans for so long, the war represented a veritable promotion in the social scale that would have been unthinkable in peacetime. Two facts especially left their imprint upon the African combatants: in battle a white bullet did the same job as a black bullet, and a dead white man was the same as a dead black. Although the Germans had proved to Africans before the war that they were stronger, now they had been beaten by other whites without having ever suffered an obvious defeat in the field. And the idea implanted in the African mind that the whites were not invincible was to play a significant role in the campaign for the independence of Tanganyika.

BIBLIOGRAPHY

Bouchaud, J. *Histoire et géographie du Cameroun sous mandat français*. New ed. Douala, 1944.

Bridgman, Jon, and David E. Clarke. *German Africa: a select annotated bibliography*. Stanford, Calif., Hoover Institution, 1965.

Brunschwig, Henri. *L'expansion allemande outre-mer du XVe siècle à nos jours*. Paris, 1957.

Byern, Georg von. *Deutsch-Ostafrika und seine weissen und schwarzen Bewohner*. Berlin, 1913.

Calvert, Albert F. *German East Africa*. London, 1917.

Chéradame, André. *La colonisation et les colonies allemandes*. Paris, 1905.

Comité de l'Afrique Française, Paris. *Les crimes allemands en Afrique*. Paris, 1917.

Cornevin, Robert. *Histoire du Togo*. 3rd ed. Paris, 1969.
Togo: nation-pilote. Paris, 1963.

Debrunner, Hans W. *A church between colonial powers*. London, 1965.

Decharme, Pierre. *Compagnies et sociétés coloniales allemandes*. Paris, 1903.

Deutscher Kolonialkongress, Berlin. *Verhandlungen des Deutschen Kolonialkongresses 1902 zu Berlin am 10. und 11. Oktober 1902*. Berlin, 1903.
Verhandlungen des Deutschen Kolonialkongresses 1905 zu Berlin am 5., 6. und 7. Oktober 1905. Berlin, 1906.

Deutscher Kolonialkongress, Berlin. *Verhandlungen des Deutschen Kolonialkongresses 1910 zu Berlin am 6., 7. und 8. Oktober 1910*.
Verhandlungen des Deutschen Kolonialkongresses 1924 zu Berlin am 17. und 18. September 1924. Berlin, 1924.

Dove, Karl. *Die deutschen Kolonien*, vol. III: *Ostafrika*. Leipzig, 1912.

Dubois, L.-A.-P. 'Campagne des allemands dans le Sud-Ouest africain (1904–1905–1906)', *Revue des Troupes Coloniales*, July, Aug., Oct., Nov. 1910, **9**, nos. 97–8, 100–1.

First, Ruth. *South West Africa*. Harmondsworth, Middlesex and Baltimore, 1963.

Friedländer, Paul, and Harmut Schilling. *Kolonialmacht Westdeutschland: zum Wesen, zu den Besonderheiten und Methoden des westdeutschen Neokolonialismus*. [East] Berlin, 1962.

Full, August. *Fünfzig Jahre Togo*. Berlin, 1935.

Germany. Kolonialamt. *Kolonien unter der Peitsche*, Fritz Ferdinand Müller, ed. [East] Berlin, 1962.

Gifford, Prosser, and Wm. Roger Louis, eds. *Britain and Germany in Africa: imperial rivalry and colonial rule*. New Haven and London, Yale University Press, 1968.

Great Britain. Foreign Office. *Les colonies allemandes d'Afrique d'après les rapports consulaires anglais* [Diplomatic and consular reports, annual series]. Paris, Comité de l'Afrique Française, 1916.

Grosclaude, Pierre. *Menaces allemandes sur l'Afrique.* Paris, 1938.

Gulliver, P. H. 'A history of the Songea Ngoni', *Tanganyika Notes and Records*, Dec. 1955, no. 41.

Harlow, Vincent and E. M. Chilver, eds., assisted by Alison Smith. *History of East Africa*, vol. II. Oxford, Clarendon Press, 1965.

Henderson, W. O. 'German East Africa, 1884–1918', in *History of East Africa*, vol. II, Vincent Harlow and E. M. Chilver, eds., assisted by Alison Smith. Oxford, Clarendon Press, 1965.

Henkel, F. *Der Kampf um Südwestafrika.* Berlin, 1908.

Hintrager, Oskar. *Südwestafrika in der deutschen Zeit.* Munich, 1955.

Ikellé-Matiba, Jean. *Cette Afrique-là.* Paris, 1963.

Iliffe, John. 'The organization of the Maji Maji rebellion', *Journal of African History*, 1967, **8**, no. 3.

Ketchoua, Thomas. *Contribution à l'histoire du Cameroun de 450 avant Jésus-Christ à nos jours.* Yaounde, 1962.

Labouret, Henri. *Le Cameroun.* Paris, 1937.

Lagrave, R., and P. Guy. *Histoire du Cameroun.* Mulhouse, 1961.

Lembezat, Bertrand. *Le Cameroun.* Paris, 1964.

Lettow-Vorbeck, Paul Emil von. *Meine Erinnerungen aus Ostafrika.* Leipzig, 1920.

Leutwein, Paul, ed. *Dreissig Jahre deutscher Kolonialpolitik.* Berlin, 1914.

Leutwein, Theodor. *Elf Jahre Gouverneur in Deutsch-Südwestafrika.* 3rd ed. Berlin, 1908.

Lewin, Percy Evans. *German rule in Africa.* London, 1918.

Listowel, Judith. *The making of Tanganyika.* London, 1965.

Louis, William Roger. *Ruanda-Urundi, 1884–1919.* Oxford, Clarendon Press, 1963.

Metzger, O. F. *Unsere alte Kolonie Togo.* Neudamm, 1941.

Müller, Gustav. *Geschichte der Ewe-Mission.* Bremen, 1904.

Müller, Karl. *Geschichte der katholischen Kirche in Togo.* Kaldenkirchen, 1958.

Mveng, Engelbert. *Histoire du Cameroun.* Paris, 1963.

Newbury, Colin W. *The western Slave Coast and its rulers: European trade and administration among the Yoruba and Adja-speaking peoples of south-western Nigeria, southern Dahomey and Togo.* Oxford, Clarendon Press, 1961.

Nigmann, E. *Die Wahehe: ihre Geschichte, Kult-, Rechts-, Kriegs- und Jagd-Gebräuche.* Berlin, 1908.

Nussbaum, Manfred. *Togo: eine Musterkolonie?* Berlin, 1962.

Vom 'Kolonialenthusiasmus' zur Kolonialpolitik der Monopole: zur deutschen

Kolonialpolitik unter Bismarck, Caprivi, Hohenlohe. [East] Berlin, Akademie-Verlag, 1962.

Oliver, Roland. *The missionary factor in East Africa.* 2nd ed. London, 1965.

Patte, Henri. *Le Sud-Ouest africain allemand: révolte des Hereros.* Paris, 1907.

Peters, Carl Friedrich Hubert. *Lebenserinnerungen.* Hamburg, 1918.
Die Gründung von Deutsch-Ostafrika. Berlin, 1906.

Pfeil und Klein-Ellguth, Joachim Friedrich, Count von. *Die Erwerbung von Deutsch-Ostafrika: ein Beitrag zur Kolonial-Geschichte.* Berlin, 1907.

Pimienta, Robert. *L'ancienne colonie allemande du Sud-Ouest africain.* Paris, 1920.

Prussia. Armee. Grosser Generalstab. *Die Kämpfe der deutschen Truppen in Südwestafrika.* 2 vols. Berlin, 1906.

Puttkamer, Jesko Albert Eugen von. *Gouverneursjahre in Kamerun.* Berlin, 1912.

Raum, O. F. 'German East Africa: changes in African life under German administration, 1892–1914', in *History of East Africa*, vol. II, Vincent Harlow and E. M. Chilver, eds., assisted by Alison Smith. Oxford, Clarendon Press, 1965.

Rentzell, Werner von. *Unvergessenes Land: von glutvollen Tagen und silbernen Nächten in Togo.* Hamburg, 1922.

Royal Institute of International Affairs. Information Department. *Germany's claim to colonies.* London, 1938.

Rudin, Harry R. *Germans in the Cameroons, 1884–1914: a case study in modern imperialism.* New Haven, Yale University Press, 1938.

Schmidt, Rochus. *Deutschlands Kolonien: ihre Gestaltung, Entwicklung und Hilfsquellen.* 2 vols. Berlin, 1895.

Schramm, Percy Ernst. *Deutschland und Übersee.* Braunschweig, 1950.

Schwabe, Kurt. *Der Krieg in Deutsch-Südwestafrika, 1904–1906.* Berlin, 1907.

Seidel, August. *Deutsch-Kamerun: wie es ist und was es verspricht; historisch, geographisch, politisch, wirtschaftlich dargestellt.* Berlin, 1906.

Southwest Africa (Protectorate). Administrator's Office. *Report on the natives of South-West Africa and their treatment by Germany.* London, 1918.

Spieth, Jakob. *Die Ewestämme: Material zur Kunde des Ewe-Volkes in Deutsch-Togo.* Berlin, 1906.

Stoecker, Helmuth, ed. *Kamerun unter deutscher Kolonialherrschaft: Studien.* Vol. I. Berlin (East), 1960.

Townsend, Mary. *The rise and fall of Germany's colonial empire, 1884–1918.* New York, 1930.

Trierenberg, Georg. *Togo: die Aufrichtung der deutschen Schutzherrschaft und die Erschliessung des Landes.* Berlin, 1914.

Vedder, Heinrich. *Die Bergdama.* Hamburg, 1923.

Vietor, Johann Karl. *Geschichtliche und kulturelle Entwicklung unserer Schutz-
gebiete.* Berlin, 1913.

Watermeyer, J. C. *Deutsch-Südwest-Afrika: seine landwirtschaftlichen Verhält-
nisse.* Berlin, 1899.

Zache, Hans. *Deutsch-Ostafrika—Tanganjika Territory.* Berlin, 1926.

Zimmermann, Alfred. *Geschichte der deutschen Kolonialpolitik.* Berlin, 1914.

CHAPTER 13

IMPERIALISM AND EXPANSIONISM IN ETHIOPIA FROM 1865 TO 1900

by HAROLD G. MARCUS

The reign of Theodore II, 1856–68, marked a period of unification in the history of Ethiopia. Theodore attempted to break the power of the feudal chiefs by forcibly replacing them with administrators who were faithful to the imperial crown. At the same time he tried to build up a national army and to win the financial and moral support of the Orthodox Church. His charisma and military prowess enabled him to impose his will over the mountainous nation and to attempt to end the disunity of the previous century. In 1856 Theodore descended upon Shoa to overthrow King Haile Malekot, who had proved to be politically unreliable. After defeating the Shoan forces Theodore named an administrator to rule the province, and took Haile Malekot's orphaned son Menilek into his court.

Menilek was raised by Theodore as a prince. While acting as a page and courtier, he gained valuable experience in statecraft. He was trained also in the arts of manhood and war. The emperor acknowledged the potential of the young man by raising him to the rank of dejazmatch (earl) and honoured him with the hand of his daughter. Menilek, however, never forgot his origins nor his right to the Shoan throne, and in June 1865 he fled from Theodore's court. By this time, Theodore's hold over Ethiopia had become precarious because he had been unable to implement his revolutionary schemes. Menilek therefore had little difficulty in reaching Shoa, where he was generally welcomed by the people. In August 1865, with the nucleus of his new army around him, Menilek proclaimed himself King of Shoa.

A revitalized kingdom of Shoa showed up Theodore's domestic failure. His foreign policy, too, was bankrupt. Theodore wished to ally himself with Christendom in a crusade against the Turks. Such a mediaeval proposal was preposterous in terms of nineteenth-century international relations. Theodore was particularly interested in a British alliance, but London turned a deaf ear to his proposals and diplomatic manoeuvring. As more and more of Ethiopia fell into the hands of enemies, the need for an understanding with Britain became an obsession with Theodore. Such an arrangement would enable him to destroy the Moslems, but would help him to rally Ethiopia round him, to show his people the virtues of unity, and to destroy his reactionary enemies.

Because Theodore felt that Britain must ultimately be forced to become a party to the grand design, he carefully stepped on the lion's tail by imprisoning some minor diplomatic personnel. Such shock treatment only caused the British to mount an unnecessary expedition into Ethiopia in 1868 to erase the insult to British honour. The British moved against a man whose domestic politics were bankrupt and whose international policies were based on illusions. Ethiopia was unwilling to fight for such a leader, with the result that no army blocked the British advance to Theodore's fortress at Mak'dala. Britain was allowed to act as Ethiopia's hatchet-man. Betrayed by his dreams and deserted by his people, Theodore committed suicide, thus opening a period of imperial competition in Ethiopia.

As a reward to Dejazmatch Kassa of Tigre, who had given substantial aid to the British expeditionary force, Lord Napier ultimately turned over to him most of his surplus war materials—and in so doing gave him a significant advantage in modern weaponry over Menilek and Gobesie of Wag, the two pretenders to the imperial crown. Because Wag was closer to Tigre than Shoa, and the challenge accordingly greater, Kassa moved first against Gobesie. In July 1871 the two armies met at Aduwa, where Gobesie was defeated and captured. Kassa thereupon took the title of emperor, and on 21 January 1872 was crowned Yohannis IV of Ethiopia.

Menilek, now alone in his refusal to recognize the suzerainty of the newly-anointed emperor, realized that Yohannis had a distinct military superiority. The king therefore embarked on a new and dangerous policy. He decided to co-operate with Egypt, an imperialistic power, which had the modern arms to fight Yohannis's forces. Menilek planned to use Egyptian territorial ambitions in northern Ethiopia as a weapon against Yohannis. As part of a co-ordinated plan, Yohannis would be lured into central Ethiopia and would there be entrapped by the armies of Shoa and Egypt with its ally, Aussa. In 1873 Menilek raised a large army to implement the plan. From the beginning, the scheme was doomed to failure. Menilek's army could make no headway in Wollo. Then the Sultan of Aussa turned on the Egyptians and wiped out one of their units, killing Munzinger Pasha, a key personality in the plot against Yohannis. Finally, in 1875 and 1876 the emperor won decisive victories against the Egyptians. Menilek attempted to carry on alone, but only succeeded in exhausting his army in a fruitless campaign in the north. In 1877, moreover, Shoa was shaken by two rebellions that forced Menilek to return home. At Menilek's point of greatest weakness, Yohannis chose to invade Shoa to force the king to accept his suzerainty. Menilek had no option but to submit. In March 1878 the two antagonists concluded a treaty stipulating that Menilek should renounce the imperial title and be called King of Shoa; that he should pay periodic tribute; and that he should provide supplies and assistance for Yohannis's army in times of crisis. The Bashilo river in the north, the Abbai to the west and the Awash to the east and south were to form the boundaries of Menilek's domain.

The agreements with Yohannis temporarily thwarted attempts by Menilek to alter the political situation in the Abyssinian highlands. Although the way to the north was now closed, southern and eastern expansion might still shift the strategic balance within Ethiopia and could provide Menilek with a broader base from which to take advantage of future opportunities to gain the imperial crown. From 1878 to 1889, the year he became emperor, Menilek incorporated large areas into his kingdom by force of arms. From his new domains he obtained manpower for his armies and increased revenues that he used to purchase modern arms.

Menilek realized that his defeat at the hands of Yohannis had been partly a result of the Shoan inferiority in weapons. As early as 1871 he had attempted to set up an arms trade between Shoa and Europe. But the traffic in weapons only began to grow when France and Italy effectively took control of ports on the coast and when merchants pioneered new routes into Shoa. Between 1880 and 1884 trade from Italian Assab and French Obock grew rapidly, and Menilek was able to purchase weapons while expanding his exports of ivory, civet, hides, coffee and gold. By 1886, Menilek's arsenals were relatively full, and his fire-power had no doubt been considerably increased. In fact, so impressive was his new-found strength that he and Yohannis had already come to a new agreement in 1882. Yohannis officially confirmed Menilek's conquests and apparently recognized Menilek as the successor to the Ethiopian throne. In return, Menilek promised to hand on the succession to Yohannis's son, who was to marry Menilek's

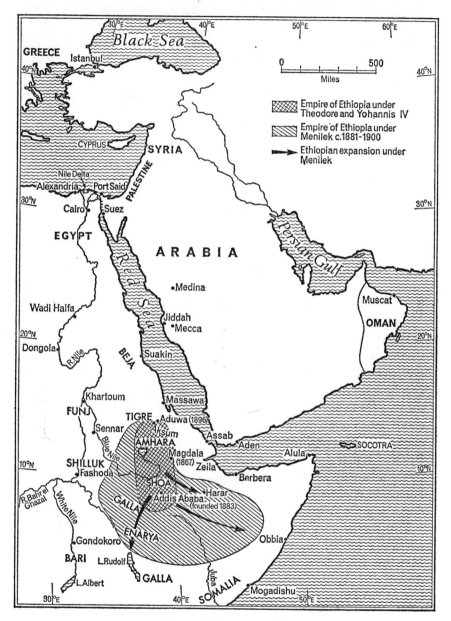

Fig. 13. Menilek's expansion.

daughter, Zawditu. The male issue of their union would, therefore, combine the two Solomonic blood lines.

With the conquest and absorption of Arussi in 1885–6 and of the city and province of Harar in 1887, Menilek controlled an area almost as large as the northern Ethiopian heartland, with excellent natural resources and a large population from which to recruit a bigger army. To gain further strength, he signed an apparently secret 'Treaty of Amity and Alliance' with Italy on 20 October 1887. By this instrument Italy virtually recognized Menilek as a sovereign power in Ethiopia and assured him 'military aid and otherwise to make good his rights' in return for a promise 'to aid the Government of His Majesty the King of Italy in all circumstances'. Menilek was granted 5,000 Remington rifles, the acquisition of which was probably his real motive for signing the treaty. The 1887 agreement can only represent an act of insubordination by Menilek against the imperial crown, since, by this time, Yohannis was warring against Italy.

Yohannis, the Italians and Menilek, 1885–9

In February 1885 the Italians had occupied the Red Sea port of Massawa, overriding protests from the Egyptian authorities but with the British government's full knowledge if not actual support. The British were deeply concerned lest the Egyptian débâcle in the Sudan should open the way for France to enter the Nile Basin from the east. They therefore chose not to interfere with the recently-awakened Italian imperialism, even though it was directed towards Egypt, their own client state. The British felt that it would be wiser to have the Massawa area controlled by the relatively weak Italians rather than by their arch-imperial enemy, France. In effect, the British decided to use the Italians as their watchdog along the Eritrean coast.

The Emperor of Ethiopia was irritated by the Italian action but raised no formal objection because the Italians had occupied only Massawa and a few adjacent villages. When the Italians moved into Arafali and Arkiko, however, the emperor and his chief lieutenant, Ras Alula of Hamasien, became uneasy. Their fears materialized when in June 1885 the Italians took Saati, a hitherto neutral zone. While the Italians had probably acted to secure the trade route into the Sudan, Ras Alula viewed the action as an affront to the integrity of Ethiopia and as a sign that the Italian government intended to expand its zone of influence and occupation. The Italians also made an insulting blunder by welcoming at Massawa with great pomp the Cantibai (or Sheik) of Habab, one of Yohannis's acknowledged vassals, and by asking him to make an independent agreement with the Italians ensuring the liberty and security of the trade route to the Sudan.

To calm Ethiopian fears, the Italian government decided to dispatch a high-ranking mission to Yohannis. In late January 1886, the members of the mission were well enough received by Ras Alula, who began arranging for their journey inland to meet Yohannis. But the emperor was otherwise occupied, and the necessary letter of safety could not be easily obtained—much to the chagrin of the Italians. Furthermore, the Italian government received intelligence of a letter written by the emperor to Menilek that showed a menacing distaste for Italians. On 8 March, therefore, the Rome government ordered the mission to return. This move insulted the emperor, who had fully intended to negotiate with the envoys. And, in terms of Ethiopian politics, such a withdrawal also seemed a sign of weakness and an admission of failure.

The Italians had not, however, given up hopes for a settlement, and dispatched a letter to Yohannis and Alula about the frontiers. In late October 1886 Ras Alula replied to Count Augusto Salimbeni, an experienced Italian agent, that discussions based upon the Italian letter should be pursued after the Ethiopian leader returned from a campaign against the Mahdists. Apparently uninformed about the diplomatic tentative, General Genè, the Italian commander at Massawa, marched to the wells at Ua-à, four hours' march from Zula—ostensibly to guarantee further the free passage of caravans into the Sudan. In reply to the immediate Ethiopian protest, Genè feebly responded that he had occupied the area out of friendship for the Ethiopians and to facilitate trade. Ras Alula, finally learning of the latest Italian encroachment, told Salimbeni that the Italian government obviously wanted to invade Abyssinian territory via the same route that the ill-fated Egyptians had followed. He was further enraged because it appeared that the Italian authorities had taken advantage of his involvement elsewhere to invade Ethiopia.

The Ras thereupon organized his forces and on 24 January 1887 left Asmara for Saati with a large army. The next morning he engaged the 500-man Italian garrison. Though the Italians fought magnificently and held their positions, they were surrounded by a vastly superior force. General Genè accordingly sent reinforcements of 550 men under the command of Lieutenant-Colonel Tommaso de Cristoforis. On 26 January at 8.00 a.m., this column was ambushed at Dogali by Ras Alula. Overwhelmed by 10,000 Ethiopians, the Italians lost 430 officers and men killed and 82 wounded. Upon word of this disaster, Genè consolidated his defence by withdrawing the garrisons at Saati, Ua-à, and Arafali.

The news of the 'massacre' at Dogali was received with consternation in Italy. The majority of deputies in Parliament voted to avenge their dead and authorized 20 million lire ($3,648,000) for a special African expeditionary corps commanded by General Alessandro Asinari di San Marzano. While this force was being trained, Italian policy-makers tried to gain Menilek's active support against the emperor, intending to weaken the latter's domestic position. Several prominent Italians had convinced the Rome government to assist Menilek's ambitions in Ethiopia so that when he became emperor he would happily make concessions out of gratitude. While Menilek probably did not understand the full implications of the Italian Shoan policy, he did realize that Italian support could be significant. He therefore negotiated with the Italians, but temporized about undertaking any potentially embarrassing obligations until he should feel strong enough to challenge the emperor's position directly. If nothing else, the Shoan–Italian treaty of October 1887 represented Menilek's feeling that he would ultimately be stronger than Yohannis and that he was now in a position to win the imperial crown.

His chance came after the Italians had humiliated Yohannis by the astute use of the expeditionary army that had arrived in November 1887. General di San Marzano had instructions to reoccupy Saati and Ua-à. Having sufficient funds and the active support of his government, the general built roads and bridges to ensure mobility; he connected Saati and Moncullo with a 27 kilometre light railway; he established good relations with the local population; and he made Massawa impregnable. Di San Marzano fondly hoped that Yohannis's army would destroy itself against the newly constructed defences of the Italian colony.

The emperor, however, realized that his undisciplined levies could not take the Italian fortifications and chose not to attack. Yohannis thereby weakened his prestige in the eyes of his chiefs, who had come from all parts of Ethiopia—except, significantly, from Shoa and Gojjam—to fight against the Europeans. After a month's confrontation, the provisions of the Ethiopian forces ran out, and the emperor began a rapid retreat on 2 April 1887.

The Italian revenge was to become even more complete when the repercussions from Yohannis's humiliation began to be felt. While Yohannis was engaged in his fruitless campaign against the Italians, the Mahdists had invaded Gojjam, had defeated King Tekle Haimanot and had sacked Gondar, the capital of Amhara. Being otherwise occupied, Yohannis could not send any assistance to Tekle Haimanot. The king was not only bitter about this lack of support, but was at the same time deeply saddened by the loss of two children who had been caught and killed by the Mahdists. Taking advantage of the Gojjami leader's disaffection, Menilek invited Tekle Haimanot to join him in a move against the authority of the emperor. Both rulers therefore refused to send Yohannis additional troops, but keeping the door open for negotiations they did not disavow their obligation to transmit tribute in money and goods. Furthermore, Menilek concluded a defensive alliance with Tekle Haimanot—a direct affront to the emperor's power. Meanwhile, Menilek signed the Treaty of Amity and Alliance with the Italians.

Late in 1888, though his own position was difficult, Yohannis moved against his rebellious vassals. Northern Ethiopia at the time was stricken by large-scale animal typhus and human dysentery epidemics. The emperor was still threatened on the north and east by the Mahdists and the Italians, and the Italian victory had lowered his prestige. Yohannis was able to move easily through Gojjam because Tekle Haimanot had gone with his army to join Menilek. But on the banks of the Abbai river, the frontier between Shoa and Gojjam, Yohannis was forced to encamp and to open negotiations. Menilek was now as strong as the emperor because Yohannis could not force his two recalcitrant chiefs to provide him with material assistance. When the Mahdists attacked in the north-west, Yohannis was forced to retire, 'leaving his rebellious vassals in triumphant possession of the field'.[1]

Emperor Menilek and the Italians, 1889–96

On the verge of a brilliant victory over the Mahdists, the Emperor Yohannis was mortally wounded at the Battle of Metemmah (9 and 10 March 1889). As he lay dying, he called together his chiefs and 'acknowledged young Ras [then Dejazmatch] Mangasha as his natural son by

[1] George Fitz-Hardinge Berkeley, 'The Abyssinian question and its history', *The Nineteenth Century and After*, Jan. 1903, **53**, no. 311, p. 93.

the wife of his own brother'. He commended Mangasha to his followers and especially to Ras Alula of Asmara, an old companion in arms. In effect, Yohannis had declared Mangasha his heir; and Ras Alula supported him in Tigre, the base from which Mangasha would have to make good his claim to the throne. Most other Ethiopian leaders tentatively accepted Menilek as the new emperor because of his military strength and the legitimacy of his claim.

Mangasha nevertheless succeeded in establishing himself as an autonomous ruler. Since Tigre bordered on the Italian holdings on the Red Sea coast, Menilek feared that Mangasha might persuade the Italians to further his ambitions. Thus, to neutralize Mangasha, as well as to regularize his own status, Menilek decided to obtain formal Italian recognition of his imperial accession.

In September 1888 Count Pietro Antonelli, the Italian plenipotentiary in Ethiopia, had drafted a new treaty that would have given Menilek increased Italian support in return for the cession of certain strategic highland areas adjacent to Massawa. Antonelli had been the main architect of Italy's Shoan policy, which aimed at assisting Menilek to become emperor in hopes that, out of gratitude, the new emperor would accept an Italian protectorate over his country. He probably failed to understand the ultimate aims of Italian policy and signed the suggested treaty on 2 May 1889 at the town of Wuchale. He thereby gained official Italian recognition as emperor[1] and the important right to bring in military supplies duty-free through the Italian port of Massawa. In return, Menilek ceded to the Italians strategic areas in Tigre—these happened to be a part of Ras Alula's domains— and granted them concessions in commerce, industry and justice.

Article 17 of the treaty seemed to implement Antonelli's policy of turning Ethiopia into an Italian dependency. The Italian text of the article read: 'the King of Kings of Ethiopia consents to use [servirsi] the Government of...the King of Italy for all the business he has with other powers or government'.[2] Menilek approved this article because

---

[1] Here I disagree with Sven Rubenson, who feels that Menilek had little further need of Italian support after his accession to the throne and that Ras Mangasha and Ras Alula were more dangerous to the Italians than to Menilek. If this analysis were correct, there would have been no real reason for Menilek to sign the Treaty of Wuchale. I cannot believe that a politician and diplomat as shrewd as Menilek would have signed a treaty that gave him no advantage. See Sven Rubenson, 'The protectorate paragraph of the Wichale treaty', *Journal of African History*, 1964, 5, no. 2, p. 278.

[2] Carlo Rossetti, *Storia diplomatica dell' Etiopia durante il regno di Menilek II* (Turin, 1910), pp. 41 ff.

its Amharic version merely suggested that he might make use of the Italian government in diplomatic matters if he wished and because Antonelli insisted that such a statement would indicate the emperor's goodwill and sincerity towards the Italian government.

Italy immediately implemented the Treaty of Wuchale when General Antonio Baldissera occupied Keren, the capital of Bogos, on 2 June 1889 and Asmara on 3 August. To obtain a defensible frontier along the Mareb, Belessa and Mai Muni rivers, the Italians then went beyond the terms of the agreement, and proceeded to take the rest of Alula's province of Hamasien and the provinces of Oculie-Cusai and Serae. These moves, coupled with the occupation of the important commercial and political Tigrean city of Aduwa on 26 January 1890, proved to be a damaging blunder. Italy's actions pushed Mangasha to improve his relations with Menilek in order to save at least a part of his patrimony, and they provided Menilek with the first clear evidence of Italy's intentions towards Tigre and possibly towards the rest of Ethiopia.

The pattern of Italian aims became even clearer when Dejatch Makonnen returned from Italy with the text of a supplementary convention to the Treaty of Wuchale, signed in Rome in October 1889. By Articles 5 and 6 of this convention, Menilek was loaned four million lire; and Article 3 provided for a rectification of territorial boundaries on the basis of *uti possidetis* to date.[1] Menilek understood Article 3 to mean territories controlled as of the date of signature of the convention. He therefore ratified it, over the opposition of some advisers, because he needed the loan to buy armaments. Later he wrote to King Humbert that he had accepted the supplementary agreement out of friendship, despite the 'many articles which are not advantageous to our country'. Regarding the original territorial concessions he had made in the Treaty of Wuchale, Menilek contended that, according to Antonelli, Italy 'only desired a site with a cool climate for the soldiers at Massawa, as a refuge in the hot months'. Menilek explained also that during a meeting in March 1890 he and Antonelli had been unable to agree on a satisfactory frontier because of his conviction that 'If I . . . [am Emperor] of Ethiopia, it is because I have added Tigre to my kingdom;

---

[1] Text of the convention, as quoted in Rossetti, *Storia diplomatica*, pp. 45 ff. For the controversy about the actual date of the signature of the supplementary convention, see Sven Rubenson, 'Professor Giglio, Antonelli and Article XVII of the Treaty of Wichalē', *Journal of African History*, 1966, **7**, no. 3, pp. 446–7; see also Professor Carlo Giglio's letter in the same issue of the *Journal of African History*, p. 542.

and if, then, you will take [land] up to the Mareb, what is left for me?'[1]

In this same letter Menilek informed the Italian king that he had been severely criticized by Shoan and Tigrean notables about giving up so much territory in the Treaty of Wuchale. When Count Augusto Salimbeni, the new Italian plenipotentiary, arrived in Shoa on 1 July 1890, he quickly discovered that Menilek was indeed in an extremely vulnerable position. His chiefs claimed that he had sold the country; the empress maliciously asked Menilek: 'How come King John never wanted to cede...territory; be battled the Italians [and] he battled the Egyptians for this [principle]; he died for it; and you, after such an example, wish to sell your country? Who will [want to] tell your history?' To diminish such criticism, Menilek could not allow any further Italian encroachment. Salimbeni quickly concluded that if Italy wished 'to maintain the Mareb frontier, we must rely only upon bayonets and cannon'.[2]

Meanwhile, the controversy about Article 17 of the Treaty of Wuchale had begun. On 11 October 1889 the Italian government, 'in conformity with the General Act of the Conference of Berlin', informed other powers of the contents of Article 17.[3] On 14 December, however, Menilek, who did not feel bound by the article, sent letters directly to the heads of state of Great Britain, France and Germany. Queen Victoria's reply to Menilek's communication not only contained the Italian version of Article 17 but the statement that 'We shall communicate to the Government of our friend His Majesty the King of Italy copies of Your Majesty's letter and of our reply'.[4] Menilek was upset by the implications of Queen Victoria's letter and instructed Alfred Ilg to compare the Italian and Amharic versions of the Treaty of Wuchale. When the mistranslation was discovered, Menilek immediately concluded that Antonelli and the Italian government had deliberately tricked him.

On 18 August 1890 Menilek wrote to Salimbeni that Ethiopia had been humiliated in Europe because of the inaccurate translation of Article 17, despite the stipulation in Article 19 that the Italian and Amharic versions of the treaty were equally faithful and valid. On 27

[1] Menilek to King Humberto, 27 Sept. 1890, as quoted in Rossetti, *Storia diplomatica*, p. 81.
[2] Carlo Zaghi, ed., *Crispi e Menelich nel diario inedito del Conte Augusto Salimbeni* (Turin, 1956), pp. 110, 124–5.
[3] Rossetti, *Storia diplomatica*, pp. 60–1.
[4] Zaghi, *Crispi*, p. 405.

September 1890 he wrote to King Humbert, spelling out his basic position: 'Having studied anew the said Article, we have established undeniably that the terms written in Amharic and the translation in Italian do not conform. . . I did not make. . . at that time, any obligatory statement, and today I am still not the man to accept it'. He hoped that Humbert would 'rectify the error. . . and announce the mistake to the friendly powers to whom you have communicated the said Article'.[1] In any event, Menilek informed Europe of the imbroglio.[2]

Because of Menilek's stubbornness regarding the northern frontier and Article 17, Salimbeni's situation became increasingly difficult. In late August 1890, he confided to General Gandolfi that, 'according to my point of view, war is the only possible solution to the Ethiopian problem'.[3] He believed that the crux of the problem was that 'in Italy they confuse, and disgracefully continue to confound, the poor King of Shoa. . . with the Emperor, who is another thing entirely'.[4] Crispi did not accept Salimbeni's analysis and sent Antonelli to Addis Ababa to solve all outstanding difficulties.

Antonelli arrived on 18 December 1890 with authority to grant Menilek the boundaries he demanded, if he would only accept the Italian version of Article 17. Salimbeni felt that 'Antonelli counts too much upon his influence with the King and hopes to persuade him [too] easily';[5] indeed, Antonelli's high expectations were dashed the first time he raised the issue of the mistranslation with Menilek and tried to place the blame on the Ethiopian interpreter, Gerazmach (Count) Joseph. 'The King and the Queen sustained the attack and responded [with great] violence, the King scolding [*imbriscola*] so much that he lost his voice.'[6] The following day, Antonelli presented a compromise that would still have treated Ethiopia as less than sovereign. This time 'the Queen was more upset than the King', saying, among other things, 'I am a woman and I do not love war; but rather than accept this, I prefer war'.[7] At still another meeting she exclaimed: 'You want. . . the other powers to consider us. . . as your protectorate, but that will never be.'[8] That all Ethiopia supported the emperor and

---

[1] As quoted in Rossetti, *Storia diplomatica*, pp. 78 ff.
[2] See, for example, Menilek to Queen Victoria, 24 Aug. 1890, as quoted in Zaghi, *Crispi*, p. 409.
[3] Salimbeni to Gandolfi, 31 Aug. 1890, in Zaghi, *Crispi*, p. 157.
[4] Salimbeni to Traversi, 6 Sept. 1890, in Zaghi, *Crispi*, p. 161.
[5] Zaghi, *Crispi*, p. 251.   [6] *Ibid.*, p. 253.   [7] *Ibid.*, p. 254.
[8] Report of Antonelli to Crispi, 29 Jan. 1891, in Zaghi, *Crispi*, p. 285, n. 31.

empress in their fight to maintain their rigid positions was made clear to Antonelli when Ras Mangasha and Ras Makonnen were included in the negotiations.

By late January 1891, Antonelli realized that his attempts were futile and sent Crispi a long dispatch. He pointed out that the bases for Italian policy in Ethiopia were primarily 'economic and peaceful'. Since Italy had already accomplished a great deal in Ethiopia, Article 17 was not necessary to safeguard its interests in the country. Although Antonelli could not bring himself to admit the real reasons for his conclusions, he suggested that the article had made it difficult for Italy to come to an accord with other powers about the Italian sphere of influence. He added, almost as an afterthought, that abrogation of the article would facilitate friendly relations with Menilek. On 2 February 1891, recognizing the futility of further discussions, Antonelli instructed Salimbeni to leave Addis Ababa as soon as possible and requested instructions from Italy regarding his own departure.

On 3 February 1891 Ras Makonnen unexpectedly transmitted to Antonelli a draft that apparently softened the Ethiopian government's position. In exchange for the territories that Italy had absorbed, the draft paradoxically stated that Menilek would accept Article 17 as it stood *in both the Italian and the Amharic texts*. The emperor claimed that this concession demonstrated his friendship for King Humbert, for whose sake he was willing to transact all his European business 'with the assistance [*appoggio*] of Italy'.[1] Antonelli, delighted by this unexpected volte-face, accepted the proposed accommodation. On 6 February he was called to the palace, where he signed various agreements even though they were as yet only partially in treaty form and the document regarding Article 17 was only in Amharic. Antonelli was assured 'that it was as had been fixed in the letter', and that as soon as a translation had been made it would be transmitted to him.

When the translation had not arrived by 8 February, Antonelli asked Salimbeni to translate the Amharic text for him. Salimbeni discovered that the Amharic text included one word which, in effect, cancelled Article 17. Antonelli rushed to the *Gibbi* (palace) where, in a stormy interview with Ras Makonnen, he pulled the seals off the documents to render them null and void. Later, in a heated discussion with Menilek, Antonelli demanded that all the signed documents, particularly the frontier agreements, be returned to him immediately. That evening,

[1] Zaghi, *Crispi*, p. 294.

he sent a letter to the *Gibbi* announcing the withdrawal of all Italian diplomatic personnel from the country because he regarded the change in the text as 'an offence against my King'. Salimbeni and Antonelli left Shoa on 12 February 1891.

The failure of the Antonelli mission provided an opportunity for several important Italian military and civil administrators in Eritrea to set forth a 'Tigrean policy', which aimed at setting Mangasha and other Tigrean chiefs against Menilek. These men felt that 'to continue to support Menilek was merely to render him all-powerful and independent'.[1] Furthermore, they considered Menilek 'a myth created by the imagination of Antonelli' and 'preferred the more modest and secure advantages of agreements made with local chiefs' to the expensive policy of supporting an independent Ethiopia. After the obvious failure of the Shoan policy, a new Italian government under the Marquis Antonio Starebbi di Rudini chose to obtain the amity of the Tigrean chiefs in hopes 'of forming a buffer between us and Shoa and establishing a permanent division between the north and south of Abyssinia, a division which could be considered necessary to the security of Eritrea'.[2] Italian authorites in Eritrea immediately opened negotiations with the important Tigrean chiefs and especially with Mangasha, who may have welcomed Italian support. Negotiations were successfully concluded on 8 December 1891 when General Gandolfi exchanged a pledge of friendship with Mangasha and several other chiefs, who formally agreed to the Italian annexation of Serae and Oculie-Cusai.

Menilek must have foreseen the possibility of war with Italy when he denounced the Treaty of Wuchale as of 1 May 1893. In a letter to the President of France, Menilek explained that the Italians were really imperialistic but that he would safeguard the independence of Ethiopia, which needed no protector.[3] The French government, which had never recognized the Italian protectorate, responded through its president that France had 'profound sympathy' for Menilek's courageous stand.[4] More encouraging to Menilek than this sympathetic

[1] George Fitz-Hardinge Berkeley, *The campaign of Adowa and the rise of Menilek* (London, 1902), p. 22.

[2] Oreste Baratieri, *Mémoires d'Afrique, 1892–1896* (Paris, 1899), p. 17.

[3] Menilek letter in Develle to Billot, 1 July 1895, France, Commission pour la publication des documents relatifs aux origines de la guerre de 1914–1918, *Documents diplomatiques français*, 1st ser. (1871–1900), x (Paris, 1945), 515.

[4] Carnot to Menilek, 22 Sept. 1893, *Documents diplomatiques français*, 1st ser., xi (Paris, 1947), 6.

reply, however, was the continuing stream of munitions that came through Djibouti into Ethiopia from France and from its ally in Africa, Russia. While bolstering Menilek's strength and morale,[1] these arms shipments caused growing concern to Italy.[2]

The Italian government did not, of course, admit that Menilek's unilateral denunciation of the Treaty of Wuchale had abrogated its claimed protectorate.[3] Italy always hoped for Menilek's recognition of Article 17, and in February 1893 sent another mission to gain his acceptance. Ironically, the mission's gift of two million cartridges seems to have so strengthened Menilek's position that he was able to denounce the treaty all the sooner. Furthermore, the mission injured Italian–Tigrean relations, which reached a nadir when General Baratieri, the Governor of Eritrea, was instructed to obtain from Mangasha a letter that would include a statement to the following effect: 'Obedient to the supreme will of His Majesty the King of Italy, I declare my readiness to recognize Menilek, King of Shoa, as Negus Negast ["King of Kings"].'[4] Thus, Mangasha was again robbed of using Italian support to gain the imperial throne, or even of remaining independent. The Italians now appeared as treacherous to the Tigreans as they did to Menilek, and a nationwide feeling against white men developed in Ethiopia and 'stimulated the fear of conquest'.[5]

'Tired of his profitless alliance with Italy' and pushed by the growing national revulsion against the Italians, Mangasha had to submit to Menilek if he wanted to save himself from becoming a pawn in the Italian policy of chasing 'the phantom of Uccialli'.[6] On the morning of 9 June 1894 Mangasha appeared at the palace in Addis Ababa carrying 'upon his shoulder a rock...to place, as a sign of submission, at the foot of the Negus'.[7] Menilek accepted the submission and apparently intimated that the Ras might later become Negus of Tigre if he assisted in the impending struggle against the Italians. Spurred on by his ambitions, Mangasha had by December 1894 concentrated enough forces in Tigre to cause Italy grave concern. On 17 December General Baratieri ordered Mangasha to disband his men, and when Mangasha refused, the Italians marched across the Mareb frontier on 30 December.

[1] Lagarde to Marty, 25 Feb. 1894, *Documents diplomatiques français*, XI, 85.
[2] Report of Italian Government in Ford to Kimberley, 9 June 1895, PRO, F.O. 403/221.
[3] Note from the Italian Embassy, 10 Jan. 1894, *Documents diplomatiques français*, XI, 11.
[4] Baratieri, *Mémoires*, pp. 37–8.
[5] *Ibid.*, p. 75.   [6] *Ibid.*, p. 77.
[7] J. G. Vanderheym, *Une expédition avec le négous Ménélik* (Paris, 1896), p. 130.

During the following month's campaign against Mangasha, the Italian colonial army established garrisons at the towns of Senafe and Saganeiti and at the strong points of Addis Adi and Adi Kaie. General Baratieri then faced two alternatives: to advance farther into Tigre and risk war; or to retire from the areas conquered, a politically difficult decision. By March 1895, however, there was no longer any choice. Mangasha had raised new forces. To forestall him Baratieri had to take the strategic Tigrean town of Adi Grat, which commanded the 'natural route of invasion for Shoa'. When he then occupied the important military, political and commercial city of Aduwa, war with Ethiopia could no longer be avoided.

A series of easy and quick victories caused the Italians to under-estimate Menilek's strength. They could not foresee that when Menilek issued his mobilization proclamation, 'every *tucul* [hut] and village in every far-off glen of Ethiopia... [would send] out its warrior'.[1]

On 7 and 8 December 1895 Ras Makonnen opened the war with a victory over the Italians at Amba Alagi. While this defeat was not a military disaster for Italy, it did undermine its colonial 'political edifice'.[2] Many chieftains who had had doubts about the outcome of the war now joined Menilek's forces.

Ras Makonnen followed the retreating Italians and besieged them at Mek'ele from 8 December, until they surrendered on 23 January 1896. He then allowed them to evacuate the fort with the honours of war and to join General Baratieri at Idaga Hamus. The Italian forces thereupon crossed the Mareb and took up defensive positions from Adi Grat to Inticho and Adi Quala.[3]

The Italian army numbered about 20,000 men and officers, of whom Baratieri would be able to rely upon 17,700 effectives for the impending battle. His forces included 10,596 Europeans, and the remainder were largely African regular troops. His overall fire-power was 14,519 rifles and 56 artillery and machine-gun units. Opposed to Baratieri's army was an Ethiopian force of nearly 110,000 men, composed of 80,000 riflemen, 8,600 cavalry, 42 artillery and machine-gun batteries, and about 20,000 hangers-on armed only with spears, lances and swords, but who were ready to take over the rifles of those who might fall in action. Unlike the Italian army, Menilek's forces had no provision for commissariat and transport. This weakness almost cost him the war

---

[1] Berkeley, *Adowa*, p. 126.   [2] Baratieri, *Mémoires*, p. 281.
[3] Ford to Salisbury, 25 Jan. 1896, F.O. 403/239.

because, even though he advanced to Hawzen and Aduwa in late January 1896, he would not attack the fortified Italian positions and was forced to encamp.

Until the end of February he attempted to entice the Italians out of their forts where his superior numbers could envelop the smaller army. Like Yohannis, Menelik daily watched his prestige diminish, while, more importantly, the forage disappeared. Had General Baratieri not decided to attack, 'Menelik might have been compelled to retire, possibly to disband his army; and then in the course of years we should have seen the ancient empire of Ethiopia, ruled over by a set of vassal Ras, gradually succumbing to the domination, and becoming imbued with the Latin civilization, of Italy'. The Italian commander, however, under severe pressure from his government and urged on by his over-confident generals, ordered an advance upon the Ethiopian camp at Aduwa.

Baratieri intended to march close to Aduwa and occupy three hills in a row that formed a barrier between the Italian positions at Sauria and the Ethiopian encampment. To the left of the three was another hill that had to be taken to secure the Italian left flank. Baratieri incorrectly called this hill Kidane Mehret, the name of a different location; and most of his misfortunes arose from this error because his Ethiopian guides led the Italian left wing to a hill of a similar name four miles in advance of the rest of the army. Baratieri's left flank was therefore uncovered; one brigade of his army could take no part in the great battle about to take place and was indeed completely vulnerable.

Baratieri's strategy was sound in principle. His army was to occupy the high points and to deploy in strong defensive positions on the front slopes. If the Ethiopians chose to attack, Baratieri felt he would win; if Menilek did not commit his troops, the Italians would have gained a psychological victory. A third possibility, hoped for but not expected, was that the Ethiopians would take fright and retreat. But the plan did not work.

The Italians marched through the night of 29 February; 'the night was black and there was a profound silence'. Around 4.00 a.m. on Sunday, while most of the warriors in the Ethiopian camp still slept, Menilek and the Empress Taitu were at divine services with Ras Mikail, Ras Makonnen and Ras Wolie of Yejju (Taitu's brother). During the beginning of the service, 'a courier rushed up at full speed, and stopped in front of the emperor. He had come from the outposts.' He reported that much noise had been heard but that it was too dark to identify the source of the disturbance. 'One had become so accustomed to similar alerts over the previous month that John Hoi [the emperor] smiled, shrugged his shoulders, dismissed the messenger and continued worshipping.' Only after the arrival of four other couriers did it become clear that the Italians were approaching in force. 'He [the enemy] had watched all night, hoping to surprise us at the time when our soldiers worshipped God. Many hesitated to believe [that the Italians could have] so much audacity but the multiplicity of couriers dispelled all doubts'.

'The Emperor appreciated the imminence of the peril. The Rases were informed.' Special trumpeters were ordered to sound the call to arms. Priests dashed about giving Holy Communion to the troops. 'The mass of humble Abyssinians beseeched the God of combat: "for the Motherland!" "for the Emperor!" "for the Faith!"' By 5.30 a.m., the Ethiopian forces were ready to fight an already tired enemy which had not yet consolidated its line of defence, which was already outflanked, and which had no idea of the fire-power and size of the Ethiopian army. Moving out of their encampments, the Ethiopians began their attack at 6.00 a.m., and by mid-day they had already enveloped and overwhelmed the smaller Italian force. 'The machine guns of the Negus, the Remingtons [and], the Gras [rifles]...[had done] their work of death.'

The Italians paid dearly for their audacity. About 4,000 European men and officers and 2,000 askari (Eritrean troops) had died; 1,428 European and Eritrean soldiers were wounded. Italian casualties were approximately 7,500, or nearly 43 per cent of the force engaged! Ethiopian losses have been estimated at 7,000 killed and 10,000 wounded, or 14 per cent of the emperor's army if a 120,000 figure be accepted as its probable size. Over 1,800 Italians were captured, later to become bargaining pawns in the peace negotiations. The battle of Aduwa was a decisive victory for Ethiopia, and five days later the Italians sued for peace.[1]

Menilek's prime condition was the abrogation of the Treaty of Wuchale, although he conceded the need for a new agreement; and he surprisingly allowed the Mareb–Belessa–Mai Muni frontier to stand.

[1] The material specifically quoted in the last three paragraphs concerning the Ethiopian view of the engagement comes from 'La bataille d'Adowa d'après un récit Abyssin', *Revue Française de l'Etranger et des Colonies: Exploration et Gazette Géographique*, Nov. 1896, **21**, no. 215, pp. 656–8.

The repatriation of Italian prisoners of war was put off until the conclusion of the formal treaty because Menilek apparently wished to have bargaining strength during the final negotiations; and because he wished to consult with his advisers in Addis Ababa before making binding commitments.[1] The Italian government found it impossible to obtain from Menilek any preliminary statement that would pledge him to refuse the protection of any other European power.[2] These problems were resolved in the final treaty negotiations, which were completed in Addis Ababa on 26 October 1896.

The Addis Ababa treaty affirmed Ethiopia's historic independence and represented a major victory for Menilek's foreign policy. Article 1 declared the war over. Article 2 annulled the Treaty of Wuchale. By Article 3, Italy recognized the full sovereignty and independence of Ethiopia. Articles 4 and 5 retained the *status quo ante* on the frontiers and left the question open for future negotiations.

There are several explanations for Menilek's decision to accept the *status quo* on the frontier instead of driving the Italians out of Ethiopia. If he had pressed the Italian government too hard, national pride might have compelled Rome to mount a larger military effort. Menilek knew, from experience, that his army could not overcome the heavily fortified positions into which the Italians had retired. He did not wish to risk his reputation as an astute military leader and his army's hard-won prestige. Nor did he have any desire to lead his army, short of rations as it now was, through the poor and already ravaged country south of Eritrea, especially in view of the impending long rainy season. His men had now been in the field for a longer period of time than was usual in Ethiopian warfare and were becoming restive. In addition, Menilek probably felt that the incorporation of further Tigre-speaking areas into the empire would unnecessarily strengthen the position of Ras Mangasha, whose loyalty to the imperial crown remained questionable. Furthermore, the emperor had won the essential object of the war, and the peace treaty formally ended the first period of active Italian imperialism in Ethiopia. Menilek's victory gave Ethiopia another one and a half generations of independence and established the country as a power in eastern Africa.

[1] Baldissera to Ricotti, 19 March 1896, in Italy, Commissione per la Publicazione dei Documenti Diplomatici, *I Documenti Diplomatici Italiani*, 3rd ser. (1896–1907), I (Rome, 1953), 24.

[2] Rudini, Ricotti, and Caetani to Baldissera, 20 March 1896, 22 March 1896, and 24 March 1896, *Documenti diplomatici italiani*, I, 23, 26, 28.

Diplomacy, 1896–8

The Italian threat having been eliminated, Menilek wanted to gain formal recognition of his independent status from the adjacent European colonial powers. British possessions flanked Ethiopia in the east and south, and British authority might soon establish itself in the Sudan. Before Aduwa, British policy-makers had considered Menilek's empire as an 'Italian Sphere of Influence'[1] and had relied upon Italy to act as their watchdog against a possible French sally into the Nile Valley from the east. The British therefore reacted swiftly to the Italian defeat; on 12 March 1896 Egyptian army units marched on Dongola 'to relieve the pressure on the Italians'[2] because Lord Salisbury's cabinet felt 'that the collapse of Italy...and Dervish success would jeopardize British interests'.[3]

The Mahdist state under the rule of the Khalifa Abdallahi still seemed powerful; neither British nor Ethiopian policy-makers could discount the possibility of an English defeat. Menilek also had to face the complications arising from the French desire to gain control of the upper Nile Valley as a lever to force British concessions in Egypt. France hoped to gain Ethiopian co-operation and assistance in this plan[4] but in mid-1896 had dispatched a mission under Major Marchand into the Nile Valley from the west. Regardless of what course he followed, therefore, Menilek had to envisage a possible French success in the Sudan.

Menilek's long-run interest in the Nile basin derived as much from the need to protect his empire as from the desire to expand it westward. He did not, therefore, care to alienate any of the three powers who might control that area. Diplomacy would be required to guarantee and enhance his position irrespective of the outcome of the Sudanese struggle.

[1] Until 1896, official British maps called Ethiopia 'The Italian Sphere of Influence'; later, however, this designation was lined out and replaced by 'Abyssinian Boundaries'. See F.O. 1/32, map of East Africa, May 1897.
[2] William Leonard Langer, *The diplomacy of imperialism, 1890–1902*, 2nd ed., reprinted (New York, 1956), p. 537.
[3] John Ashley Soames Grenville, *Lord Salisbury and foreign policy: the close of the nineteenth century* (London, 1964), p. 118. This recent study clearly proves—contrary to Langer's opinion (p. 537)—that fear of a French thrust into the Nile Valley was not a significant factor in the decision to mount the Egyptian advance on Dongola.
[4] France had always considered Ethiopian assistance necessary for the success of its policy in the Nile basin. See C. Maistre, 'Le Président Carnot et le plan d'action sur le Nil en 1893', *L'Afrique Française*, March 1932, **42**, no. 3, p. 156.

The French port of Djibouti was the major entrepôt for Ethiopia's trade in arms. Open failure to support the French could result in the enmity of Menilek's main supporter against the Italians. The emperor, moreover, might again need French help to checkmate Great Britain if that country desired to secure *all* the Nile sources for Egypt. On the other hand, if Menilek openly supported either France or the Sudan, Great Britain could regard him as an enemy. If victorious against the khalifa, Britain might extend its campaign into Ethiopia. Finally, open support of either one of the European powers might arouse the khalifa, who would be a most dangerous neighbour, should he successfully retain his country's independence.

To solve his dilemma, Menilek began by improving relations with the Sudan on the basis of their common interest in withstanding European imperialism and securing their common frontier. Menilek and Abdullahi exchanged some information and assured each other of their good intentions, but there was apparently no formal agreement. From the emperor's point of view, it was politic merely to buoy up the khalifa's morale without making any commitments.[1]

The Ethiopians had greater difficulty in retaining the friendship of France. After the battle of Aduwa, French authorities felt the time had come for a grateful Ethiopia to support France's policy in the upper Nile Valley. On 24 November 1896 the French Cabinet therefore decided to send a mission led by M. Leonce Lagarde, the Governor of French Somaliland, to undertake negotiations.[2] On 29 and 30 January 1897 Lagarde and Ras Makonnen signed two agreements which specified, respectively, that Menilek would consider Djibouti as the official outlet for Ethiopian commerce and that armaments for the Ethiopian government would pass through Djibouti duty-free.[3] Two more important treaties were signed by Menilek and Lagarde on 20 March. The first, a frontier treaty, ceded to Ethiopia a large part of France's Somaliland holdings, thus diminishing that colony to its present small size.[4] In return for this concession, Menilek signed the agreement described by

1 G. N. Sanderson, 'Contributions from African sources to the history of European competition in the upper valley of the Nile', *Journal of African History*, 1962, 3, no. 1, pp. 70, 84–6.
2 Menilek had suggested such a treaty in March 1895 when he sought French aid against the Italian claim to protectorate over Ethiopia. Note from the Political Director, 30 Sept. 1896, *Documents diplomatiques français*, 1st ser., XIII (Paris, 1953), f.n., 62; and Menilek to Felix Faure, March 1895, *Documents diplomatiques français*, XIII, 133.
3 Agreements of 29 Jan. and 30 Jan. 1897, *Documents diplomatiques français*, XIII, 147.
4 Frontier Treaty, 20 March 1897, *Documents diplomatiques français*, XIII, 277.

French authorities as 'a real treaty of alliance'.[1] The 'Convention for the White Nile' pledged Menilek to establish 'his authority on the right bank of the White Nile from 14° south' and to aid, 'as much as possible, the agents of the French government, who will be on the left bank between 14° and 5° 30'.[2] The first three agreements gave Menilek major territorial, political and economic concessions. But the secret treaty pledged him to actions that would have damaged his détente with the Sudan and might even have brought him into direct conflict with Great Britain. Menilek therefore embarked on a policy of subtle evasion. He allowed the French to use Ethiopia as a jumping-off place in the east for several expeditions sent to meet the Marchand mission. At the same time he issued his men 'ambiguous instructions... [provided] guides who misled the French, and... [permitted] his agents to frustrate the missions by every possible means...'[3] When the French complained, the emperor apologized for the 'imbeciles' who disobeyed his instructions and prepared new letters of authorization. None the less, so much time and human resource had been expended that the ill-equipped French missions failed. Menilek had protected himself against all eventualities: he had shown enough goodwill toward France that, 'had the French succeeded in their schemes for the upper Nile, he would doubtless have found ways of turning their success to his advantage';[4] he had not hurt his détente with the khalifa, who did not know about the secret Nile convention; and he had not damaged his relations with Great Britain.

Meanwhile, the British had become uneasy about Ethiopia's relations with France and the Sudan. In December 1896 they learned that Ethiopian envoys had recently been in Omdurman and that the trade routes via Gallabat and Gedaref had been reopened. The British knew that Menilek and the khalifa had well-established contacts, but London

---

[1] François Julien Pierre-Alype, *Sous la couronne de Salomon: l'empire des négus, de la reine de Saba à la Société des Nations* (Paris, 1925).

[2] Convention for the White Nile, 20 March 1897, *Documents diplomatiques français*, XIII, 278.

[3] G. N. Sanderson, 'The foreign policy of the Negus Menilek, 1896–1898', *Journal of African History*, 1964, 5, no. 1, p. 88.

[4] Sanderson, 'Foreign policy', p. 93. In this article, Professor Sanderson takes me to task for making precisely this same point, but in another way: 'Had the whole venture been successful, there seems little doubt that Menilek would have made territorial claims from the French.' I find it difficult, therefore, to see the basis for that complaint. See Harold G. Marcus, 'Ethio-British negotiations concerning the western border with Sudan', *Journal of African History*, 1963, 4, no. 1, p. 86.

viewed this recent mission as particularly ominous and decided to forestall a possible arms trade between the two countries.[1] Furthermore, the British now realized that the military operations in the Sudan would require the administration of the upper Nile region. Besides, Ethiopian infiltration into the hinterland of Britain's Somaliland Protectorate was becoming serious.[2]

These problems could only be solved by the opening of direct diplomatic relations with Ethiopia. Britain's Ethiopian policy was therefore defensive rather than offensive. The British mission to Menilek, headed by Rennell Rodd, Cromer's chief lieutenant in Egypt, had three major objectives, none objectionable to Menilek: first, Rodd sought Menilek's agreement not to assist the Mahdists in the Sudan; second, he hoped to regularize the British Somaliland–Ethiopian border; and third, he wished to obtain a commercial treaty embodying the most-favoured-nation principle.[3]

In a treaty signed on 14 May 1897, Menilek promised to 'halt to the best of his ability the passage across his Empire of arms and munitions to the Mahdists, whom he declares the enemies of his empire'.[4] His willingness to sign such a statement indicates that Menilek had never intended to give material aid to the khalifa; he therefore felt that he could afford a pledge of nonintervention in the Sudan in return for concessions in British Somaliland. Furthermore, in exchange for a most-favoured-nation agreement satisfactory to Lord Salisbury, Menilek forced Rodd to concede the duty-free transit of goods passing through Zeila.[5]

The most difficult negotiations for the treaty concerned the Somaliland border. These were concluded at Harar by Rodd and Ras Makonnen, after the actual signature of the treaty and were annexed to it. Britain ceded to Ethiopia 13,500 square miles of Somali territory,[6] thereby giving Menilek control of the Gadabursi and Zeila–Jildessa trade routes and putting him in good strategic position to march on

[1] Cromer to Salisbury, 1 Dec. 1896; Wingate to Intelligence Division, 23 Nov. 1896 and 6 Dec. 1896, F.O. 403/289.
[2] Ferris to Rodd, 1 Sept. 1896, F.O. 403/289.
[3] Salisbury to Rodd, 24 and 25 Feb. 1897, F.O. 403/255.
[4] Italy, Treaties, etc., *Trattati e convenzioni fra il regno d'Italia e gli stati esteri, raccolti per cura del Ministero degli Affari Esteri...*, 1 (Rome, 1906), 556; see also Rodd's draft treaty and Menilek's counter-draft, 13 May 1897, F.O. 403/255.
[5] F.O. 403/255.
[6] Memorandum by J. C. Ardagh, Director of Military Intelligence, 28 Feb. 1898, F.O. 403/274.

Berbera.[1] There was little the British could have done to avoid this large cession since the Ethiopians had controlled most of it for years, and only force could have dislodged them. Most important, 'failure to reach a settlement would have prejudiced our certainty of securing friendly neutrality on the western side'.[2]

G. N. Sanderson, a modern historian, is thus correct in writing that 'Menilek was...a subtle and far-sighted diplomatist with, at times, an almost Bismarckian capacity for keeping several irons in the fire'.[3] But we cannot concur with Sanderson's statement, 'down to the collapse of the Mahdist state itself, the Mahdist alliance was the central feature of Menilek's diplomacy'.[4] The détente with the Sudan was only one of many aspects of a complex foreign policy that protected Ethiopia against all eventualities; its brilliant success is a measure of Menilek's statesmanship.

Economic Progress, 1896–7

Having secured his country's independence, Menilek turned to Ethiopia's modernization. Greatly interested in contemporary technology, he made numerous innovations. At his invitation, foreign workmen constructed modern buildings in Addis Ababa. In 1886 the first engineered bridge over the Awash was erected, followed by other spans throughout the empire. Menilek pioneered a real postal system for the country, which gained it admittance to the International Postal Union in 1908. Foreign engineers installed two telegraph and telephone systems. These ensured rapid communication with the outside world and facilitated the administration of the empire and the dissemination of information within the country. In 1894 Menilek issued Ethiopia's first national currency, and in 1903 he installed a mint in Addis Ababa. In 1905 he chartered the Bank of Abyssinia, an affiliate of the National Bank of Egypt. Advances in education and health were made with the opening of hospitals and schools, the founding of an Amharic newspaper and the establishment of a government printing press.

The most significant feature of Menilek's policy of modernization, however, was the construction of the Djibouti–Addis Ababa railway. The complex story of the Ethiopian railway began when Alfred Ilg

---

[1] Government of India to Lord Hamilton, 28 July 1897, F.O. 403/255.
[2] James Rennel Rodd (Baron Rennel), *Social and diplomatic memories (second series) 1894–1901: Egypt and Abyssinia* (London, 1923), pp. 182–3.
[3] *Ibid.*, p. 93.   [4] *Ibid.*

constructed a model to show Menilek what rail transportation could mean for the future of Shoa. Remembering, however, the small railway which the British had built during the Mak'dala expedition, Menilek at this time felt that he should not build anything so strategically dangerous. He believed also that Yohannis would never agree to a project that would greatly strengthen Shoa. After Menilek had become emperor, Ilg again suggested that rail possibilities be investigated. Menilek, now anxious to enhance his strategic position *vis-à-vis* the Italians, issued a decree on 11 February 1893 authorizing Ilg to undertake a feasibility study. Later that year, Ilg reported that his plans were workable and that funds could be obtained in France.

On 9 March 1894 the emperor granted Ilg a ninety-nine-year concession, allowing him to form a company to build a railway in three stages: Djibouti to Harar; Harar to Addis Ababa; and Addis Ababa to Kaffa and the White Nile. The concession, however, dealt in detail only with the first part of the line and guaranteed that no competing lines would be built from the Indian Ocean or the Red Sea.[1] In January 1896 a contract for the railway construction was signed with a Paris firm. In 1897 the French government formally permitted the Imperial Railway Company of Ethiopia to lay the line over French Somali territory and to build appurtenances in Djibouti.[2]

The railway company 'casually assumed that they could procure with ease the large sum required' for the construction.[3] But it soon ran into financial difficulties, and in 1899 and 1900 was forced to invite British capital to invest in the venture. As a result, a British holding company gained control of the French railway company by the middle of 1901.[4] Greatly concerned, French colonial circles immediately began a vigorous campaign to secure governmental intervention to keep the railway French.

The British had meanwhile become concerned that the 'French should not occupy the predominant position in Abyssinia, which the railway will probably give them'.[5] Sir John Lane Harrington, the

---

[1] Conrad Keller, *Alfred Ilg: sein Leben und seine Werke* (Frauenfeld and Leipzig, 1918), pp. 133–4; Railway Concession, Oct. 1900, F.O. 403/299; Law Officers of the Crown to Foreign Office, 16 Feb. 1903, F.O. 403/334; Italy, Treaties, etc., *Tratatti*, p. 415.

[2] Rossetti, *Storia diplomatica*, pp. 139–40.

[3] John B. Christopher, 'Ethiopia, the Jibuti railway and the powers, 1899–1906' (Ph.D. thesis, Harvard University, 1942), p. 26.

[4] Memorandum by Lansdowne to Salisbury, 26 June 1901, F.O. 1/41.

[5] Crowe to Foreign Office, 15 May 1900, F.O. 403/298.

British plenipotentiary, indeed suggested to the emperor that the railway 'had placed practically the whole future commercial development of his country in the hands of the French'.[1] While the emperor denied this interpretation, Harrington's action did arouse Menilek's suspicions of France, whose motives he had not hitherto seriously questioned.[2] That Britain's concern and Menilek's suspicions were not unfounded became clear on 6 February 1902,[3] when the French government and the railway company signed a remarkable convention.

It embodies an agreement between a European government and a company domiciled in Europe, by which the Government agreed to financial assistance to the company for the purpose of constructing...a railway in the territory of an independent foreign state, the sovereign of which had granted a concession...to the company as a commercial enterprise.[4]

As a result of this convention, 'a private enterprise suddenly became the official protégé of one state, operating in another equally sovereign state, but without the consent of the second party'.[5]

Menilek was furious about the convention. If the French wanted to control the railway, he felt 'they might as well tell me to prepare for war at once...Why don't they say they will buy Abyssinia?' The emperor recognized that the final article of the convention, which required his agreement before the Ethiopian section of the line could be constructed, was only 'to smooth it all over'. Had the French really wanted his consent, they could have shown him the convention before signing it; 'this is only to cover our eyes'. To counter this French manoeuvre, Menilek turned to Great Britain for assistance.[6] In view of Harrington's concern, the emperor expected speedy British action. But the London government felt that 'King Menilek's proposals ...would involve...heavy expenditure and...far-reaching responsibilities' [to build his own railway].[7] After further study, the London government concluded that 'the issues are scarcely of sufficient gravity to warrant expenditure of millions'.[8]

Thereafter, try as he might,[9] the emperor could not obtain British

[1] Harrington to Salisbury, 30 May 1900, F.O. 403/299.
[2] *Ibid.*   [3] Monson to Lansdowne, 7 Feb. 1902, F.O. 403/322.
[4] Thomas Gilmour, *Abyssinia: the Ethiopian railway and the powers* (London, 1906), p. 22.
[5] Christopher, 'Ethiopia', p. 140.   [6] Harrington to Boyle, 5 April 1902, F.O. 1/40.
[7] Lansdowne to Cromer, 14 April 1902, F.O. 403/322.
[8] Sanderson to Cromer, 17 March 1903, F.O. 1/43.
[9] Menilek to Harrington in Harrington to Cromer, 10 April 1903, F.O. 403/334; Menilek to Harrington, 18 June 1903, F.O. 1/43.

financial aid.[1] He continued, however, to enjoy considerable British diplomatic backing and was therefore able to block railway construction under the terms of the 1902 Convention. He had earlier shown his displeasure with the railway company by refusing to attend the inauguration of the Djibouti–Dirri Dawa section of the line finished in December 1902.[2] He then damaged the company's borrowing power by abrogating its right to collect a 10 per cent levy on merchandise in transit. He also broke his promise to channel goods shipped between Djibouti and Dirri Dawa toward the company, thus causing railway traffic to drop below the level where receipts could cover current expenses and pay interest on bonds. Finally, Menilek refused to sanction the construction of the second section of line, and the company was forced to stand by, idly eating up its capital.

The railway company now faced another financial crisis. The 1902 Convention had broken the domination of British capital; the subvention granted by the convention had been discounted to obtain the cash necessary to buy out British interests and to finish the first section of the line. The company had expected more capital from the Paris money market. But faced with Menilek's refusal to recognize the convention and with his obstructionist behaviour, it could procure no further funds in Paris and faced an annual deficit of more than one million francs. The situation was further complicated when France, Britain and Italy began negotiations to define their interests in Ethiopia. All work on the railway therefore ceased for several years until the financial and political problems could be solved.

On 4 July 1906 a tripartite treaty, reconciling the differences between England, France, and Italy in Ethiopia, was initialled.[3] The treaty recognized the right of the French company to continue the railway from Dirri Dawa on condition that it should practise no discrimination 'in...matters of trade and transit'.[4] The treaty did not, however, reconcile Menilek's differences with France, and he still would not permit the resumption of the company's operations.

In early 1907 the French government therefore sent a special envoy to Ethiopia to negotiate another agreement. On 30 January 1908, after months of hard bargaining, Menilek granted the French company a

[1] Sanderson to Cromer, 17 March 1903, F.O. 1/43.
[2] Monson to Lansdowne, 24 Feb. 1903, F.O. 403/334.
[3] Grey to Lister, 4 July 1906, F.O. 401/9.
[4] Tripartite Agreement, 13 Dec. 1906, F.O. 401/9; *Documents on international affairs, 1935*, vol. II, Stephen Heald, ed. (London, Oxford University Press, 1937), pp. 556–60.

new concession that strengthened Ethiopia's control over its section of the line. Unfortunately, Menilek never saw the completed railway; he became paralysed shortly after the signature of the new concession; and, owing to further complications over the construction,[1] the line was not completed until 1917. None the less, the construction of the railway, which opened up Ethiopia to the outside world, can be attributed largely to the persistence and foresight of Menilek.

The building of a new Ethiopian empire

Another of Menilek's great achievements was the formation of a greater Ethiopia that he had begun even while King of Shoa. He continued this process when he became emperor and ultimately advanced into European-claimed areas. In July 1890 Germany had recognized British holdings in East Africa as 'coterminous' with the Italian-influenced areas in Gallaland and Abyssinia. Britain and Italy then signed the Protocol of 29 March 1891, which stipulated that Italian control extended to 6° N. latitude, or over most of northern and central Ethiopia. Had this agreement been implemented, Britain would have obtained most of Sidamo-Borena, part of Gemu Gofa, and a small but strategically important area of the south-eastern Ogaden. By a Protocol of 15 April 1891, Italy gave Great Britain the guarantees it wanted concerning the Ethiopian sources of the Nile.

In reaction to these claims and, ironically enough, at the suggestion of the Italian government, Menilek sent the European powers a circular in April 1891 claiming that the boundaries of Ethiopia formed a rough circle defined by the Gulf of Arafali (just below Massawa), Fashoda, Lake Rudolph and Assab. Menilek included not only large areas already claimed by the British and the Italians but also territory defined as French by the Anglo-French treaty of 9 February 1888.

The major European powers received Menilek's circular but paid it little heed, probably because they assumed that Ethiopia would soon become an Italian colony.[2] Menilek's neighbours made no protest, therefore, when, before 1896, he acted upon his letter by energetically expanding his power into southern Arussi and Wallega and by infil-

---

[1] Hervey to Grey, 19 Feb. 1909, F.O. 401/12.

[2] Circular letter of 1891, April 1891, F.O. 403/155. For the original Amharic version of the letter see Menilek to Rodd, 13 May 1897, F.O. 1/32; Italy, Treaties, etc., *Trattati*, p. 191; Somalia, Information Services, *The Somali Peninsula: a new light on imperial motives* (Mogadiscio, 1962), p. 10; Zaghi, *Crispi*, pp. 151–2.

trating into those parts of the Ogaden claimed—*but not occupied*—by the Europeans. After Aduwa, Menilek's policy was to construct a protective buffer zone around the highlands. To implement this plan he sent units of his army into the border regions of today's Ethiopian empire. Between 1896 and 1907 his men infiltrated the Ogaden and Borena and strengthened Ethiopian control over hitherto loosely-governed areas along the Sudanese border.

Menilek's concern about the security of the highlands was a feature of the negotiations of 1897 regarding the extent of the British Somaliland protectorate. Sir Rennell Rodd pointed out that Menilek claimed more than half of the British protectorate as hitherto defined, and the Englishman insisted that the frontier run near Jijiga. Menilek exclaimed, 'but you are advancing right up to the gates of Harar'. Rodd felt, however, that 'it was Abyssinia which had advanced up to us'. It was quite clear that the emperor's major preoccupation was the British proximity to Harar.[1] The Ethiopians moreover effectively controlled a large part of the British-claimed Ogaden. Rodd was forced to sign the treaty of 14 May 1897, by which Britain ceded 13,500 square miles of Somali territory. The treaty created a large, sparsely-settled arid buffer zone, approximately 110 miles in width, between an important strategic area of Ethiopia and the British protectorate.[2]

For the most part Menilek used force to enlarge his territory, though local rulers were usually given the opportunity of submitting peacefully to his overlordship. Since many such offers were rejected, full-scale military efforts were sometimes required to integrate countries into the empire. In all cases the Shoans had the great advantage of modern weaponry. One European observer wrote that the Galla were 'conquered, and...held in subjection by the help of firearms which... [the Shoans] take care they do not obtain'.[3] In a Galla area north of Lake Stephanie, a British officer was 'begged...to stop...and show them [the Galla] how to make guns, that they might resist the Abyssinian raids'.[4] An informant from Kaffa, conquered in 1897, thought

[1] Rodd to Salisbury, 13 May 1897, F.O. 403/255; see also Menilek to Rodd and Rodd to Menilek, 14 May 1897, F.O. 403/255.
[2] Memorandum by J. C. Ardagh, 28 Feb.1898, F.O. 403/274; Rodd, *Memories*, pp. 182–3.
[3] Reginald Koettlitz, 'Appendix to Herbert Weld Blundell's "A journey through Abyssinia to the Nile"', *Geographical Journal*, March 1900, **15**, no. 3, p. 270.
[4] Montagu Sinclair Wellby, 'King Menilek's dominions and the country between Lake Gallop (Rudolph) and the Nile Valley', *Geographical Journal*, Sept. 1900, **16**, no. 3, p. 298.

that the Shoans came with 20,000 rifles against the 300 of the King of Kaffa.[1] As a matter of fact, because some Europeans were selling modern weapons to Menilek, the King of Kaffa regarded all foreigners as Menilek's agents and closed his country to them, thereby preventing them from strengthening Kaffa's military position.

We are fortunate to have an excellent description regarding the actual mechanism of Shoan conquests, by J. G. Vanderheym, a French commercial agent. He accompanied Menilek on an expedition into Wollamo in December 1894. Wollamo Galla raiding into the empire was threatening to become more serious because several punitive expeditions had failed. Menilek decided that only a personally led campaign would succeed in subduing the Wollamos. On a Saturday in August 1894 the royal drums announced the impending venture; a royal edict commanded each soldier to prepare for war. For three months thereafter Addis Ababa had an air of 'unaccustomed activity', and on 1 November Ras Mikail with 10,000 troops joined the waiting armies of the emperor and Ras Wolde Giorgis in the capital. The next day long files of women started for the first camp, each one carrying something or driving cattle and sheep. The soldiers left one day later, followed by Menilek on 15 November. By this time the roads had been repaired and Menilek quickly caught up with his armies. On 1 December they arrived in Wollamo where 'the army of the advance guard had already burnt the houses abandoned by the Wollamos, fleeing before the invasion'.

From the evening of 1 December, when the Shoans fought some skirmishes, the soldiers chanted songs of war and self-praise 'every day and every hour. These cries never ceased to resound and became a veritable obsession'. To force the country into submission, the Shoans ravaged the land.[2] Every day the conquerors came back to camp with slaves and booty. With their superior weapons, the Shoans slaughtered many Wollamos: 'It was a terrible butchery of living or dead flesh... by the soldiers drunk from blood.' As the Galla warriors left cover to throw their spears, they would be shot dead by Shoan riflemen. By

[1] Friedrich J. Bieber, 'Geschichte des kaffaisch-äthiopischen Krieges: eine Überlieferung der Kaffitscho oder Gonga', Berlin, Universität, Seminar für orientalische Sprachen, *Mitteilungen*, 1922, **23/25**, pt. 26.
[2] Charles Michel, *Vers Fachoda: mission de Bonchamps* (Paris, 1901), p. 121. Leopoldo Traversi, 'Viaggi negli Arussi, Guraghi, ecc.', Società Geografica Italiana, *Bollettino*, April 1887, **24**, no. 4, p. 270. Louis de Gonzague, 'Mgr. Massaja et l'empereur Joannes', *L'Exploration*, 17 June 1880, **10**, no. 176, p. 72.

11 December, Wollamo resistance had been broken, and on the march that day, 'our mules turned aside continuously from recently killed corpses which encumbered the country. The wounded, horribly mutilated, were trampled by the cavalry men.' On that same day the seriously wounded King Tona of the Wollamos was captured, thus ending the war. After the booty had been divided up, Menilek returned triumphantly to Addis Ababa with King Tona.

One feature of the process of conquest, apparently found only in pagan areas and in territories directly administered by the northerners, was the infiltration of Ethiopian Christianity. A Catholic cleric travelling through Ethiopia in 1896 reported that Menilek was always eager to foster Christianity, and that he did 'not always employ to that end the method of persuasion'.[1] Furthermore, Christian officials brought their clergy and religion into newly conquered areas. In 1901 a British officer wrote that, in Gore, 'in addition to a large council-chamber, workshops, arsenal, storerooms, etc., the...Abyssinians have built a small church here'.[2] In many areas the Christians apparently placed their churches 'in...spots where the pagans honoured their cults'.[3]

In Moslem countries with traditions of statehood, not adjacent to Christian areas, Menilek, however, allowed no proselytizing and did not hinder local religious practices. He controlled church construction in the Moslem areas of south-western Ethiopia, with the result that by 1911, 'except for chapels in the camps of chiefs, only one Church had been built in Limmu'.[4] Menilek probably felt that a policy of religious persecution added to political subjugation would result in rebellion.

Most new converts had only a superficial commitment to Christianity. For some of them, however, conversion began a process of acculturation and accommodation that led to political assimilation into the Ethiopian state. The northerners practised various kinds of indirect rule. Hence the ruling classes of the subject peoples came into closer contact with the relatively sophisticated Christians, particularly in the

[1] Kyrillos Maçaire, 'Mon voyage en Abyssinie', Société Khédivale de Géographie, *Bulletin*, March 1897, **4**, no. 11, p. 719.
[2] Herbert Henry Austin, 'Survey of the Sobat region', *Geographical Journal*, May 1901, **17**, no. 5, pp. 507–8.
[3] Guèbrè Sellassié, *Chronique du règne de Ménélik II, roi des rois d'Ethiopie*, vol. 1, trans. from Amharic by Tèsfa Sellassié, Maurice de Coppet, ed. (Paris, 1930), p. 281. This process of Christianization was remarkably similar to the methods used in Ethiopian expansion in the fourteenth and fifteenth centuries.
[4] Enrico Cerulli, 'L'Islam nei Regni Galla Independenti', *L'Africa Italiana*, May–June 1916, **35**, nos. 5–6, p. 117.

strategic and administrative centres. An Italian, travelling in 1880, observed that members of the ruling classes of the Soddo Galla were affecting Shoan dress and mannerisms, even though Amharic was not generally spoken. In 1903, a Frenchman observed that recently conquered Gofa, in south-western Ethiopia, was nominally governed by a princess who had 'entirely adopted the manners of the Abyssinians'.[1] A British visitor to Kaffa in 1900 noticed that the people no longer wore national costumes but dressed like Shoans. Another traveller discovered that this outward conformity extended even to the cord around the neck, one of the identifying marks of the Christian Ethiopian. In Wollamo, some time after 1896, this same traveller was accosted by a boy who wanted a cord, not because he wished to convert but because, as an apparent Christian, he would be better treated by the northerners.

Over an extended period such superficial effects of northern rule on traditional life were bound to deepen. In 1904 a British explorer who visited a Galla area near the confluence of the Nile and the Didessa reported great changes in the life of the local people because of their contact with the Shoans. Their ruler had formerly been named Gumsa. When the Abyssinians came, he was made a dejazmatch and had been baptized Gebre Egzabhier. Most of his followers had taken similar names. While the people maintained the forms and ceremonies of their traditional government, 'the power of the Luba [the governing age set]...has been merged with that of officials appointed by the King [Menilek]'.

Menilek's policy toward the Abajifar (Sultan) of Jimma portrays a significant variation in the Ethiopian method of expansion. Before invading the state, Menilek offered its ruler terms that 'secured complete local control...in return for an annual tribute and assistance in the war against Kaffa'. Since Kaffa was Jimma's enemy, and since the sultan knew that he could not defeat Menilek's army, he readily submitted. Kaffa, however, refused similar terms and was invaded, devastated and depopulated, while Jimma survived and flourished.

The Galla of Wollega yielded to Menilek because they feared his greater strength. Roba, an Arussi Galla chieftain, similarly realized that his people could not withstand the Shoan armies; hence he accepted Menilek's offer to submit and pay taxes. Five years later, however,

---

[1] Pierre Marie Robert du Bourg de Bozas, 'D'Addis Abbabá au Nil par le lac Rodolphe', *La Géographie*, 15 Feb. 1903, **7**, no. 2, p. 96.

Roba still dreamt of independence: 'The hour has not come, but it will come; perhaps our children will see the departure of the oppressor.'[1]

The Ethiopians extended their territory also by infiltration, followed by effective occupation. This method was particularly useful where European governments had merely based their claims upon treaties signed among themselves but not recognized by the Ethiopian government. As a matter of fact, European governments had not bothered to inform Menilek about the treaties they had concluded with each other affecting his empire. Accordingly, when he was asked to recognize the Anglo-German Agreement of 1890, he refused, complaining, 'Myself, I have never heard of it until you told me. Neither of the two Governments have sent it to me'.[2]

In 1896, shortly after Aduwa, Ras Makonnen quickened the pace of infiltration into the Ogaden, which the British claimed for their protectorate. The Ethiopians established military posts, causing the British Consul at Berbera to complain in a dispatch that 'Ras Makunan ignores the delimitation...between Italy and Britain, and lays claims ...to a considerable portion of the British Protectorate'.[3] Upon British protest, Makonnen replied that he was implementing Menilek's territorial declaration of 1891.[4] Consul Ferris knew that the Ethiopians would stop only if faced with an effective British administration or a garrison.[5] London, however, refused to act, and the Ethiopians continued their occupation. When the British ultimately signed a treaty with Ethiopia, they therefore had to surrender much of the Ethiopian-occupied territory. Menilek used infiltration and occupation with equal effectiveness in the areas of Somaliland claimed by France and Italy and in British-claimed areas of southern and western Ethiopia. Infiltration was useful for the most part only in sparsely settled areas where the peoples were militarily weak.

Once the Ethiopian government had effectively occupied an area, it governed its subjects by establishing *ketemas*, or fortified garrison towns. 'Many of the villages...are really permanent corps of armed men. These are always perched high upon the summit of the loftiest

[1] Pierre Marie Robert du Bourg de Bozas, *Mission scientifique Du Bourg de Bozas: de la mer Rouge à l'Atlantique à travers l'Afrique tropicale...* (Paris, 1906), pp. 122, 125.
[2] Menilek to Rodd, 14 May 1897, F.O. 403/255.
[3] Ferris to Rodd, 1 Sept. 1896, F.O. 403/239.
[4] Makonnen to Ferris, 27 Aug. 1896, F.O. 403/239.
[5] Ferris to Cunningham, 28 Oct. 1896, F.O. 403/239.

hills, and are quite a feature here'.[1] Such 'skillfully planted Abyssinian posts'[2] achieved strategic control over the adjacent countryside. For example, from Arero in Borena, 'the Abyssinians control[led] the whole of Dirri, Tertale, and the inhabited part of Liban'.[3] These centres not only governed the empire but also 'form[ed]...a line of defence around Shoa'. A communication system between the posts made it possible for forces to be rapidly concentrated at any point. Thus, these *ketemas* effectively controlled subject peoples and represented to the Europeans the visible evidence of 'effective occupation'.[4]

The results of Menilek's expansion were beneficial to Ethiopia over the long run even though the methods of empire building may at first have been destructive. A British officer travelling through Arussi in 1899 pointed out a significant decrease of intertribal strife. He noted, however, that 'the tribes vary considerably in their condition, according as they accept their ruler with good or ill grace'. He had no doubt that Menilek, 'aims at, and for the most part succeeds in governing with justice'.[5] Another traveller found that the Ethiopians 'seemed just and not oppressive' rulers; as long as taxes were paid and there was no rebellion, the northerners scarcely interfered in local matters. One army officer felt that 'although their methods leave much to be desired, they undoubtedly manage to rule their territories with an organization and a rough justice which, all things considered, are surprising'.[6] Although there were abuses in Menilek's empire, these usually occurred in newly conquered areas where the enmity between conquered and conqueror was still strong; in the traditional slave-raiding Negro areas along the western border; or on the empire's marches, which were inhabited by easily exploited and badly organized tribal peoples such as the Anuak. None the less, law and order usually prevailed among the subject

---

[1] Reginald Koettlitz, 'A journey through Somali Land and Southern Abyssinia to the Berta or Shangalla country and the Blue Nile, and through the Sudan to Egypt', Tyneside Geographical Society, *Journal*, Jan. 1901, **4**, no. 5, p. 337. Again, this use of military colonization was very similar to the methods used in Ethiopian expansion in the fourteenth and fifteenth centuries.

[2] Wellby, 'King Menilek's dominions', p. 297.

[3] Philip Maud, 'Exploration in the southern borderland of Abyssinia', *Geographical Journal*, May 1904, **23**, no. 5, p. 565.

[4] Henri Dehérain, 'Les Katamas dans les provinces méridionales de l'Abyssinie pendant le règne de l'empereur Ménélik', Ministère de l'Instruction Publique et des Beaux Arts, Comité des Travaux Historiques et Scientifiques, Section de Géographie, *Bulletin*, 1914, **29**, 239, 241.

[5] Wellby, 'King Menilek's dominions', p. 295.

[6] Sir Alfred Edward Pease, *Travel and sport in Africa* (London, 1902), III, 6.

peoples. A French journalist wrote in glowing terms about the 'absolute safety with regard to one's life and one's belongings', no matter where you were in the empire.[1] During his journey an American traveller observed that 'the name of Menilek meant safety, and the rulers of provinces rose to show respect when they saw the seal of the King'.[2] An Englishman 'could not help being impressed by the security... which, indeed is not so common in more civilized lands'.[3]

The territorial integration, the decrease in intertribal strife and the increased security allowed greater areas to be exploited and led directly to an increase in commerce. Perhaps the most important single result of Ethiopian expansion was the creation of a unitary economy centred in Addis Ababa. To this market-place came products from every part of the empire. As one British sportsman put it: 'here you can feel the commercial pulse of Abyssinia, gain some insight into the present state of her civilization, and gather what she wants to offer in exchange'.[4]

Robert Skinner, the head of the first American diplomatic mission to Menilek, came to Addis Ababa in 1903 to sign a commercial treaty ensuring American commercial interests in Ethiopia. His conclusions about Menilek and his empire provide us with a very competent appraisal of the man and his work. 'Menilek', he wrote, 'has created the United States of Abyssinia—a work for which he was endowed by Nature with the constructive intelligence of a Bismarck, and the faculty for handling men... [with the] sheer amiability of a McKinley.'[5]

The smashing victory at Aduwa in March 1896 forced Europe to recognize Ethiopian power in north-eastern Africa. The defeat of European imperialism gave Ethiopia another forty years of independence, if not total freedom of action. During this period Menilek continued the expansion, consolidation and integration of his empire. Like Peter the Great, he opened a window to the outside world and was responsible for many innovations. He established a unitary economy and set the preconditions for modernization. He led a conservative

[1] Oscar Neumann, 'From the Somali coast through Southern Ethiopia to the Sudan', Tyneside Geographical Society, *Journal*, Jan. 1903, **5**, no. 1, p. 392.
[2] Hughes le Roux, 'New trails in Abyssinia', *Century Magazine*, April 1902, **63**, no. 6, p. 894.
[3] Oscar T. Crosby, 'Personal impressions of Menilek', *Century Magazine*, April 1902, **63**, no. 6, pp. 883–4.
[4] Father Anastase, 'La station de Lafto en pays Galla', *Le Semeur d'Ethiopie*, Sept. 1906, **2**, 80.
[5] Robert P. Skinner, *Abyssinia of today* (London and New York, 1906), p. 141.

nobility, a reactionary clergy and a traditionalist peasantry toward a new age. When Menilek became incapacitated, however, the momentum was lost. The nature of the Ethiopian state required a strong charismatic leader; and in the absence of such a man Ethiopia marked time until the reign of Haile Selassie. In the meantime, the lack of strong leadership had made Ethiopia again a prey for Italian imperialism.

BIBLIOGRAPHY

Afeworq, Gebre Yesus. *Dagmawi Menilek (Emperor Menilek)*. Rome, 1901.

Anastase, Father. 'La station de Lafto en pays Galla', *Le Semeur d'Ethiopie*, Sept. 1906, **2**.

Angoulvant, Gabriel Louis, and Sylvain Vignères. *Djibouti, mer Rouge, Abyssinie*. Paris, 1902.

Antinori, Orazio. 'La spedizione in Africa', Società Geografica Italiana, *Bollettino*, May 1880, **18**, no. 5.

Antonelli, Pietro. 'Lettere', Società Geografica Italiana, *Bollettino*, Nov. 1882, **20**, no. 11.

   'Il mio viaggio da Assab allo Scioa', Società Geografica Italiana, *Bollettino*, Dec. 1883, **20**, no. 12.

   'Scioa e Scioani, lettere del Conte P. Antonelli', Società Geografica Italiana, *Bollettino*, Jan. 1882, **19**, no. 1.

Aubry, Alphonse. 'Une mission au Choa et dans les Pays Galla', Société de Géographie de Paris, *Bulletin*, 1889, **8**, no. 4.

Audon, Henry. 'Voyage au Choa', *Le Tour du Monde*, 1889, **58**.

Austin, Herbert Henry. 'Survey of the Sobat region', *Geographical Journal*, May 1901, **17**, no. 5.

Baratier, Albert Ernest Augustin. *Souvenirs de la mission Marchand*. Paris, 1941.

Baratieri, Oreste. *Mémoires d'Afrique, 1892–1896*. Paris, 1899.

'La bataille d'Adowa d'après un récit Abyssin', *Revue Française de l'Etranger et des Colonies: Exploration et Gazette Géographique*, Nov. 1896, **21**, no. 215.

Berkeley, George Fitz-Hardinge. 'The Abyssinian question and its history', *The Nineteenth Century and After*, Jan. 1903, **53**, no. 311.

   The campaign of Adowa and the rise of Menelik. London, 1902.

Bianchi, Gustavo. 'Fra i Soddo-Galla', *Africa*, July 1882, **1**, no. 1.

Bieber, Friedrich J. 'Geschichte des kaffaisch-äthiopischen Krieges: eine Überlieferung der Kaffitscho oder Gonga', Berlin, Universität, Seminar für orientalische Sprachen, *Mitteilungen*, 1922, **23/25**, pt. 26.

Borelli, Jules. *Ethiopie méridionale*. Paris, 1890.

Carre, Jean-Marie. 'Arthur Rimbaud en Ethiopie: lettres inédites', *La Revue de France*, June 1915, **16**, no. 2.

Carry, François. 'La captivité des italiens en Abyssinie, d'après des publications récentes', *Le Correspondant*, 10 Aug. 1897, **188**, no. 3.

Castonnet des Fosses, Henri Louis. *L'Abyssinie et les italiens*. Paris, 1897.

Castro, Lincoln de. *Nella terra dei Negus: pagine raccolte in Abissinia*. 2 vols. Milan, 1915.

Cecchi, Antonio. *Da Zeila alle frontiere del Caffa*. 3 vols. Rome, 1886.

Cerulli, Enrico. 'The folk-literature of the Galla of Southern Abyssinia', in *Harvard African studies*, vol. III (*Varia Africana*, III). Cambridge, Mass., African Department of the Peabody Museum of Harvard University, 1922.

'L'Islam nei Regni Galla Independenti', *L'Africa Italiana*, May–June 1916, **35**, nos. 5–6.

Chiarini, Giovanni. 'Memorie sulla storia recente dello Scioa, della morte de Sahle Salassie sino ad oggi (novembre 1877)', Società Geografica Italiana, *Memorie*, 1878, vol. **I**.

Christopher, John B. 'Ethiopia, the Jibuti railway and the powers, 1899–1906.' Ph.D. thesis, Harvard University, 1942.

Cicognani, Luigi. 'Attraverso il paese dei Danachili', Società Africana d'Italia, *Bollettino*, July–Aug. 1887, **6**, nos. 7–8.

'Sulle condizione odierne dell'Abissinia', Società Africana d'Italia, *Bollettino*, Jan.–Feb. 1887, **6**, nos. 1–2.

Crispi, Francesco. *La prima guerra d'Africa*. Milan, 1914.

Crosby, Oscar T. 'Abyssinia—the country and the people', *National Geographic Magazine*, March 1901, **12**, no. 3.

'Personal impressions of Menilek', *Century Magazine*, April 1902, **63**, no. 6.

Cucca, Carlo. 'In Africa', *Africa*, Jan.–Feb. 1887, **6**, nos. 1–2.

'Dallo Scioa', Società Africana d'Italia, *Bollettino*, March–April 1889, **8**, nos. 3–4.

Dehérain, Henri. 'Les Katamas dans les provinces méridionales de l'Abyssinie pendant le règne de l'empereur Ménélik', Ministère de l'Instruction Publique et des Beaux Arts, Comité de Travaux Historiques et Scientifiques, Section de Géographie, *Bulletin*, 1914, **29**.

Dimotheos, Father. *Deux ans de séjour en Abyssinie, ou Vie morale, politique et religieuse des abyssiniens*. 2 vols. Jerusalem, 1871.

Documents on international affairs, 1935, vol. **II**, Stephen Heald, ed. London, Oxford University Press, 1937.

Du Bourg de Bozas, Pierre Marie Robert, viscount. 'D'Addis Abbabá au Nil par le lac Rodolphe', *La Géographie*, 15 Feb. 1903, **7**, no. 2.

Mission scientifique Du Bourg de Bozas: de la mer Rouge à l'Atlantique à travers l'Afrique tropicale (octobre 1900–mai 1903); carnets de routes. Preface by R. de Saint Arroman. Paris, 1906.

Dye, William M. *Moslem Egypt and Christian Ethiopia*. New York, 1880.

Effendi, X. 'Le Maahdi, l'Egypte et l'Abyssinie', *Revue Brittanique*, Feb. 1884, **60**, no. 2.

Ferrand, Gabriel. 'Notes sur la situation politique, commerciale et religieuse du Pachalik de Harrar et de ses dépendances', Société de Géographie de l'Est, *Bulletin*, 1886, **8**, no. 2.

Florio-Sartori, Florindo. 'I capi ribelli Abissini', Società Africana d'Italia, *Bollettino*, 1887, **6**, nos. 9–10.

France. Commission pour la Publication des Documents Relatifs aux Origines de la Guerre de 1914–1918. *Documents diplomatiques français*, 1st ser. (1871–1900), vols. X, XI, XIII. Paris, 1945, 1947, 1953.

France, Tribunal Civil (Seine). *La concession du chemin de fer franco-éthiopien*. Paris, 1924.

Gebre Hiwot, Baykedane. 'Atze Menilek ya-Etiopia (the Emperor Menilek of Ethiopia)'. Unpublished manuscript.

Giffen, Morrison Beall. *Fashoda: the incident and its diplomatic setting*. University of Chicago Press, 1930.

Giglio, Carlo. *L'impresa di Massawa (1884–1885)*. Rome, Istituto Italiano per l'Africa, 1955.

[Letter to the Editor], *Journal of African History*, 1966, **7**, no. 3.

La politica africana dell'Inghilterra nel XIX secolo. Padua, 1950.

Gilmour, Thomas Lennox. *Abyssinia: the Ethiopian railway and the powers*. London, 1906.

Gonzague, Louis de. 'Mgr. Massaja et l'empereur Joannes', *L'Exploration*, 17 June 1880, **10**, no. 176.

Grenville, John Ashley Soames. *Lord Salisbury and foreign policy: the close of the nineteenth century*. London, 1964.

Guèbrè Sellassié. *Chronique du règne de Ménélik II, roi des rois d'Ethiopie*, tr. from Amharic by Tèsfa Sellassié; Maurice de Coppet, ed. 2 vols. and atlas. Paris, 1930–2.

Gwynn, Sir Charles William. 'A journey in Southern Abyssinia', *Geographical Journal*, Aug. 1911, **38**, no. 2.

Hans, Albert. 'L'armée de Ménélik', *Revue des Deux Mondes*, 15 June 1896, **135**.

Holland, Trevenen J., and Henry Hozier. *Record of the expedition to Abyssinia*. 3 vols. London, 1870.

Ilg, Alfred. 'Über die Verkehrsentwicklung in Äthiopien', Geographisch-Ethnographische Gesellschaft, Zürich, *Jahresbericht*, 1899–1900, **47**.

'Italiani in Africa', *Africa*, Dec. 1882, **1**, no. 6.

Italy. Commissione per la Pubblicazione dei Documenti Diplomatici. *I documenti diplomatici italiani*, 3rd ser. (1896–1907), vol. I. Rome, 1953.

Italy. Treaties, etc. *Trattati e convenzioni fra il regno d'Italia e gli stati esteri, raccolti per cura del Ministero degli Affari Esteri...*, vol. I. Rome, 1906.

Jesman, C. 'The tragedy of Mak'dala', *Ethiopia Observer*, 1966, 10, no. 2.

Keller, Conrad. *Alfred Ilg: sein Leben und seine Werke*. Frauenfeld and Leipzig, 1918.

Koettlitz, Reginald. 'Appendix to Herbert Weld Blundell's "A journey through Abyssinia to the Nile"', *Geographical Journal*, March 1900, 15, no. 3.

'A journey through Somali Land and Southern Abyssinia to the Berta or Shangalla country and the Blue Nile, and through the Sudan to Egypt', Tyneside Geographical Society, *Journal*, Jan. 1901, 4, no. 5.

Landor, Arnold Henry Savage. *Across widest Africa: an account of the country and people of Eastern, Central, and Western Africa as seen during a twelve months' journey from Djibuti to Cape Verde*. 2 vols. New York, 1907.

Langer, William Leonard. *The diplomacy of imperialism, 1890–1902*. 2nd ed. New York, 1951; reprinted, 1956, 1960.

Le Roux, Hughes. 'New trails in Abyssinia', *Century Magazine*, April 1902, 63, no. 6.

Lewandowski, Herbert. *Ein Leben für Afrika*. Zürich, 1954.

Louis-Lande, M. L. 'Un voyageur français dans l'Ethiopie méridionale', *Revue des Deux Mondes*, 15 Dec. 1878, 30; 15 Jan. 1879, 31.

Luzeux, Alexandre-Charles. *Etudes critiques sur la guerre entre l'Italie et l'Abyssinie*. Paris, 1896.

Maçaire, Kyrillos. 'Mon voyage en Abyssinie', Société Khédivale de Géographie, *Bulletin*, March 1897, 4, no. 11.

Maheteme-Sillasse, Wolde Meskal. *Zikre neger (Remembrance of things)*. Addis Ababa, 1950.

Maistre, C. 'Le président Carnot et le plan d'action sur le Nil en 1893', *L'Afrique Française*, March 1932, 42, no. 3.

Marcus, Harold G. 'A background to direct British diplomatic involvement in Ethiopia, 1894–1896', *Journal of Ethiopian Studies*, July 1963, I, no. 2.

'Ethio-British negotiations concerning the western border with Sudan', *Journal of African History*, 1963, 4, no. 1.

'The foreign policy of the Emperor Menilek, 1896–1898: a rejoinder', *Journal of African History*, 1966, 7, no. 1.

'A history of the negotiations concerning the border between Ethiopia and British East Africa, 1897–1914', in *Boston University Papers on Africa*, vol. II: *African History*, Jeffrey Butler, ed. Boston University Press, 1966.

'A preliminary history of the Tripartite Treaty of December 13, 1906', *Journal of Ethiopian Studies*, 1965, 2.

Massaia, Guglielmo, cardinal. *I miei trentacinque anni di missione nell'Alta Etiopia*. 12 vols. Rome, 1921–30.

Maud, Philip. 'Exploration in the southern borderland of Abyssinia', *Geographical Journal*, May 1904, **23**, no. 5.

Michel, Charles. *Vers Fachoda: mission de Bonchamps*. Paris, 1901.

Montandon, Georges. 'Alfred Ilg', *Le Globe: Journal Géographique*, 1916, **55**. 'A journey in south-western Abyssinia', *Geographical Journal*, Oct. 1912, **40**, no. 4.

Morié, Louis J. *Les civilisations africaines: histoire de l'Ethiopie (Nubie et Abyssinie) depuis les temps les plus reculés jusqu'à nos jours*. 2 vols. Paris, 1904.

Naretti, Giacomo. 'Exploratori ed avvenimenti in Abissinia', Società Geografica Italiana, *Bollettino*, Oct. 1882, **19**, no. 10.

Neumann, Oscar. 'From the Somali coast through Southern Ethiopia to the Sudan', Tyneside Geographical Society, *Journal*, Jan. 1903, **11**, no. 1.

'Nostra correspondenza dallo Scioa', Società Africana d'Italia, *Bollettino*, Nov.–Dec. 1887, **6**, nos. 11–12.

Pankhurst, Estelle Sylvia. 'The beginning of modern transport in Ethiopia: the Franco-Ethiopian railway and its history', *Ethiopia Observer*, Nov. 1957, **I**, no. 12.

Pankhurst, Richard K. 'The battle of Adowa', *Ethiopia Observer*, special issue, Oct. 1957, **I**, no. 11.

'Fire-arms in Ethiopian history (1800–1935)', *Ethiopia Observer*, 1962, **6**, no. 2.

'Misoneism and innovation in Ethiopian history', *Ethiopia Observer*, 1964, **7**, no. 4.

Pease, Sir Alfred Edward. *Travel and sport in Africa*. 3 vols. London, 1902.

Pierre-Alype, François Julien. *Sous la couronne de Salomon: l'empire des Négus, de la reine de Saba à la Société des Nations*. Paris, 1925.

Plowden, Walter Chichele. *Travels in Abyssinia and the Galla country, with an account of a mission to Ras Ali in 1848*. Trevor Chichele Plowden, ed. London, 1868.

Porena, Filippo. 'Sulle condizione odierne dell'Abissinia a proposito di un libro de G. Rohlfs', Società Geografica Italiana, *Bollettino*, Aug. 1888, **21**, no. 8.

Ragazzi, Vincenzo. 'Lettera', Società Geografica Italiana, *Bollettino*, Dec. 1889, **26**, no. 12.

Rawson, Sir Rawson W. 'European territorial claims on the coasts of the Red Sea and its southern approaches in 1885', Royal Geographical Society, *Proceedings*, Feb. 1885, **7**, no. 2.

Rennel, James Rennel Rodd, baron. *Social and diplomatic memories (second series), 1894–1901: Egypt and Abyssinia*. London, 1923.

Riola, G. 'Da Saati a Metemma', Società Africana d'Italia, *Bollettino*, March–April 1889, **8**, nos. 3–4.

Robinson, Ronald E., and John Gallagher, with Alice Denny. *Africa and the Victorians: the climax of imperialism in the dark continent.* London, 1961.

Rohlfs, Gerhard. *Meine Mission nach Abessinien.* Leipzig, 1883.

Rossetti, Carlo. *Storia diplomatica dell'Etiopia durante il regno di Menilek II.* Turin, 1910.

Rubenson, Sven. *King of kings, Tewodros of Ethiopia.* Addis Ababa and Nairobi, Haile Sellassie I University Press, 1966.

'Professor Giglio, Antonelli and Article XVII of the Treaty of Wiçhalē', *Journal of African History*, 1966, **7**, no. 3.

'The protectorate paragraph of the Wiçhalē treaty', *Journal of African History*, 1964, **5**, no. 2.

'Some aspects of the survival of Ethiopian independence in the period of the scramble for Africa', University College of Addis Ababa, *Review*, 1961, **1**.

Sabelli, Luca dei. *Storia di Abissinia.* 4 vols. Rome, 1936–8.

Sanderson, G. N. 'Contributions from African sources to the history of European competition in the upper valley of the Nile', *Journal of African History*, 1962, **3**, no. 1.

'The foreign policy of the Negus Menilek, 1896–1898', *Journal of African History*, 1964, **5**, no. 1.

Silberman, Leo. 'Why the Haud was ceded', *Cahiers d'Etudes Africaines*, 1961, **2**, no. 5.

Skinner, Robert P. *Abyssinia of today.* London and New York, 1906.

Smith, Donaldson. 'Expedition to Somaliland', *Geographical Journal*, Feb. 1895, **5**, no. 2.

Soleillet, Paul. 'Obock et le Choa', Société Normande de Géographie, *Bulletin*, Nov.–Dec. 1884, **6**.

'Rapport adressé à M. le Ministre des Affaires Etrangères à Paris sur la possession française d'Obokh et le royaume de Choa', Société Normande de Géographie, *Bulletin*, Sept.–Oct. 1883, **5**.

Voyages en Ethiopie. Rouen, 1886.

Somalia. Information Services. *The Somali Peninsula: a new light on imperial motives.* Mogadiscio, 1962.

'La spedizione Salembeni', Società Geografica Italiana, *Bollettino*, March 1887, **24**, no. 3.

Starkie, Enid. *Arthur Rimbaud in Abyssinia.* Oxford, Clarendon Press, 1937.

Stern, Henry A. *The captive missionary.* London, 1868[?].

Wanderings among the Falashas in Abyssinia. London, 1862.

Stigand, Chauncy Hugh. *To Abyssinia through an unknown land.* London, 1910.

Swayne, Harold George Carlos. 'A trip to Harrar and Ime', *Geographical Journal*, Sept. 1893, **2**, no. 3.

'I territori dipendati dallo Scioa', Società Geografica Italiana, *Bollettino*, July 1886, **23**, no. 7.

Traversi, Leopoldo. 'Escursione nel Gimma', Società Geografica Italiana, *Bollettino*, Oct.–Nov. 1888, **25**, nos. 10–11.

'Viaggi negli Arussi, Guraghi, ecc.', Società Geografica Italiana, *Bollettino*, April 1887, **24**, no. 4.

Underhill, G. E. 'Abyssinia under Menelik and after', *Quarterly Review*, Jan. 1922, **273**, no. 470.

Vanderheym, J. G. *Une expédition avec le négous Ménélik*. Paris, 1896.

'Il viaggio di Antonelli e Ragazzi allo Scioa', Società Geografica Italiana, *Bollettino*, Dec. 1884, **21**, no. 12.

Walda, Maryam. 'The history of King Theodore', tr. H. Weld-Blundell, *Journal of the African Society*, Oct. 1909, **6**, no. 21.

Waldmeier, Theophilus. *Autobiography*. London, 1888.

Weld-Blundell, Herbert Joseph. 'Exploration in the Abai Basin, Abyssinia', *Geographical Journal*, June 1906, **27**, no. 6.

Wellby, Montagu Sinclair. 'King Menilek's dominions and the country between Lake Gallop (Rudolph) and the Nile Valley', *Geographical Journal*, Sept. 1900, **16**, no. 3.

Woolf, Leonard. *Empire and commerce in Africa*. London, n.d.

Wylde, Augustus B. *'83 to '87 in the Soudan, with an account of Sir William Hewett's mission to King John of Abyssinia*. 2nd ed. 2 vols. London, 1888.
Modern Abyssinia. London, 1901.

Yaltasamma (pseud.). *Les amis de Ménélik II*. Paris, 1899.

Zaghi, Carlo. *Le origini della colonia Eritrea*. Bologna, 1934.
ed. *Crispi e Menelich nel diario inedito del Conte Augusto Salimbeni*. Turin, 1956.

CHAPTER 14

MISSIONARY AND HUMANITARIAN ASPECTS OF IMPERIALISM FROM 1870 TO 1914

by CHARLES PELHAM GROVES

The first pioneers of the Gospel in tropical Africa were the Portuguese. For many decades, Portuguese priests laboured in the kingdom of Kongo, in the realm of Monomotapa and elsewhere; but in the long run, their labours proved of little avail. The eighteenth century, however, witnessed a series of religious revivals. A new religiosity, often popular and emotional in character, swept over many parts of northern Europe, affecting people as diverse as poverty-stricken peasants in Germany, disinherited Jewish hawkers in Poland and factory workers in England.

This reformist creed, with its intense desire to uplift and convert the masses at home, soon spilled over into the foreign field. In 1787 the Methodists set up a regular system of overseas missions, followed subsequently by the Baptist Missionary Society, the interdenominational London Missionary Society, the evangelical Church Missionary Society and other bodies in Great Britain and the United States. The bulk of the early mission work was developed by English-speaking groups whose evangelical labours benefited from the expansion of British and American commerce and, in the case of British societies, from British territorial expansion.

But continental Protestantism did not lag far behind. Germany played a major part in the evangelical revival, and in the 1820s and 1830s German benefactors founded several important mission groups, including the Berlin, the Rhenish, the Leipzig and the Bremen societies. Partly under Scottish inspiration, the evangelical revival spread also to Switzerland, and from there to France. In France, particularly, the movement benefited from the post-revolutionary revulsion against atheism as well as from the demand for a socially constructive, rather than a purely negative, creed. In 1828 the Paris Evangelical Society came into existence, together with other charitable institutions, and received support from Protestants in Italy, Switzerland and Britain as well as in France.

After some delay, the Catholic Church also joined the race. The Catholic hierarchy met the new opportunities of European expansion overseas in its traditional manner, by redeploying older orders and creating new ones. Among the new orders were the White Fathers, founded in 1868 by Archbishop (later Cardinal) Lavigerie. Like nearly all other great ecclesiastical leaders of the time, Lavigerie was a firm believer in colonial expansion as an engine of progress. He regarded European rule in Africa as essential to crush the African slave-trade, to pacify strife-torn lands and to spread the faith. Catholic Christianity thus also came to play an essential role in the evangelization of Africa, and Catholic missions received widespread support from France, Italy, Germany, Ireland, Canada, Belgium and elsewhere.

Seen purely in territorial terms, Christianity had by 1870 not made much of an impact on Africa. The great landmass was still 'a continent of outposts'. Outside of the settler colonies in South Africa and Algeria, European penetration—religious and secular alike—was largely confined to the coasts. Christian endeavour had, however, played a major part in reshaping the pattern of trade in tropical Africa. The evangelical conscience detested not only slave-raiders and slave-traders, but slave- and plantation-owners as well, regarding them all as representatives of a backward economy, a reactionary social order and a sinful way of life. Evangelical preachers, like secular middle-class economists, believed in a free labour market and 'legitimate commerce'. Traffic in tropical produce should replace the traffic in man, and benefit both the metropolitan and the colonial countries.

The parliamentary activities of William Wilberforce and his colleagues—many being members of the Clapham Sect—thus received widespread support among Dissenters and Anglicans alike. The evangelical conscience became a force in politics; and in 1807 Great Britain forbade the slave-trade to all her subjects. Within a few days, the United States Congress also enacted a law prohibiting the traffic as of 1808. Whereas the American law remained largely ineffective, however, British legislation was backed by the mightiest navy in the world. British, and to a lesser extent American and French, vessels, gradually reduced the volume of the transatlantic slave traffic, and thereby helped to bring about an economic revolution in Africa.

The antislavery campaign unwittingly helped to draw the Western powers into Africa. The Sierra Leone Company, a philanthropic venture to provide a home for repatriated Africans from the New World and from the destitute black poor in England, established a settlement in Sierra Leone in 1787. The new colony struggled on with varying fortunes until 1807, when it was transferred to the Crown— the first British Crown Colony in West Africa. It now became the reception centre for discharged slave cargoes captured by British gunboats on patrol. The British tried to rehabilitate the Africans from many tribes who had been torn from hearth and home. Cultural assimilation produced a new kind of African, the Creole—English by language, Protestant by religion, well adjusted to the world of trade and religion. The Creoles themselves began to play an important part in the religious and commercial penetration of West Africa.

Farther along the Guinea Coast, Lagos, which had been for some time a great emporium of the slave-trade, was occupied partially in pursuit of the same antislavery policy. The town and its defences were in due course reduced, and in 1852 the King of Lagos accepted a treaty for the abolition of the traffic. Another decade passed, however, before the trade through Lagos was finally rooted out by British annexation on 6 August 1861.

Evangelically-minded Americans also shared the humanitarian interest in ending slavery, the slave-trade and the complex socioeconomic institutions that depended on this form of bondage. In 1816 a group of distinguished Americans founded the American Colonization Society to promote the colonization of Africa by free American Negroes. American emigrants established a settlement in 1820, and in 1847 the new state of Liberia declared its independence. The Republic was formally recognized by the United States in 1862. But even before, the Liberian government, which was based on a narrow ruling stratum of Afro-American settlers and their descendants, had drawn moral strength, missionary support and sometimes physical aid from the parent country. The presence of American warships enabled the struggling Liberian government to act decisively against slavers, and sometimes against indigenous African chiefs. The antislavery issue affected also French colonization in tropical Africa, with French vessels participating in the eradication of the traffic. In 1839 the French established a territorial foothold on the northern Gabon coast, and ten years later Negroes freed from a slave-ship founded a new settlement, significantly named Libreville. The French had long been established

464

also around the mouth of the Senegal. The somnolent settlement obtained a great economic impetus from the developing trade in peanuts; and it was stirred into political activity in 1854 by the arrival of General Faidherbe as governor. By 1870 the colony of Senegal was organized, and footholds were secured also on the Ivory Coast and Dahomey. After 1870 the great spaces of the hinterland offered both an ample training ground for the military, and untapped resources for commercial development.

In East Africa, on the other hand, the story had a different setting. The bulk of the East African slave-trade was conducted by Muslim merchants, with Zanzibar as one of the main centres. But again, the Western humanitarian conscience intervened—backed by British sea power. In 1866 John Kirk, David Livingstone's medical colleague on the Zambezi expedition, was appointed vice-consul at Zanzibar and later consul. He actively promoted negotiations for the abolition of the slave-trade. An Anglo-Zanzibar treaty drawn up in 1873 ended the trade in the sultan's dominion and closed the slave-markets. In South Africa too, where the Cape had fallen to the British in the comprehensive settlement following the Napoleonic Wars, the antislavery policy was effectively applied. No more slaves were landed at the Cape after 1807. In 1834 the British abolished the status of slavery throughout their dominions, with the result that many Boer farmers, who were already labouring under other grievances, decided to emigrate. Between 1836 and 1840 they embarked on their Great Trek inland and established the Orange Free State and the Transvaal. Thus one unintended effect of the abolition of slavery was to encourage white settlement in the interior.

The humanitarian conscience, without doubt, played an essential part in early Western colonial policy. Abolitionist sentiments, of course, were combined with more mundane political and economic considerations. But even when full allowance is made for the secular aspects of the movement, a great residue of unselfish idealism remains. The British, more than any other nation, backed philanthropy by hard cash. They disbursed vast sums in compensation to slave-holders in the West Indies and the Cape; they made extensive grants to Spain and Portugal in return for engagements to end the traffic; they shouldered heavy financial responsibilities in founding Sierra Leone; they spent vast amounts of money to patrol the coasts of Africa. British, and also American and French, sailors, faced all kinds of hardship and sometimes death to break the stranglehold of the slave commerce on Africa. Humanitarian impulses thereby profoundly affected the internal balance of power through vast portions of the continent.

The battle against the slave-trade gave a new impetus also to mission work. By 1870, some missions had been established on the West African coast from the Gambia to the Cameroons. In the Cape Colony and the adjoining regions, penetration had already become more effective and competitive. Protestant societies pioneered the way, with Catholic missionaries following by mid-century. By 1870 there were eight societies from the continent of Europe, seven from Great Britain, and seven from the United States, while three had their headquarters in Cape Colony. Of the total, more than half (thirteen) were at work in South Africa, including six of the eight continental societies. The master motive of the service was not national, but an earnest desire to offer, in the Christian name, some restitution to Africa for the evils of the slave-trade.

The subsequent expansion of European missionary enterprise depended on a great variety of local factors. European churchmen generally wanted to build schools and churches in populous villages. But there is no consistent correlation between the size of indigenous population clusters and the location of Christian missions because some of Africa's most densely settled regions were Muslim. The power of Islam accounted for the small number of stations found in the Sudanic belt and along the East African coast, in contrast to the West African shoreline. The relatively densely populated highland of Ethiopia proved hard to penetrate because of the presence of two rival religions, Islam and Coptic Christianity. The intensive missionary occupation of Uganda came about not only because of the presence of a highly developed and populous society (though this was certainly present), but also because of the desire to prevent the advance of Islam. The frequency of missions in Rwanda and Burundi coincided with heavy population densities, but was related also to Protestant and Catholic competition in a region on which missionary pioneers converged from north, east and west.

Most mission concentrations in highland regions may be attributed to their climatic and scenic attractions for Europeans, as well as to their dense populations or strategic location for defence. Missionary settlements in the Akwapim–Togo ranges in West Africa, the Jos Plateau in Nigeria, the Kilimanjaro and Usambara regions in Tanzania, the Shire

Highlands in Malawi and the central highlands of Kenya provide examples for this rule. Numerous older stations in Sierra Leone and Liberia and the Cross river region of Nigeria owed much to the existence of naval and trading-posts in these regions. The saturation of South Africa with mission stations resulted from a favourable climate and the promise of evangelization work among both Africans and white settlers in Cape Colony and on the frontier under conditions that tended to favour Protestant societies. Missionaries moreover had exalted visions of bringing the Bible's pastoral message to grazing peoples. Nomadism in fact proved to be one of the hardest obstacles to overcome; yet some very impressive stations were founded in sparsely settled pastoral regions.

In addition, logistics played a vital role in missionary strategy. All missionaries came to sub-Saharan African by sea; to a greater or lesser extent they all depended for their maintenance on imports from the coastal ports. Two of the most important relay points for the trans-atlantic exchange were Freetown and Fernando Po. Both played a major role in shaping missionary strategy. So did Libreville and above all Cape Town, the stopover point for coastal expansion as far as the Inhambane district of Moçambique. Cape Town was the starting-point for overland advance to South West Africa as far as Ovamboland and, with trans-shipments to Port Elizabeth, to what is now Botswana along the 'Missionaries' Road'. From Cape Town emanated even the fatal mission sent to the Shire Highlands by the Universities Mission to Central Africa. Zanzibar, the island entrepôt for East African and Indian trade, served as the point of departure for the first mission stations north of the Rovuma river. Zanzibar continued to be an important port of call even when the missionaries had begun to outfit in Mombasa, though the island never became a base for missionary work in East Africa.[1]

Limitations of space forbid a more detailed discussion, but four representative case histories illustrate particular situations. In Sierra Leone the missionaries found their hands more than full with the landing, after 1807, of captured slave cargoes. Villages were established for the reception and rehabilitation of the liberated Africans, and lay schoolmasters, as well as ordained men, were recruited for the service.

---

[1] For detailed treatment from the geographic point of view see Hildegard Binder Johnson, 'The location of Christian missions in Africa', in Geographical Review, April 1965, 57, no. 2, pp. 168–202.

After ten years, one report stated, 'We have now masons, bricklayers, carpenters, shinglemakers, sawyers, smiths, tailors, and brickmakers'.[1] They had completed a road two miles long to the capital in one month. Most significant in a mixed community of liberated Africans but recently torn from home and family was the tribute paid, after ten years, by the Chief Justice at Quarter Sessions in Freetown. He remarked that when the population of the colony numbered 4,000, he had had forty cases for trial; now it was 16,000 and he had only six, and added it was remarkable 'that there was not a single case from any of the villages under the superintendence of a missionary or schoolmaster'.[2]

Another mission centre was situated in the city of Abeokuta, some 100 miles inland from Lagos. Here, missionaries from Sierra Leone came in the forties at the invitation of Christian Yorubas among the liberated in Sierra Leone who had sought their homeland once more. This was an African-ruled city, and missionaries had to rely upon African goodwill. With the British occupation of Lagos, the missionaries encouraged trade in palm-oil, for which there had been no adequate outlet before. They hoped thereby to promote legitimate commerce to replace the traffic in slaves. Samuel Crowther, the eminent African Christian leader, reported of a Yoruba clan:

Their head chiefs could not help confessing to me, that they, aged persons, never remembered any time of the slave trade that so much wealth was brought to their country as has been since the commencement of the palm-oil trade for the last four years; that they were perfectly satisfied with legitimate trade and with proceedings of the British government [in prohibiting the slave-trade through Lagos].[3]

The missionaries went further; they encouraged the growing of cotton by providing an institution where were taught the cleaning and packing of the crop for export and care of the requisite machinery. Friends of the Church Missionary Society, eager to see legitimate trade replace the slave-trade, financed the enterprise. In 1859 four cotton merchants from Manchester, England, arrived in Abeokuta prepared to buy as much cotton as could be offered. The mission was active on lines that harmonized well with British policy, but it cannot on that account be considered imperialist.

[1] *A memoir of the Rev. W. A. B. Johnson* (London, 1852), p. 51.
[2] *Memoir...Johnson*, p. 316.
[3] *Proceedings of the Church Missionary Society* (London, 1857), p. 38.

Turning back to South Africa, we find a sharp contrast. Here were a majority of Boer farmers, descendants of the Dutch and other settlers of the seventeenth century, with a minority of English artisans who had arrived after the Napoleonic Wars. The Boers, deprived of fresh slave-labour after 1807, became dependent on the local Hottentots of the Western Cape, with the result that the Hottentots' condition as free people rapidly deteriorated. Dr John Philip, who served in the Colony for thirty years as General Superintendent of the London Missionary Society, courageously took up the cause of the oppressed and censured compulsory labour and the pass system as two of their more severe abuses. The situation was brought to the notice of William Wilberforce, who asked, 'Why does not Dr Philip appeal to the Colonial Government?' only to be told, 'It is with them the oppression rests'. Crown Commissioners were appointed to visit the Cape, and Philip co-operated actively. 'I am at one object', he wrote, 'the question is... in what way I can most certainly and effectually secure the emancipation of the poor natives from their dreadful thraldom, the Missions from the oppressive system they are groaning under, and to give permanency to the cause of God in South Africa.'[1] By 1828 the object had finally been achieved, and a local ordinance (secured against change or cancellation by Order in Council) guaranteed to the Hottentots their status as free men. But Philip paid a heavy price: he became the most hated man in the Colony, and a distorted picture of his activities long persisted among local historians. He is today recognized to have been a Christian statesman with a wide view of his missionary calling.

Daniel Lindley, pioneer missionary to Zululand of the American Board of Commissioners for Foreign Missions, who served in South Africa from 1835 to 1873, illustrates still another facet of the situation at the Cape. He saw the exodus from the Cape of the emigrant Boers as a serious ecclesiastical problem. The Dutch Reformed Church authorities had condemned the Trek and had made no pastoral provision for the trekkers. Hence, Lindley argued, 'the whites *must be provided for*, or we labour in vain to make Christians of the blacks'.[2] By opening a school for young Boers and by learning Afrikaans, he won the regard and affection of the Boers. Moreover, he was received as an American, where a Britisher might have been rejected out of hand. When, later,

[1] William Miller Macmillan, *Bantu, Boer and Briton: the making of the South African problem* (London, 1929), p. 139.
[2] Edwin William Smith, *The life and times of Daniel Lindley* (London, 1949), p. 160.

consideration was given to a pastor for the community, Lindley received the call. He accepted conditionally, with the approval of the Board, seeing the new service as an integral part of the total missionary plan. With headquarters in Pietermaritzburg, he was the only ordained minister for some 20,000 Dutch-speaking inhabitants of Natal, the Orange Free State and the Transvaal Republic, and has been acclaimed as the founder of the Dutch Reformed Church in those territories. For seven and a half years he served them, and then returned to work among the Zulu people. He was deeply loved, though fearless in his preaching about his people's prejudices. His biographer relates: 'When Daniel Lindley announced his decision to return to his missionary labours, it was received with consternation by his congregation. It is on record that men who time and again had faced death unflinchingly on the battlefield, shed tears in church for him that day.'[1] His example showed that missionary fervour could be effective among white and black Africans alike. He stood out as one of those many ecclesiastical pioneers who were ready to meet the needs of different contemporary societies.

No missionary, however, struck public imagination more profoundly than did David Livingstone. Outstanding alike as a preacher, as an explorer, as a student of tropical medicine and ethnography, Livingstone also made his name as a publicist. His death in Africa in 1873 made a profound impression throughout the civilized world. Protestant Christianity had found a martyr of imposing stature, and H. M. Stanley records what Livingstone's death meant for him. 'The effect which this news had upon me, after the first shock had passed away, was to fire me with a resolution to complete his work...to clear up... the secrets of the Great River throughout its course...'[2] As he resolved, so he performed. Within four months of the funeral in Westminster Abbey, Stanley was on his way to Zanzibar. Three years later, on the 999th day from Zanzibar, he emerged from the great Congo journey on the Atlantic shore. He landed in Europe in January 1878.

Meanwhile, Lieutenant W. L. Cameron, R.N., had led an expedition across Africa from east to west by a more southerly land-route and published his record of it in 1877. He made treaties with African chiefs giving Great Britain the option of declaring a protectorate over the inner Congo basin. He even ventured to issue a proclamation in these terms, urging that this would deal a deathblow to the local slave-trade. When the British, however, refused to commit themselves, Leopold II

[1] Smith, *Lindley*, p. 202.   [2] *Through the dark continent* (London, 1878), I, I.

stepped in. Colonization in the Congo, in turn, played a major part in setting off the scramble for Africa.

The politics of partition, with its complex economic, political and strategic strands, forms the subject of an extensive literature and need not concern us here. But missionary and humanitarian impulses also had a profound effect on the story. An attempt at international action took place between 1884 and 1885 when fourteen European powers, as well as the United States, assembled at an international conference at Berlin. The General Act of the Conference embodied the classical demands of nineteenth-century missionaries and humanitarians. The signatories agreed that there should be freedom of trade in the Congo basin and freedom of navigation on the Congo and Niger rivers. They pledged themselves also to freedom of religion—evangelical work, in other words, was not to be impeded by missionary mono-polies. The Act put forward also a doctrine of trusteeship for the peoples of Africa, recognized by international agreement. The powers promised to 'watch over the preservation of the native tribes and to care for the improvement of their moral and material well being, and to help in suppressing slavery and especially the Slave Trade'.[1]

These provisions may be interpreted in many different ways. Treaty obligations were often disregarded. Even when observed, they can justifiably be seen in mundane terms. Free trade and navigation, for instance, benefited the stronger industrial countries, especially Great Britain. The condemnation of the slave-trade served political as well as humanitarian requirements. No colonial power could countenance armed slave-traders as rivals for political supremacy within the colonial dominions. All European governments had an obvious military interest in preventing the uncontrolled influx of arms into their spheres of in-fluence. The international approach of the Berlin Conference—dear to the hearts of reformers—itself represented a diplomatic compromise, based on the assumption that the colonizers could co-operate to a limited extent in Africa. But the Act expressed also purely humanitarian aspira-tions, and set up standards by which the white rulers would them-selves evaluate or condemn one another's record on the African continent.

While diplomatic partition of Africa was largely completed during the 1880s and 1890s, effective pacification and occupation took a good

[1] Great Britain, *Parliamentary papers*, vol. XLVII, C. 4739, *General Act of the Conference of Berlin* (London, 1886).

deal longer and involved missionaries at almost every stage. In many parts of Africa, such as in Uganda, Nyasaland and Barotseland, white clergymen had pioneered the trail, and the flag followed the Cross. Imperial expansion faced the white preachers with questions of extreme difficulty. By and large, the missionaries welcomed European protection for the people whom they considered their wards. In addition, many clergymen were affected by the nationalism of their own respective countries. This was perhaps most marked, though not exclusively so, in the German colonies. Advocates of German imperial expansion saw the Christian missions from the Fatherland as a means of impressing the German image upon colonial peoples; and many French imperialists took a similar view of the missionary role in the French empire. Advocates of such a kind, however, were not friends of the missions in the accepted sense, since they lacked an understanding of the supra-national character of the Christian religion. Hence, some Germans seriously demanded that all German mission work should be concentrated in the German colonies, or that non-German missions should be eliminated from the possessions of the Reich. In 1886, for instance, the Berliner Evangelische Missionsgesellschaft für Ostafrika was founded for exclusive service in German East Africa—with Carl Peters among its patrons. Happily for the Christian cause, there were able and experienced missionary leaders who effectively countered such proposals. Gustav Warneck, a missionary statesman of pre-eminent authority, exposed the fundamental fallacies of this appeal, and commended the British for allowing equal entry to all missions. But, generally speaking, British societies would gravitate to British territories and Belgian Catholic orders were attracted to the Congo, although American missions went into all colonial areas.

Such national identification tended to make missionaries appear in African eyes not merely as members of the European ruling race, but also, more specifically, as citizens of the new colonial power. Not that governments and missions ever became wholly coterminous in national terms. Missionaries and government officials sometimes clashed and sometimes collaborated with one another. Hence the relationship between the two groups raised complex problems. At the same time, we must distinguish between a society's policy at headquarters and the personal attitude of its agents on the spot. An able and likable German missionary, repatriated from a German colony in the Great War, once said later, in the writer's presence: 'I am a German first and a Christian second';

but as the author knows, this was far from being the outlook of the German missionary body in question.

The problem of government-mission relations may usefully be considered under two distinct headings: first, the influence of the missions on colonial governments; and secondly, the impact of governments on the missions. Not only was the general character of the scramble modified by the Christian impact, but mission enterprise also influenced the local direction of the imperial thrust. In Barotseland in what is now Zambia, for instance, the Paris Evangelical Society was directly involved in imperial annexation. François Coillard, a French Protestant of outstanding stature, was sincerely convinced that only British protection would stop Barotse civil strife at home and would end Matabele threats abroad; only the British could save the Barotse from the future depredations of white gold-seekers and from the intrigues of foreign powers. Coillard refused an offer from Rhodes to act as the British South Africa Company's local resident, but took an active part in the negotiations that placed Barotseland under British protection.

In Uganda the position was even more complex. Here, representatives of the Church Missionary Society, a British body, had arrived in 1877 by the 800-mile overland route. The British missionaries, like their French colleages in Barotseland, had to operate within the framework of a highly organized, quasi-feudal state, with a strong royal house. The goodwill of the king was essential not only to the preachers' success, but to their very survival. The emissaries of Christianity had to compete with Muslim Arabs from the coast. Subsequently, two members of Lavigerie's White Fathers arrived in the country. To complicate matters further, there was a German irruption in 1889 when Carl Peters, treaty gathering, reached Uganda, and secured an agreement. This instrument, however, became invalid, since Great Britain and Germany had meanwhile reached a comprehensive settlement of their East African affairs. The Imperial British East African Company (IBEA Co.), administering the territory between Lake Victoria and the coast, was about to breathe more freely when the British government asked it to deal with the Uganda situation. This involved an expedition (which threatened to overtax the company's resources). Captain F. D. Lugard, the commander, was successful in securing the king's acceptance of a treaty with the company. Internal rivalries, however, again flared up, and the financial cost of occupation was so alarming that Lugard was instructed to retire.

At this point, Bishop Tucker of Uganda, together with the Church Missionary Society, took action to delay withdrawal for one year, during which time it was hoped to induce the British government to declare a protectorate over Uganda based on the existing treaty with the company. Since society funds could not be used for such a purpose, a special campaign was initiated under dramatic circumstances. Bishop Tucker was guest at a country house in the Scottish Highlands when Sir William Mackinnon, Chairman of IBEA Co., unexpectedly arrived. When the question of the company's retirement from Uganda was raised, Mackinnon stated plainly the financial drain on their resources: 'Uganda is costing us £40,000 a year. Help us to raise a sum of £30,000, and we will undertake to continue in the country for at least another year. If you will raise £15,000,' he generously added, 'I will myself give £10,000 and will try to raise another £5,000 amongst my friends.'[1] The offer was accepted. The £15,000 was raised within two weeks. The public campaign to induce the government to take over from the company responsibility for Uganda aroused great enthusiasm throughout the country, by no means in Anglican circles alone. The government yielded to public opinion, and a protectorate was proclaimed on 18 June 1894.

Not unnaturally, this unusual episcopal operation, together with the society's action, has since been, and was even at the time, the subject of critical comment. The missionaries were said to be imperialists after all. Tucker countered the charge by reviewing Uganda's recent history. The missionaries had entered Uganda with no official protection or thought of it, confident in the Divine call that took them there, and on the human side dependent upon the king. Through thirteen years they had laboured thus.

One day, a drum beat is heard—a caravan arrives at the head of which is an Englishman...They turn to the mission for advice. 'Here is a man', they say, 'who says he is an Englishman—is it so?' The answer is 'yes', 'he also says that he represents a great company—is that true?' 'Yes.' 'He wants us to sign a treaty with him—we cannot understand it. What shall we do? Will you explain it to us and advise us what to do?' The answer is 'Certainly we will'— and they do so. This is the whole case of the so-called interference of missionaries in the politics of Uganda.[2]

The Church Missionary Society having thus become identified with the British cause, any withdrawal would expose it and its people to reprisals

[1] A. R. Tucker, *Eighteen years in Uganda and East Africa* (London, 1908), I, 144-6.
[2] *Ibid.*

from its rivals in that troubled country, so that circumstances themselves conspired to drive the missionaries into an unintended course of action.

The instances of Barotseland and Uganda illustrate the part played by the missions as allies of government. Their role was, however, never clear-cut. Most churchmen shared certain basic assumptions with secular advocates of empire. They generally believed that only European rule could guide Africa into the path of progress. But power, in their view, entailed moral responsibility; and the missionary thus became a censor, as well as an ally of the colonial régimes. For this task, the mission societies were peculiarly well suited. Since they obtained all or most of their funds from independent well-wishers overseas, they were not in the early years financially dependent on the support of local governments. The missionaries were men of education; and, especially in the early phase of the imperial epoch, they were often the only highly literate people outside the ranks of the government service. The missions had their own means of publicity overseas, and mission bodies—in alliance with secular humanitarian groups—could often exert political pressure on metropolitan governments in the style of the old antislavery campaigns.

The most famous instance of such a campaign was the 'Red Rubber' agitation against the Congo Free State.[1] The Congo administration, short of funds and pressed with administrative and military tasks beyond its resources, tried to make ends meet by embarking on a restrictive concessionary policy and by imposing forced labour on Africans. Local agents of the administration, few in numbers, widely scattered geographically, and poorly supervised, often committed acts of extreme cruelty; and many Africans suffered from the vicious brutality of soldiers and officials and their African assistants.

Humanitarian organizations provided a platform for missionary criticism, until Leopold could no longer ignore the scandal. In such unsavoury situations, where vested interests are deeply involved, the main problem is to ascertain the facts of the case from trustworthy witnesses. Here the various missionaries, living in the midst of the people, with knowledge of their languages and aware of their activities, were in a key position. Not all the mission agents were equally communicative and not all were working in the worst concession areas. But enough evidence was forthcoming, mainly from American, British and Swedish missionaries, to furnish a damning indictment of Leopold's

---

[1] For details see the article by Stengers in this volume, pp. 261–92.

rule. Roger Casement, British Consul in the Congo State, carried out personal investigations of great value. George Grenfell, the distinguished Baptist missionary and explorer, found himself at first in a difficult position. Few men, if any, knew the Congo as well as he. He began with full confidence in the bona fides of Leopold, whom he knew personally and had served as boundary commissioner. But he soon changed his mind. As his biographer quotes him: 'It was with nothing less than consternation that I was compelled to accept the evidence and to believe what looked like the incredible.'[1]

Members of the Belgian Roman Catholic orders remained more complacent; and when in 1906 Leopold made over to these missions, and these alone (despite the Berlin Act), liberal land grants in full ownership, there were some raised eyebrows. The missionaries and their humanitarian coadjutors supplied the ammunition that was used with such effect by experienced publicists in Britain—Grattan Guiness, W. T. Stead, E. D. Morel, H. R. Fox Bourne and others—that the British government eventually brought heavy pressure to bear on Belgium. The 'Red Rubber' campaign, together with the activities of Belgian reformers, led to the transfer of the Congo Free State under direct Belgian rule in 1908; and a more enlightened régime subsequently introduced far-reaching improvements.

Missionaries acted as censors of government also in less spectacular fashions. The missionaries commonly resisted the imposition of what they regarded as the excessive taxation of Africans. In 1903, for instance, the Southern Rhodesian administration planned to increase sharply the fiscal burdens on the black people in the colony. An increased tax, in their view, would stimulate African agricultural production for the market, and would also force more Africans into wage labour. But Father R. P. Richartz, head of the Jesuit mission at Chishawasha, came out strongly against the project on the grounds that Africans could not afford to pay so much. The imperially appointed Resident Commissioner agreed with Richartz, with the result that the imperial government subsequently refused to give its assent to a local ordinance putting up the tax. Missionary opinion, in other words, helped to act as a brake on local lobbies.

[1] Harry Lathey Hemmens, *George Grenfell, pioneer in Congo* (London, 1927), p. 211. See also Ruth M. Slade, *English-speaking missions in the Congo Independent State (1878–1908)* (Brussels, Académie Royale des Sciences Coloniales, 1959); and *King Leopold's Congo: aspects of the development of race relations in the Congo Independent State* (London, Oxford University Press, 1962).

The Rhodesian example was only one of numerous comparable instances where the missionary acted as the *tribunus populi*, pleading the cause of the subjects against their rulers in matters as varied as fiscal impositions, labour conditions and similar questions. Missionary opinion, though not generally opposed to white settlement as such, would censure also what clergymen regarded as the abuses of white colonists. In Rhodesia, for instance, Africans found doughty champions of their cause in the Reverend John White and Arthur S. Cripps; and the Missionary Conference of Southern Rhodesia, like similar bodies elsewhere, played an important part in ventilating, and sometimes in redressing, African grievances.

Missionaries sometimes incurred the hostility of government officials also by criticizing the rulers' private morals. Missionary pressure may well thereby have played some part in raising the general tone of the colonial state machinery. In British possessions, the clergyman's role as a watchdog often became institutionalized through formal representation on the legislative council. After the creation of the Nyasaland Legislative Council in 1908, the British governors in time made a practice of always appointing one unofficial (that is to say a non-government) member from one of the mission societies, thus in the government's view providing the African people with a form of indirect representation.

The effects of government activities on the missions were equally complex. The attitudes of administrations varied considerably from territory to territory, and state–church relations in the colonies raised just as many problems as they did at home. But governments were overwhelmingly secular in outlook. The missions stood for a religious faith; hence mission–government relationship had many contradictions. In some cases, mission societies from a foreign country were altogether excluded from a colony for nationalist reasons. This most extreme step may be illustrated from German Cameroun. The British Baptists had been established in the country for forty years when the German government took over. The German rulers were naturally sensitive to the attachment manifested by chiefs and people to the British, whose protectorate they had confidently expected. As a result conflict broke out; and the German governor finally offered the Baptists conditions that were tantamount to an invitation to leave. The Swiss Basel Mission (with missionaries recruited also from South Germany), having been assured of the goodwill of the Baptists in the transaction, then took over their stations. The African members of the Baptists, however, were restive at being transferred in this way to other pastors, and some time passed before the rift was healed.

A less drastic type of control was exercised where Islam was the prevailing religion. Two British territories fell into this category: the Anglo-Egyptian Sudan and Northern Nigeria. In each case the territory had been occupied by virtue of conquest, and the commanding officers —Kitchener and Lugard, respectively—were responsible for the initial settlement. The assumed hostility of Islamic peoples to alien religious propaganda led to closing the Muslim zone of each territory to Christian missions. In the official view, government permission for Christian evangelists to enter the country would be regarded by African Muslims as government encouragement, and would bring disastrous results. Later, however, there was some relaxation of this policy. In Northern Nigeria, pioneers of the Church Missionary Society had already arrived in advance of the British force. They were not disturbed, but Lugard made his policy clear:

At the time of the conquest of the Mohammedan Emirates in 1903, I declared that the British government would not interfere with the religion of the people, and every man should be free to worship God as he chose. The Emirs, though they have not been very consistent in the matter, no doubt view with dislike and distrust the efforts of Europeans to convert their people to Christianity, the more so that the administrative and judicial systems and the social life of the people is to such a large extent based on the teaching of the Koran, and so intimately associated with religion, that the Emirs not unnaturally fear a weakening of their authority and a breakup of the social system if their religion is undermined. The government in these circumstances has considered it right to be guided by the wishes of the Emirs and their counsellors.

And a few years later, he stated:

The reply of the administrator, however reluctantly given, can only be what it has always been in Nigeria: that the government will offer no objection if the ruling chief concurs; that in a matter solely concerned with religion, the government does not feel justified in compelling a Moslem ruler to grant permission which but for government intervention he would refuse.[1]

In such situations, however, a policy justifiable in the original circumstances stood in danger of fossilizing, without regard to changing

[1] Frederick John Dealtry Lugard, 1st baron, *The dual mandate in British tropical Africa* (London, 1929), pp. 593–4.

conditions. The people of Northern Nigeria thus had to pay a heavy price in educational terms for a policy of partial exclusion.

Governments also imposed linguistic restrictions on mission bodies under their local control. All colonial administrators were alike in this respect. They insisted that their own tongue should be used as the official medium of instruction—not that of the missionaries if it differed from the language of the government. This was not an unnatural requirement, but could not be complied with overnight. One mission on which this pressed to the point of transfer of its work was that of the Board of Foreign Missions of the Presbyterian Church in the United States of America. The field in question lay in Equatorial West Africa in Gabon and on the Ogooué (Ogowe). The French administration of Gabon was intensified during the eighties at the time of the scramble, and the requirement of the use of French in all schools was strictly enforced.

By and large, however, the positive effects of governmental action on mission work far outweighed its negative side. For all their numerous and sometimes bitter internal differences, officials and missionaries believed themselves engaged in the same battle. The missions in late nineteenth-century Africa, like the mediaeval church in Europe, always had a natural interest in strong government. The missionaries passion-ately supported the liquidation of the slave-trade. The rapid and comprehensive extension of European political control during the scramble presented a hitherto unequalled opportunity for its suppression. Happily, this opportunity was promptly seized. From the French side, Cardinal Lavigerie entered with characteristic enthusiasm upon an antislavery campaign, and secured a federation of the various anti-slavery societies of Europe in L'Œuvre antiesclavagiste, for which he won considerable commendation, tempered by the observation that he gave scant credit to the Protestant pioneers of the movement. Germany, Britain and Belgium also entered wholeheartedly upon the campaign in their respective territories. By the beginning of the present century, the problem had been largely solved; and the slave-trade, one of Africa's earliest and most onerous forms of labour migration, had generally become a thing of the past.

Pacification involved also the suppression of internecine warfare—a policy resented by the strong but welcomed by the weak. This equiva-lent of a Pax et Imperium was an elementary necessity both for the economic development of a territory and for its evangelization. In Matabeleland, for instance, a predatory warrior state with rigid social stratification, Christian missionaries were not allowed to preach the Gospel, though the Matabele aristocracy was willing enough to admit white clergymen as technical experts. The Matabele held, quite correctly, that Christianity was incompatible with the social constitution of their kingdom. They objected to the missionaries' criticism of raiding, and also to the Christians' implicit message of social equality between the conquerors and their subjects. The military occupation of Matabeleland in 1893 by the British South Africa Company, however, opened up a vast new area where missionaries could safely preach, and the Europeans' new prestige attracted many converts. Pacification followed close upon a strict control of the arms traffic, whereby in the past, unprincipled free-lance European traders had made large profits. The Berlin Conference had given particular attention to this point in view of the part played by fire-arms in the prosecution of the slave-trade and the promotion of intertribal conflict.

In addition to such provisions for security dealing collectively with the people, consideration was given, as in all civilized communities, to the safeguarding of human life. The colonizers stamped out inter-tribal warfare. They also combated the practice of cannibalism. In this matter the people of the Guinea coast and the Congo basin were the two worst offenders. Stanley and his men on the great Congo journey had to run the gauntlet of cannibal riverine tribes out, not for their blood, but for their flesh. At the time of the Arab war in the eastern Congo, the continuing practice was unveiled. The writer knows of up-country Ibos in Nigeria who, seeking education in the south, would not travel in groups of fewer than half a dozen armed with spears, because of passing through cannibal country.

Bound up with tribal beliefs concerning the world of the departed was the killing of slaves and others to serve in the world of shades as a retinue for the deceased. Large numbers might be involved, according to the status of the dead chief, for he was still a chief in the other world. H. M. Bentley gave the figure for the Upper Kasai in the Congo on such occasions as 300 slaves. Then again, there was killing for magical medicines or ritual murder, as it is termed. For the lowly there was little security of life.[1]

---

[1] The question of cannibalism in the Guinea coastlands is a difficult matter to judge. There was a tendency to impute cannibalism to peoples thought to be more primitive and to strangers whom one feared. Europeans sometimes were misled by the fact that many African languages used words which literally meant 'to eat' but might better

Governments supported by the missionaries decreed that all this must stop. The ban was by no means without effect, though some hidden survivals were to be expected. Trial by poison ordeal for those accused of witchcraft was in the same category, as the European judiciary did not recognize death by alleged witchcraft as involving a criminal act. While African law and custom were widely countenanced, imposition of the death penalty was nevertheless reserved to the colonial government. The laws governing these customs were all in the nature of negative injunctions, in the 'Thou shalt not' category under the new régime, and were soon understood, and obeyed in public at least. But the greater security of the person had many beneficial effects. Life became more humane, trade increased, travel became safer, and new ideas circulated through the various African countries.

The colonizers also made a major contribution to Africa through the development of communications, for example, boats on the Great Lakes and the Stevenson Road. Here again, commercial, humanitarian and missionary interests converged. Men like Livingstone had long held not only that the development of railways and steam navigation would benefit Africa by developing legitimate trade in place of the slave-traffic; but they also showed that only steam-power would eliminate the drudgery of slave porters. The tropical regions of precolonial Africa had depended solely on muscle-power. Travel was impeded also by internecine warfare, and in many regions villagers dared not go more than a few miles from their homes. Winding bushpaths were not so aligned by accident: they made escape easier for men in flight. The new colonial governments built for their own purposes of oversight and defence, wide thoroughfares, straight as an arrow often for miles on end, known everywhere as 'government roads'. It was the first decade of the twentieth century before these began to appear in any number, and they bound the territory together as roads did for the Roman empire.

Another positive feature of the new régimes was the creation of supratribal political units in which, in due time, Africans served, not only as clerks, but also in positions of some responsibility as they became equipped to do so. This policy was preparation for a day not then on the horizon, but an important one for the long-term view.

have been translated 'to destroy'. In West Africa there seems to have been the custom of killing people for the use of certain parts of their body for ritual or religious purposes rather than for meat or cannibalism. [*The Editors.*]

The colonial governments varied, of course, in the extent to which they appointed Africans to higher posts, but the administrative training was an important aspect of colonial rule. Western democratic procedures were involved in processes such as the nomination by the governor of British West Africans to a seat on the legislative council, where the governor-in-council represented the highest authority delegated by the home government. These were simple beginnings, but as important as the acorn to the oak. Similarly, with judicial procedure on a Western model, the higher courts were at first served by Europeans only; but as West Africans qualified in their legal studies in Europe, they were admitted to a share in the legal profession.

The emergent African intelligentsia played an essential part in colonial government as clerks, court interpreters and junior inspectors. They performed an equally important economic function as clerks and storekeepers, often though not always in European employment. They had an essential role in the work of missions as teachers and evangelists. All of them had one thing in common—they owed their education to mission enterprise. White clergymen pioneered the great majority of modern social services for the indigenous people in tropical Africa, and education came high on the list. The missionaries wished to teach a new religion, but they were the 'People of the Book'. What was the use of preaching, if prospective converts could neither read the Bible nor the prayer book? The majority of missionaries also saw education as a means of integrating the faithful into a wider social framework that would transcend the narrow limits of a tribal community. The missions accordingly laid the foundations of modern school systems through nearly the whole of non-Muslim Africa. They generally began their labours in the villages, following the educational maxim: Put the bottom rung of the ladder where the man is. The pressure on missionary resources for this service in the decade before World War I was truly remarkable. A tabular presentation of some of the increases, as shown on the following page, will best express it.

This spectacular increase was partly due to African initiative. (One is reminded of the stampede to get to school in the southern states of the United States after emancipation.) In school was to be found the opening to a better life (in material terms) under the new colonial order. With schools demanding teachers, training institutions began to spring up in commensurate numbers. Governments varied in the support they offered by grants-in-aid. They were most generous in

British colonies, where 90 per cent of primary education was in mission hands. Higher education, as more expensive to provide, was sometimes, though by no means always, a government provision. But the official concern tended to be rather self-regarding, seeking clerical staff for official service. In the early days, British colonies in West Africa recruited clerical staff from Sierra Leone—the colony's top export— but this was costly. Hence, in the Education Code of 1911 in Southern Nigeria, both shorthand and typewriting were optional subjects for primary schools, while at high-school level, shorthand was compulsory. In this educational progress, there was a valuable mingling of the population. Thus, in training institutions, almost always serving more than a tribal area, students with different vernaculars and from different traditional backgrounds would meet and gain a better understanding of their African neighbours by living together, for at this level institutes were usually residential.

	Year	Primary Schools	Scholars
Cameroons (all)	1913	631	40,461
Nyasaland (DRC)	1903	110	10,000
	1910	865	25,706
German East Africa (Berlin)	1910	89	3,395
	1912	135	6,074
Uganda (CMS)	1900	72	7,682
	1913	331	32,458

On occasion, in the mission educational service, teachers might be transferred from one territory to another—real migration to a foreign land. When James Stewart of Lovedale, South Africa, went to the Scottish Presbyterian Mission in Livingstonia, he took with him four Lovedale students, chosen from thirteen who had volunteered for Nyasaland. The four who went in 1877 were of Bantu stock from the Xosa and Fingo tribes, one-time mutual enemies. It was a dramatic stroke to combine them in pioneer Christian service, symbolic of a happier future for Africa. One became a pioneer to the warrior Ngoni of Nyasaland. The Paris Mission in its pioneer work in Barotseland north of the Zambezi similarly drew African agents from its base in Basutoland, to be fellow workers with the French missionaries in Lewanika's country. They were all devoted men. François Coillard has recorded that the first Mosuto to die so far from home—a sore trial to a pagan African—had bravely said: 'When you go back to my country, tell my wife and fellow Christians not to weep as heaven is as near on the Zambezi as in Basutoland.'[1]

Both educational and evangelical work required linguistic qualifications, and one of the missionaries' greatest contributions to Africa was the systematic study of indigenous tongues. South of the Sahara, before the arrival of the missionaries, hardly any of the vernaculars had a written form.[2] Within the period under consideration, missionaries delved into no fewer than 192 languages and major dialects. These they supplied with a written form, and provided the beginnings of a translated literature, in addition to school texts. It was naturally with biblical literature that the missionary translators began, the Gospel of Mark being easily the first choice.

This study of their language by the missionaries gave the tribesmen a feeling that they themselves were worthy of understanding and respect. An illuminating incident occurred in South West Africa in days of stress under German rule. After the disastrous Hottentot and Herero revolts of 1904–5, these communities were broken and scattered. Subsequently, there was a marked increase of non-Christians attending inquirers' classes, without being themselves inquirers. The missionaries attributed this to the use of the vernacular, this being, in their defeat, still an expression of their unity as a people. This was wisely fostered by the Rhenish missionaries in the establishment of two indigenous monthly papers, in Herero and Nama, respectively, which achieved marked success in binding the scattered people together.

The study of the language inevitably gave the missionary a more intimate understanding of the social structure of the people and of their outlook on life and the world. Not all who came by this knowledge, of course, evaluated it in the same way. Some were rather scornfully condemnatory, while others discovered positive values they wished to preserve. According to Dr L. S. B. Leakey, the archaeologist, the scorners carried their own Western social background in one package with the Christian gospel, and so failed to appreciate the functional value of much behaviour in African societies. But others took a more enlightened view. To them, Africa owes the pioneer studies of social systems and forms of religious belief—a world apart from the mere museum items picked up by passing travellers—which are accepted as standard mono-

[1] *Annual report of the Primitive Methodist Missionary Society* (London, 1897), p. xlv.
[2] The only exception known to the writer is Vai of Liberia, first discovered in 1848. See A. Klingenheben, 'The Vai script', *Africa*, 1933, 6, pp. 158–71.

graphs of the peoples concerned. Three of these, produced in our period, are outstanding: *The Baganda* (London, 1911) by James Roscoe; *The life of a South African tribe* (London, 1912) by Henri A. Junod; and the *Ila-speaking peoples of Northern Rhodesia* (London, 1920—publication delayed by war) by Edwin William Smith and Andrew Murray Dale. All were written by working missionaries (save that Dale, who collaborated with E. W. Smith for about 10 per cent of the study, was a political officer). Professor W. H. R. Rivers of Cambridge, England, once declared in his lecture-room that these three monographs were the only first-class African tribal studies in the early twenties. A group of professional social anthropologists paid this tribute in 1951 to *The Ila-speaking peoples* a generation after its appearance: 'It founded modern anthropological research in British Central Africa.'[1] Edwin W. Smith, missionary though he was, was elected president of the Royal Anthropological Institute of Great Britain for 1933–5. African students have since entered the academic lists with valuable Ph.D. theses, but let it not be forgotten that missionary students blazed the trail.

Missionaries made a contribution also in the economic sphere. Many mission societies developed industrial training for Africans. Tribal collectivism, white churchmen believed, must be replaced by individual effort. African enterprise should produce more food as well as cash crops such as cotton, indigo, and dyes for the world market. Commercial farming would put an end to the slave-trade, to intertribal raiding and internal violence. The salvation of Africa, Livingstone insisted, would come through 'Commerce and Christianity'. According to Thomas Fowell Buxton, an eloquent advocate of the antislavery cause, Africa would be redeemed by 'the Bible and the Plow'. The plough would not only make agriculture more efficient; it would also release women from hoe cultivation and thereby, the missionaries argued, help to break down the sinful shackles of polygamy. The missionaries therefore had a major interest in trying to change traditional modes of African production. But missionary values thereby clashed with those of the indigenous people. As long as any successful and wealthy African might be accused of witchcraft, there could be no progress, spiritual or material. The missionaries were used to a system of wage-labour and the standards of an urban European economy. Hence many clergymen

---

[1] Elizabeth Colson and Max Gluckman, *Seven tribes of British Central Africa* (London, Oxford University Press, 1951), p. ix.

believed that Africans lived in idleness. This sloth, they commonly suspected, depended on the servitude of women, which in turn encouraged the evils of polygamy. As one missionary puts it, Africa was a nation of unemployed.

Practical as well as moral reasons made industrial training necessary. Since the missions were poor, they had to rely on local labour for their buildings and furniture. Sometimes they also had to engage in trade. This meant that they had to train their own storekeepers and workmen. European missionaries would then be set free for the more urgent tasks of evangelization; and spiritual work would benefit. Many missions thus gave some training in bricklaying and carpentry, skills essential for the building of stations. Some, like the Nyasaland missions, went farther, building up centralized training institutes where specialized courses were given in smithing, carpentry, printing, bookbinding, telegraphy and other arts. Since there was little demand in native villages for such skills, the mission pupils did not stay in the village. They entered European employment and found work with government agencies when these came into existence. The black craftsman also became a member of the new African middle class, living in contact with the European and forming an important auxiliary to European penetration. Nyasaland, for instance, became an exporter of skilled labour, and many migrants made their way into the Rhodesias.

Missionaries made their mark also in the medical field, where their humanitarian work had a universal appeal and won support even from men who looked askance at the missionaries' evangelical role. Not only did the missionaries wish to help the sick, but they saw therapeutical work as a means of combating the influence of the traditional medicine man, whose arts played a vital part in indigenous culture and religion. In their medical service, the missions had abundant scope in tropical Africa, concentrating at first on curative medicine, and subsequently developing some research and preventive measures. The literature on the subject is considerable, but we may select a few representative examples.

The distinguished doctor brothers, A. R. and J. H. Cook, were the first to identify sleeping-sickness in Uganda in 1901. A medical pioneer of another type was Neil Macvicar of the Victoria Hospital, Lovedale, whose contribution to African welfare was far-reaching. Among his concerns were the arousing of the government to the tuberculosis situation, health teaching in schools, the training of African girls as nurses, and the social effects of migration of the men for labour. John W. Hitchcock, a gentle doctor, became the spearhead of the Scottish Presbyterian Mission in Southern Nigeria in an unsubjugated region of the Protectorate. He won his way amazingly among a backward people as a beloved physician.

The missions made significant contributions also to medical knowledge. I am able to adduce one instance from my own experience: W. C. W. Eakin, of the Qua Iboe Mission in south-east Nigeria, was the first to identify sleeping-sickness in the Eket District where his station lay. He discovered that the disease was recognized in its two stages by the local African 'doctors' and that they even operated in the first stage of swelling of the cervical glands, by excision. He met healthy survivors with scarification as evidence of the operation. Combined with this rational treatment, of course, there was more of magical character. When Eakin felt his diagnosis warranted the step, he reported the situation to the government medical authorities in 1911. A medical officer visited the station and confirmed the diagnosis by finding trypanosomes in the gland-juice of several patients. Prompt action was then taken. A qualified medical man was appointed for research on the spot and was placed in charge of an isolation camp to be provided with hospital and dispensary for some 130 patients. Thanks to the regard in which Eakin was held by his people, the chiefs voluntarily gave land for the camp and erected all necessary buildings. The number of cases identified by the end of 1913 was 222.

A survey of the 600 square miles of the Eket District for the type of tsetse fly (*Glossina tachincides*) found to be the local vector of the trypanosome, revealed that in some places the fly was abundant but not infected; hence, no cases of the disease. But warning was given that once these flies became carriers, the disease threatened to escalate. Thanks to the isolation camp, where known cases were segregated, areas like this were protected. This co-operation between missionary and government officer proved abundantly fruitful. The extent of such collaboration, arising from missionary initiative, through the farflung colonial territories of tropical Africa is hard to evaluate because the evidence is scanty. But it is safe to assume that the work was not insignificant.

The overall effects of mission work were of immense complexity. I shall limit myself here to a few general remarks. The missionaries came both as the apostles of a new faith and as the representatives of a new way of life. They believed in individual salvation instead of in tribal collectivism, hallowed by beliefs in ancestral spirits and the magic of chiefs. They stood for a creed of individual economic effort and advanced productive techniques, rather than for a system of local co-operation generally based on a fairly low level of technical efficiency. They represented the values of the Christian and monogamous family as against those of extended kinship groups practising polygamy. The missionaries, in other words, came as censors of the Africans; and in preaching their ideals, the emissaries of the Gospel were usually fortified by an unquestioning belief not only in their own rightness, but also in the depravity of so many indigenous institutions. Tribal collectivism, the power of the spirit mediums, witchcraft beliefs and ancestral worship had to go, for all were impure. In order to be saved, the African must acquire a sense of sin, but this sense of sin could not come into being until the shackles of collectivism were broken. The African had to become a new man. In order to bring about this spiritual regeneration, the early missionaries were willing to risk incredible hardships and death. Only men of an inflexible cast of character were prepared to take these risks; and once they had settled down on their stations, they often became even more convinced of the wickedness of paganism by what they saw of it. Many of the early missionaries displayed a strong streak of cultural intolerance, explicable to some extent by the conditions under which they worked. It is perhaps not entirely fanciful to see a connexion between today's more liberal, more hesitant approach toward the heathen on the one hand, and improved communications and better living conditions enjoyed by modern missionaries on the other.

The number of genuine conversions achieved by missionaries during the period under survey remains impossible to document. Conditions varied widely from place to place, and the surviving statistics are often incomplete as well as unreliable. Church historians moreover have not yet produced sufficient comparative studies explaining why certain communities proved more receptive to missionary teaching than others. At this point we can only indicate in general terms some of the factors that influenced evangelization. Militaristic pastoral communities were hard to convert. Proud warriors such as the Matabele had too great a vested interest in the traditional social order to accept an alien faith that looked askance at raiding and rapine. Wandering herdsmen such as the Somali would put their trust in the tenets of Islam, a faith originally elaborated by pastoral peoples in the arid lands of Arabia and apt therefore to make a considerable appeal to herdsmen living in similar conditions elsewhere. The Christian churches were all organized on a territorial basis; hence they were unable to reach roving hunters and food-gatherers such as the Bushmen. Christianity, on the other hand, often made an appeal to aristocrats such as the leaders of Barotseland, Basutoland, Buganda or Bechuanaland. They were used to running fairly complex states organized on the territorial principle. They would often look to the white evangelists for a new faith, for new literary and technical skills to meet unaccustomed challenges from within or without their respective societies. Alternatively, the first Christian converts would derive from the opposite end of the social spectrum, among runaway slaves and outcasts, who would flock to missionary stations such as those established by the London Missionary Society in what is now north-eastern Zambia. In conditions of general disorder, the missionaries would offer a new creed, physical protection and new bonds of social cohesion.

Again, much depended on the size of the missionary investment. Nyasaland and Basutoland, both of them mountain countries, were relatively deficient in natural resources. In time many Nyasalanders and Basuto were forced to look for work abroad. But in relation to the small extent of the territories concerned, the local missionary societies in both regions made a very considerable effort, with the result that Nyasaland and Basutoland alike supplied their neighbours with many skilled and literate emigrants, while both countries in turn became centres of further ecclesiastical expansion.

The impact of European military victory, subsequent white land settlement and mining or industrial enterprise would often shatter many traditional institutions and thereby produce a spiritual vacuum which Christianity might fill. Evangelization thus made a great deal of headway in South Africa and also in Rhodesia, where the defeat of the Matabele in 1893 removed a major stumbling-block to Christian expansion. Evangelization might derive similar benefits from the impact of black settlers in Sierra Leone or Liberia. The development of trade might similarly facilitate religious and cultural penetration. Southern Nigeria, for instance, had a long history of trading contacts with the West. And as Emmanuel A. Ayandele, a modern African historian, puts it:

For more than a century Southern Nigeria has been one of the best examples —in many respects *the* best example—of the success of Christian evangelization on the African continent. In no other part of Africa was African agency encouraged by Christian missions as early and as vigorously as in Southern Nigeria; in no other part of Africa did the wards of missions exert themselves so much to spread the Christianity of the Bible in their country; in no other part of the continent did the 'African' churches, largely modelled on the pattern of the established churches, grow in such a way that has persuaded the latter to recognize them as legitimate Christian bodies. In terms of statistics, it is perhaps only in South Africa that there has been a greater response to Christian appeal than in Southern Nigeria.[1]

Religious change, of course, cannot be measured in statistical terms alone. Many converts were attracted to the missions only by the cate-chumens' desire to learn the white man's secular skills. But the missions also made converts of a very different stamp—men like Bernard Mitzeki in Rhodesia—who were willing to sacrifice their lives for the faith. These new Africans, men with new loyalties that went beyond the confines of a local or ethnic patriotism, incurred bitter criticism from the start. The back numbers of settler newspapers such as the *Livingstone Mail* and the *Rhodesia Herald* are full of complaints of the real or alleged misdoings of 'mission boys' who were censured variously for 'improper' egalitarianism or moral nihilism.

A subsequent generation of sociologically trained scholars criticized the missionaries on different grounds. They pointed out the damage done to African society by the destruction of traditional customs and beliefs. They also blamed the missionaries' general ethos, together with the whole system of values supposedly associated with the Victorian age. There is some substance in these charges. The missionary movement, as we have seen, was to some extent an overspill of evangelization carried out among the disinherited poor in the metropolitan countries. Victorian missionaries in Africa had much in common with their colleagues at home, who frequently denounced the brutal and depraved mores rampant in the slums of England. Victorian preachers often pre-sented their faith in terms either melodramatic or mawkish; their faith was strong, their language commonly intemperate. As G. Kitson Clark, a modern British historian, writes of the Victorian clergy in England:

They were inspired by widely different historic traditions, so much so that often enough they saw each other as the enemy quite as much as were the forces of Belial and mere animalism. But it does not seem to be extravagant

[1] 'Christianity in Nigeria' (book review), in *Journal of African History*, 1967, 8, no. 2, p. 363.

to see them in the light of history as one movement; the response of Christians to the challenge of the conditions of the nineteenth century.

The evils of Victorian England were real enough. Skeptics of a critical and analytical cast of mind were not likely to penetrate to 'the savagery and ignorance of the neglected and indifferent' in England. 'The mass of the people would in all probability only be moved by men imbued with strong missionary zeal who would act in ways that were pro-foundly shocking to men not equally inspired.'[1] Missionaries in Africa were faced with problems even greater than those that faced their brethren in England. If we criticize them for their approach, we must always consider at least what alternatives were available to them under the objective conditions of their work, and temper our censure with a due measure of sociological understanding.

The missionaries became involved also in a complex process of interaction with other agencies of Europen power. Seen from a political point of view alone, evangelical labour became—in a certain sense—a valuable complement to the European administrator's work. Africans in many parts of the continent learned to look on Europeans as their authority in spiritual affairs, just as they came to regard white men as their political overlords. Mission schools and training establishments prepared a whole army of intermediaries, clerks, teachers, telegraphists and interpreters, without whose assistance the imperial machinery could not have functioned. Missionaries trained teachers and evangelists, who became the first representatives of a new black intelligentsia. This group in turn produced the critics, and ultimately the heirs, of European empire in Africa. Almost from the beginning, there were educated dissidents like John Chilembwe in Nyasaland who wished to shake off white control in church and state.

African reactions in the religious sphere took many different forms. There were nativists who preached a return to ancient ways and others who wished to break away from European churches but insisted on keeping the white man's ecclesiastical and administrative innovations. Their initial role can, however, be exaggerated. In the first stage of imperial penetration, the majority of educated Africans looked to the imperial powers for progress and reform. E. J. Hobsbawm, a modern British historian, aptly says of the emergent Asian bourgeosie that their first task was to westernize against the united resistance of traditional

[1] *The making of Victorian England* (Cambridge, Mass., Harvard University Press, 1962), pp. 181, 191.

rulers and traditional ruled. They were therefore doubly cut off from their people. Africa presents certain parallels to the different Asian situations. We may therefore agree with Hobsbawm when he argues that 'nationalist mythology has often obscured this divorce, partly by suppressing the links between colonialism and the early native middle classes, partly by lending to earlier antiforeign resistance the colours of a later nationalist movement'.[1] The same was true in the religious field; and during the period under consideration the majority of African teachers and evangelists sided with the orthodox churches.

Mission activity, in a wider sense, helped to provide standards of judgement by which black men judged the whites, and the whites judged one another. True enough, the colonizers' self-criticism did not go very far. On the eve of World War I, the European on the whole seemed placidly content with the benefits he was conferring on the underdeveloped peoples, or to use the terms then current, on the backward peoples and the lower races. His self-satisfaction with his civilizing mission tended to rest on his ideals rather than on his practice. But it was European practice that shaped the African view of what was happening. He often saw the European as greedy for material gain. There was the saying on the west coast: You preach the golden rule but practise the rule of gold. And in South Africa, the charge was current: When you came here we had the land and you had the Bible; now we've got the Bible; you have the land. And so it was.

Another fundamental difference between the European and African points of view arose from the fact that the European had his base in Europe, even if domiciled in Africa, and could with some equanimity feel that he was protected at his back as if a strong wall had existed behind which he could retreat if need be. The African, on the other hand, not only had to remain relatively passive, in contrast to the ener-getic, adventurous European, but had his base in Africa itself, so that in changing times for him everything was at stake. If he lost in Africa, he lost all. There was no wall to which he might retreat for shelter. This produced situations with a deep emotional content. For the European to argue about the advantages he is conferring—and to argue sincerely—missed the point of the African's emotional concern. As George Grenfell observed in 1894:

The present system is wasting the resources of the country, for the people are destroying the rubber vines, not only needlessly as they take the juice,

[1] *The age of revolution, 1789–1848* (Cleveland, 1962), pp. 143–4.

but also of set purpose, so as to destroy (as they think) the value of the country in the eyes of the white man.[1]

In brief, the European tended to *see* the assets on the balance sheet, but the African to *feel* the liabilities.

The missionary could not avoid becoming himself an actor in this drama of white–black collaboration and conflict. He became, in many respects, an agent of Europe's presence in Africa. But he helped also to humanize imperialism. Missionary strains thus played their part in shaping the doctrine of the dual mandate. As stated by Lugard, it runs:

For the civilized nations have at last recognized that while on the one hand the abounding wealth of the tropical regions of the earth must be developed and used for the benefit of mankind, on the other hand, an obligation rests on the controlling power not only to safeguard the material rights of the natives, but to promote their moral and educational progress.[2]

Here, once more, we have the ideal. How far short practice has fallen during our period has been demonstrated by Bronislaw Malinowski in analysing the situation from the scientist's point of view. He contends that while the exploitation of Africa's resources has gone ahead, we have only carried out piecemeal the second mandate, to share benefits. Our sharing has been extremely selective. He lists among the elements we have held back our instruments of physical power, our economic supremacy with its advantages, a full social interchange on a cultural level, education that would go beyond what European service required. He argues, he says, not as a philanthropist but as a scientist: 'To ignore the fact that there is a selective giving on the part of the Europeans makes for a distortion of evidence, and this is a sin against science.'[3] Africa was drawn unwittingly into the political struggles of Europe. These struggles in turn produced a world conflagration, from which Africans learned much more about white men—that they were not themselves brothers after all.

[1] Sir Harry H. Johnston, *George Grenfell and the Congo: a history and description of the Congo Independent State and adjoining regions...* (London, 1908), I, 486.
[2] *Dual mandate*, p. 18.
[3] *The dynamics of culture change* (New Haven, 1945), pp. 56–8.

BIBLIOGRAPHY

Annales de la Propagation de la Foi, 1888, **60**.

Ayandele, Emmanuel A. 'Christianity in Nigeria' (book review), *Journal of African History*, 1967, **8**, no. 2.

Bentley, William Holman. *Pioneering on the Congo*. 2 vols. London, 1900.

Bracq, J. C. 'Cardinal Lavigerie and his anti-slavery work', *Missionary Review of the World*, 1890, o.s. **13**, n.s. **3**.

Burns, Sir Alan Cuthbert. *History of Nigeria*. 3rd ed. London, 1942.

Cameron, Verney Lovett. *Across Africa*. London, 1877.

Church Missionary Society. *Proceedings*. London, 1857.

Clarke, Richard Frederick, the Younger, ed. *Cardinal Lavigerie and the African slave trade*. London, 1889.

Clendenen, Clarence C., and Peter Duignan. *Americans in black Africa up to 1865*. Stanford, Calif., Hoover Institution, 1964.

Colson, Elizabeth, and Max Gluckman. *Seven tribes of British Central Africa*. London, Oxford University Press, 1951.

Cook, Albert R. *Uganda memories (1897–1940)*. Kampala, The Uganda Society, 1945.

Coupland, Sir Reginald. *The exploitation of East Africa, 1856–1890: the slave trade and the scramble*. London, 1939.

Crowther, Samuel Adjai, and John Christopher Taylor. *The Gospel on the banks of the Niger*. London, 1859.

Du Plessis, Johannes. *The evangelisation of pagan Africa*. Cape Town, 1930.

Gann, Lewis H. *The birth of a plural society: the development of Northern Rhodesia under the British South Africa Company, 1894–1914*. Manchester University Press, 1958.

    A history of Northern Rhodesia: early days to 1953. London, 1964.

    A history of Southern Rhodesia: early days to 1934. London, 1965.

Great Britain. *Parliamentary papers*, vol. XLVII, C. 4739. *General Act of the Conference of Berlin*. London, 1886.

Groves, C. P. 'The impact of Christianity upon African life', *Optima*, June 1960, **10**, no. 2.

Hemmens, Harry Lathey. *George Grenfell, pioneer in Congo*. London, 1927.

Hinde, Sidney Langford. *The fall of the Congo Arabs*. London, 1897.

Hobsbawn, E. J. *The age of revolution, 1789–1848*. Cleveland, 1962.

Hutchinson, Thomas Joseph. *Ten years' wanderings among the Ethiopians*. London, 1861.

Johnson, Hildegard Binder. 'The location of Christian missions in Africa', *Geographical Review*, April 1967, **57**, no. 2.

Johnston, Sir Harry H. *George Grenfell and the Congo: a history and description of the Congo Independent State and adjoining districts . . . diaries and researches of the late Rev. George Grenfell and records of the British Baptist Missionary Society*. 2 vols. London, 1908.

Junod, Henri Alexandre. *The life of a South African tribe*. 2 vols. London, 1912–13.

Keith, Arthur Berriedale. *The Belgian Congo and the Berlin Act*. Oxford, Clarendon Press, 1919.

Kitson Clark, George Sidney Roberts. *The making of Victorian England*. Cambridge, Mass., Harvard University Press, 1962.

Klingenheben, A. 'The Vai script', *Africa*, 1933, **6**, no. 2.

Koelle, Sigismund W. *Polyglotta Africana, or a comparative vocabulary of nearly 300 words and phrases in more than 100 African languages*. London, 1854.

Kopytoff, Jean Herskovits. *A preface to modern Nigeria: the 'Sierra Leonians' in Yoruba, 1830–1890*. Madison, University of Wisconsin Press, 1965.

Leakey, Louis S. B. *Kenya: contrasts and problems*. London, 1936.

Lugard, Frederick John Dealtry Lugard, 1st baron. *The dual mandate in British tropical Africa*. Edinburgh and London, 1922.

—— *The rise of our East African empire: early efforts in Nyasaland and Uganda*. 2 vols. Edinburgh and London, 1893.

Macfie, G. W. Scott. 'Sleeping sickness in the Eket district of Nigeria', *Annals of Tropical Medicine and Parasitology*, 1914, **8**.

Macmillan, William Miller. *Bantu, Boer and Briton: the making of the South African problem*. London, 1929.

Malinowski, Bronislaw. *The dynamics of culture change*. New Haven, Yale University Press, 1945.

A Memoir of the Rev. W. A. B. Johnson. London, 1852.

Missionary Review of the World, 1910, **23**; 1911, **24**.

Morel, E. D. *King Leopold's rule in Africa*. London, 1904.

Primitive Methodist Missionary Society. *Annual report*. London, 1897.

Roscoe, John. *The Baganda*. London, 1911.

Rudin, Harry R. *Germans in the Cameroons, 1884–1914: a case study in modern imperialism*. New Haven, Yale University Press, 1938.

Schlatter, Wilhelm. *Geschichte der Basler Mission, 1815–1915*, vol. III: *Die Geschichte der Basler Mission in Afrika*. Basel, 1916.

Shepherd, Robert Henry Wishart. *Lovedale, South Africa: the story of a century, 1841–1941*. Lovedale, C.P., South Africa, 1940.

—— *A South African medical pioneer: the life of Neil Macvicar*. Lovedale, C.P., South Africa, 1952[?].

Shepperson, George, and Thomas Price. *Independent African: John Chilembwe and the origins, setting and significance of the Nyasaland native rising of 1915*. Edinburgh University Press, 1958.

Slade, Ruth M. *English-speaking missions in the Congo Independent State (1878–1908)*. Brussels, Académie Royale des Sciences Coloniales, 1959.

Slade, Ruth M. *King Leopold's Congo: aspects of the development of race relations in the Congo Independent State.* London, Oxford University Press, 1962.

Smith, Edwin William. *The life and times of Daniel Lindley.* London, 1949.
The religion of lower races, as illustrated by the African Bantu. New York, 1923.
The way of the white fields in Northern and Southern Rhodesia. London, 1928.

Smith, Edwin William, and Andrew Murray Dale. *The Ila-speaking peoples of Northern Rhodesia.* London, 1920.

Stanley, Henry Morton. *Through the dark continent.* 2 vols. London, 1878.

Steiner, Paul. *Kamerun als Kolonie und Missionsfeld*, vol. II of *Handbücher zur Missionskunde.* Basel, 1909.

Trimingham, John Spencer. *The Christian approach to Islam in the Sudan.* London, Oxford University Press, 1948.

Tucker, A. R. *Eighteen years in Uganda and East Africa.* 2 vols. London, 1908.

Ward, Herbert. *Five years with the Congo cannibals.* London, 1891.

Warneck, Gustav. [Articles in] *Allgemeine Missionszeitschrift*, 1886, **13**.

Warren, Max Alexander Cunningham. *The missionary movement from Britain in modern history.* London, 1965.

Williams, Eric. *Capitalism and slavery.* Chapel Hill, University of North Carolina Press, 1944.

CHAPTER 15

COLONIALISM:
AN EPISODE IN AFRICAN HISTORY

by J. F. A. AJAYI

Sir Harry H. Johnston was one of the most sophisticated of the builders of European empires in Africa. He saw the European invasion and conquest of Africa in the late nineteenth century not as an isolated event but as the last of a whole series of invasions following after those of the Phoenicians, the Greeks and the Romans, the Arabs, the Turks and others from the Middle and Far East. He envisaged it, too, as a culmination of the activities of Europeans in Africa which began with the Portuguese explorations of the fifteenth century. His *History of the colonization of Africa by alien races*[1] was a pioneering effort to view the partition of Africa in a time perspective, and is therefore a useful starting-point for this discussion of the significance of European colonialism in African history.

Johnston did not share the romantic illusions of many of his contemporaries, particularly of those military leaders of 'punitive expeditions' who looked upon themselves as new *conquistadores* in the posture of gods destined to exterminate a backward or decadent people in order to clear the ground for an entirely new civilization. Nevertheless, he shared the Victorian belief that Europeans were not like other men, and that of all humanity, it was 'the white-skinned sub-species which alone has evolved beauty of facial features and originality of invention in thought and deed'.[2]

Inevitably, therefore, he saw in the European intervention in African affairs a historic finality that was lacking in previous invasions, a historic finality such as Christian historiography reserves only for divine intervention. He believed that Europeans were the harbingers of a new civilization, and that they were destined to leave their mark on the physical and mental nature of man in Africa.

We need not give any consideration to these quaint ideas, except to

---

[1] Cambridge University Press, 1899; 2nd ed., 1913; reprinted, 1930.
[2] Johnston, *Colonization of Africa*, 2nd ed., p. 450.

the extent that they represent one facet of colonization in the period between partition and the First World War that now tends to be ignored. While there was a good deal of continuity in European involvement both before and after the Congress of Berlin, particularly in West Africa, the change-over from an informal empire to a formal one necessitated significant shifts in attitude on the part of the European. There was not merely an increase in racial feeling,[1] but also a belief that colonization ideally should mean colonization as practised in the Americas and Australasia, involving significant European immigration, settlement and miscegenation. Johnston realized that this was feasible only in the temperate zones and in the highlands. He held that in the tropical areas, where the climate and the prevalent diseases discouraged large-scale European settlement, the presence of Africans could not be ignored. But this did not destroy his belief that European rule in Africa would have permanent racial and demographic results. It was possible, he said, that science might 'annul the unhealthy effects of a tropical climate' or 'A new disease may break out which destroys the negro and leaves the white man standing'.[2] But even without such extreme possibilities, he believed that European colonialism would somehow affect the physical features of Africans. 'No doubt', he said, 'as in Asia and South America, the eventual outcome of the colonization of Africa by alien peoples will be a compromise—a dark-skinned race with a white man's features and a white man's brain.'[3]

Apart from this racist obsession with physical features, Johnston saw the establishment of colonial rule as the beginning of a long process of educating Africans in the technologies of a new civilization. Since large-scale European settlement was not immediately possible and the African presence could not be ignored, Africans had to be taught, if necessary by Asians, to take the initiative in their own development. He envisaged a prolonged process of tutelage to be measured in centuries, but he did not rule out eventual African initiative. In the 1899 edition of the book, he said:

just as it would need some amazing and stupendous event to cause all Asia to rise as one man against the invasion of Europe, so it is difficult to conceive

[1] See, for example, J. F. A. Ajayi, *Christian missions in Nigeria, 1841–1891: the making of a new élite* (London, 1965), ch. 8.
[2] Johnston, *Colonization of Africa*, 2nd ed., pp. 445, 450.
[3] *Ibid.*, p. 451. Compare the missionary view that 'the African had to become a new man' (C. P. Groves, 'Missionary and humanitarian aspects of imperialism from 1870 to 1914', p. 488 in this volume).

that the black man will eventually form one united negro people demanding autonomy, and putting an end to the control of the white man, and to the immigration, settlement, and intercourse of superior races from Europe and Asia.

In the 1913 edition, he added that this conception was 'Difficult...but not impossible....All predictions as to the future of the Dark Continent seem futile in face of the unexpected, the strange, the unlooked for which arises in Africa itself.'[1]

We have moved a good deal farther than Johnston in our approach to the study of African history; we know that his analysis must be faulty because the European intervention has proved far less permanent than he had thought it would be. Johnston did not believe that Africans had any history beyond the activities of European and Asian invaders. Though our knowledge of the internal history of Africa is still very fragmentary, at least few responsible people will now deny that the Dark Continent does in fact have a history that needs to be studied and understood. In our study of European activities in Africa we are also now more conscious of the presence of Africans and we pay some attention to their reactions to European activities. But we still tend to think that we can understand colonialism and its impact on African peoples merely by studying the European impact and the reactions of African peoples to Europeans as such without relating these to the internal history of Africa and of the African peoples.

A full assessment of the impact of colonialism on Africa and on African peoples must, however, be made in a historical context. So much Johnston has shown. But the proper historical context is not the history of the colonization of Africa or the history of African reactions to European colonization, but African history as such. As even Johnston himself said in a moment of historical perception, the factors that were likely to affect the future of colonialism were not merely the external ones we so often emphasize—for example, the World Wars, the Russian Revolution and nationalism in South-East Asia—but 'the unexpected, the strange, the unlooked for which arises in Africa itself'. We need only add that so-called African reactions to European activities appear unexpected and strange only when their roots in African history are not examined.

[1] *Ibid.*, p. 450. See 1899 ed., p. 284.

J. F. A. AJAYI

The continuity of African history

The partition must therefore be viewed against a background of the whole of African history. The nineteenth century is probably the best known period, and the European conquest is now well placed in the general setting of nineteenth-century African history. Seen against the background of the Islamic revolutions in the Sudan, the Bantu migrations and essays in state-formation by Shaka, Moshesh and others, the various wars and adaptations going on in the coastal areas of West Africa throughout the century, the partition already assumes a more intelligible shape. It is now possible to write the history of the conquest and the establishment of European rule in Africa in terms of the interaction of two sets of human beings rather than in terms of the contemporary view of Europeans as gods dealing with sub-human natives.

However, because we know less about earlier centuries, there is a tendency to assume that the nineteenth century was an unusually active one in African history, as if it had been specially so ordained to prepare the way for the European partition. In fact, Professor Hargreaves talks of 'a sort of African partition of Africa, a radical reshaping of political structures and boundaries taking place throughout the century'.[1] Detached from the rest of African history, the nineteenth century is beginning to appear as a period when Africans themselves went out of their way to anticipate the great European invasion. But can we assume this?

Alternatively, it is sometimes suggested that the increased pace of African activities in the nineteenth century was a direct reaction to the increasing pace of European activities prior to the partition. Dr Colson holds this view and is inclined to see the major historical developments in Africa since the slave-trade era as a direct reaction to European manoeuvres, these developments being more far-reaching and significant in West than in East Africa in proportion to the intensity of European involvement.[2] This argument exaggerates the extent to which the activities of Europeans can be seen as the central events of African history from which all others derived. It equates the reactions of Africans to European activities with the totality of African history or, rather, it neglects African initiative throughout African history. The fact that we have some knowledge, often specific data, concerning the European trade and often less specific information about the internal

[1] John D. Hargreaves, 'West African states and the European conquest', p. 199.
[2] Elizabeth Colson, 'African society at the time of the scramble', p. 27, this volume.

history of West African communities does not justify the view that the rise and fall of West African states should be explained mainly in terms of the slave-trade.[1] It required the shifting of the frontier of European activities inland in the nineteenth century to cover a wider area and a considerable intensification of the pace of European advance before Europeans began to take the initiative in the making of African history. Even then, the question remains how much initiative was left to the African even during the partition when European development was most intense.

To see the partition within the proper perspective of African history, we therefore have to look beyond the nineteenth century and beyond the main centres of European activities. Just as we now stress that precolonial African society did not remain static till the Europeans began to tamper with it in the colonial period, we should emphasize also that it was not static before the coming of the nineteenth-century Islamic revolutions and the abolitionists. Nor had it been static before the coming of the Dutch in the seventeenth century or the Portuguese in the fifteenth. There were a number of African peoples like the Yoruba and Edo of Southern Nigeria who had organized states in response to their environment, their economic needs and the quality of their leadership before the coming of Europeans. In the history of such states, the entrance of Europeans on the scene and the increasing pace of European developments were only incidents. There is no need to take for granted that the colonial factor assumed dominance over all others that had previously affected their history, such as ecology, economic factors not related to the European trade, quality of leadership, political problems and opportunities at different periods. Nor is there need to assume that these elements were either not present or were always subsidiary to the European factor in the rise and fall and the nature of states that have developed in Africa since the coming of Europeans. Even in the case of states as dependent on the European trade as the Delta city-states at the beginning of the nineteenth century, the evidence seems to indicate that the impact of the European trade as such on their structural development may be grossly exaggerated.[2]

[1] See, for example, J. F. A. Ajayi and Robert S. Smith, *Yoruba warfare in the nineteenth century* (Cambridge University Press, 1964), pp. 123–7.
[2] See G. I. Jones, *Trading states of the Oil Rivers: a study of political development in Eastern Nigeria* (London, Oxford University Press, 1963).

J. F. A. AJAYI

The colonial impact

To argue that the major political movements in African history were not all necessarily inspired by European activities is not to deny that external factors have had an important impact on African history. The interrelationship of internal and external factors will for a long time arouse debate. Recent historiography so amply reflected throughout this book has been at pains to stress that particularly in the nineteenth century African political and religious leaders retained a good deal of initiative in the direction of African affairs in spite of the mounting intensity of the role of Europeans. It seems to me possible, however, to tilt the balance too much by suggesting that the partition was to a significant extent provoked by a growing nationalism in Africa that threatened to limit European enterprise in the informal empires, thus forcing the hand of Europeans in the establishment of formal rule. Similarly, while it is true that many an African revolt against European rule showed how ill-staffed and vulnerable the European régimes in Africa were, it is probably an exaggeration to suggest that the Europeans were not generally masters of the colonial situation. The ultimate superiority of European arms was an inescapable fact of life, nor could the divisions among Africans and the power of the myth of the 'invincible white man' be completely ignored.

The most fundamental aspect of the European impact was the loss of sovereignty which it entailed for practically every African people. Europeans exploited their technological superiority to establish their political dominance throughout the continent. They often crushed, suppressed or amalgamated states at will. In some cases they set up direct European rule with a conscious effort to order the day-to-day lives of the African peoples. In other areas, varying degrees of local autonomy were permitted to continue. The colonial régimes felt the weakness of all administrations that lacked popular support. But their ultimate ability to suppress rebellion was undoubted. They were able to exercise largely complete, even if haphazard, arbitrary and irresponsible control.[1]

Perhaps the most significant exercise of this sovereignty was the extent to which the act of partition was effected. The territories into

[1] See J. F. A. Ajayi, 'The continuity of African institutions under colonialism', in *Emerging themes in African history: proceedings of the International Historical Conference held at Dar es Salaam, 1965*, ed. T. O. Ranger (Nairobi, 1968).

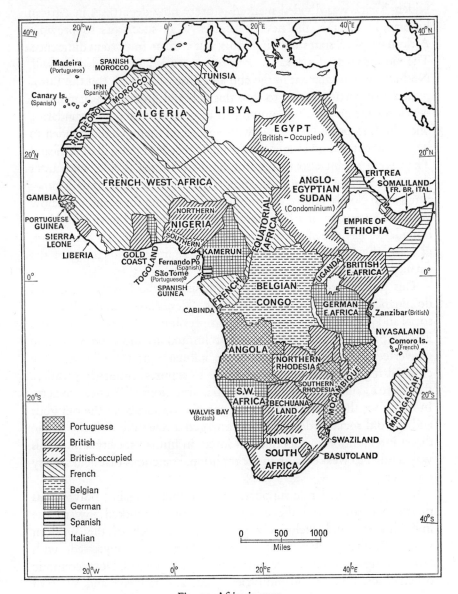

Fig. 15. Africa in 1914.

which Africa was divided marked entirely new departures in African history. In a sense, the new territories were successors to previous African empires, states and kingdoms, but with an important difference. The boundaries of previous empires expanded or receded at will. Nothing was permanent in the ebb and flow of history. But the European act of partition tried to stop this ebb and flow while channelling development into entirely unwonted directions. The new boundaries, once the Europeans themselves were agreed on them, were intended to be permanent and no longer to expand or recede at the will of Africans. They were meant also to become lines of human divide, with utter disregard for the historical destinies of hitherto contiguous and sometimes even closely related communities. For a long time, and even now with the exception of a few, notably in the mandated territories, these boundaries have been regarded as not even negotiable. To that extent, at least, the European intervention has so far had something of the finality with which Johnston credited it.

This political sovereignty was the basis for the European cultural dominance. Through this, Christianity, Western education, Western social and political ideas, made a deep impression on African institutions. The impact of Christianity was not limited to those who became converted or came under the direct influence of the Church. The colonial régimes used their sovereignty to suppress ruthlessly practices that were incompatible with the Christian traditions of Western society. In doing so, the new rulers shook people's confidence in the old gods and the old social order. They encouraged a scientific disbelief in the direct intervention of supernatural forces in human society and in this way tended to weaken faith in the traditional sanctions that held society together.

Socially, colonial rule supported the campaign against polygynous marriage customs and the extended family. It worked toward the individualistic and exclusively patrilineal approach of the Western world. Similarly, slavery and slave-trading were suppressed, with far-reaching social, economic and political consequences. New economic orientations, mining and industries, roads and railways and Western education encouraged the growth of cities. Traditional African institutions that had their roots in village and rural life had to be transformed and adapted for urban living patterns.

Far-reaching as these changes might have been, their impact on Africa was very uneven. While the lives of some communities were profoundly affected, others had hardly become aware of the Europeans' presence before they began to leave. What is more, colonial régimes were far from being uniformly radical. Just as the boundaries of colonial territories tended to put a brake on historical change, so the colonial régimes themselves tended to ally with the most conservative elements in society and to arrest the normal processes of social and political change. Once conquest had been achieved, it was the submissive chiefs, the custodians of law, order and hallowed custom, rather than radical educated élite, who became the favoured agents of European administration. No colonial régime would have hesitated to ally with the most conservative forces to topple a hostile but progressive and modernist leader. After all, the main preoccupation of those régimes was not to carry out social reform but primarily to control and to maintain law and order so as to facilitate economic exploitation. It is true that in order to control, they could make use of seemingly revolutionary forces in society so as to unseat a hostile conservative ruler. But his successor, once raised to power, would have to refrain from too much social reform. Otherwise he might risk losing the support of the colonial régime whose overriding interest, we repeat, was the maintenance of law and order, not reform. The result has been, therefore, that many of the nationalist governments today are finding that on a number of issues they have to pick up the threads of social and political reform from the point where the radical Muslim and Christian reformers of the nineteenth century left off at the coming of colonial rule.

Thus, although the Europeans were generally masters of the colonial situation and had political sovereignty, and cultural and economic dominance, they did not possess a monopoly of initiative during the colonial period. To the extent to which Africans retained initiative, the ability of Europeans to make entirely new departures in African history was limited.

African initiative

It is in this connexion that much interest has been taken recently in the history of resistance movements. These movements are interesting not merely for the extent to which they displayed African courage, strong nationalism and a talent for military organization comparable with that of Europeans. Even more remarkable is the wide variety of reactions on the part of different African communities, each faced with the challenge of conquest and European supremacy.

One fact that bears repetition is that the resistance movements cannot be taken merely to distinguish the patriotic and courageous peoples willing to oppose aggression from the diffident and opportunist ones willing to collaborate with the invaders. Rather, the issue of peace or war should be regarded as one aspect of the foreign policy of each African community. African decisions depended not only on the similar or conflicting interests at any one time of a particular African state and the invading power, but also on the relationship with the neighbour-ing African states, whose attitude to the invader was often a crucial factor. This again emphasizes that the European conquest, including the various reactions of Africans to the colonizing powers, cannot be fully understood except in the context of earlier African history.

Each African entity—village, town or kingdom—viewed the chal-lenge of European conquest as a new historical factor. Africans could either resist the white man, form alliances with the newcomers, or exploit them as far as possible in the continuous struggle for survival, wealth or power. The rulers of these states as guardians of the sov-ereignty of the people were generally hostile to whatever powers chal-lenged this sovereignty. Some of them began by believing what they were told by the missionaries and others: that European activities did not, in fact, threaten their sovereignty. A few of the weaker states, harassed by their neighbours, did welcome European rule as a form of liberation. Various communities agreed merely to co-operate or ally with the invaders and later became hostile when the extent of European ambi-tion was discovered. Others shifted from hostility to co-operation in acceptance of defeat or recognition of a force majeure. These points are fully discussed by Professor Ranger and Professor Hargreaves in their respective essays on resistance movements in East and West Africa. These changes of attitude usually came about as a result of the changing interests of the community as a whole; but sometimes they also reflected divergent attitudes among different classes or leadership groups within the same community. As such, the history of reactions to foreign rule sometimes reflected internal changes in the power structure of the community.

Of particular importance in determining the ability of communities to exploit the opportunities of the colonial period was the existence of a Western-educated élite, which was in turn dependent on missionary education, as well as on the receptiveness of the community to missionary endeavour. The educated élite were motivated by considerations different from those of the traditional rulers. They expressed general hostility to the imposition of European rule; and some of their writings, which showed exaggerated fears that European rule might mean the end of Africans as a distinct people, actually echoed the racist attitude of the invaders.[1] Yet as a group they were the ones most ready to see in the increase of European activities a great opportunity to exploit. As Professor Flint has said, perhaps with some exaggeration, 'It is a historical irony that the only people who on the eve of the scramble for Africa possessed a sense of a British "imperial mission" were the educated or semi-educated Africans'.[2]

As traders, they saw in the extension of European rule an immense increase in commercial opportunities. As teachers and clerks, they looked to opportunities for jobs. As visionaries of new African nations, they regarded the building of roads, railways, ports, hospitals, schools and other features of European technological civilization as the necessary infrastructure of the nations of their dreams. They agreed with the invaders that European tutelage would enable Africans to take the initiative in their own development. But since they had never doubted the African capacity for self-government, they did not expect the period of tutelage to be a long one. Since they were aware of a continuing African history, they did not at first perceive the historic finality in the European intervention that Johnston and others saw in it, and which most of the traditional élite feared would result from even a temporary loss of African sovereignty. They were soon to change their opinions; and while the traditional élite led the initial resistance movements against colonial rule, the 'new men' led the nationalist protests that followed.

African initiative, however, was not limited to these resistance and nationalist movements. It was displayed also in innumerable local pressures and manoeuvres, each small in itself, but having a total effect of severely restricting the extent to which the colonial régimes completely dominated the colonial period. One significant example of this is the extent to which district boundaries within the colonial territories have never achieved the permanence of the national boundaries.

[1] For example: 'The world has, perhaps never witnessed until now such highhanded a robbery on so large a scale. Africa is helpless to prevent it...It is on the cards that this "Christian" business can only end, at no distant date, in the annihilation of the natives' (*Lagos Observer*, 19 Feb. 1885, **4**, no. 2, on the conclusion of the West African Berlin Conference).

[2] John E. Flint, 'Nigeria: the colonial experience...', p. 222 in this volume.

While the colonial administrators sought the most rational units of local government, they were subjected to pressures from local communities for the adjustment of boundaries to suit either the political interests of different communities or previous historical factors hitherto ignored by foreign rulers. The British, for example, bowed to such demands in both Uganda and Northern Rhodesia. These political interests and historical factors were an aspect of the history of inter-group relations, and their importance in the colonial period is another indication of the unbroken continuity of African history from the precolonial period.[1] For, within the international boundaries the Europeans created, and occasionally across them, different communities continued their historic pattern of seeking survival and development.

Arbitrary European decisions about the siting of railways, ports, schools, hospitals, and administrative centres, affected the fortunes of these communities; to that extent the European initiative was supreme. But in so far as these decisions could be affected by the Africans themselves through war, riot, protest, or local enterprise and initiative in producing qualified personnel, Africans also retained some control over their own destinies.

This African effort and initiative represents only in part a reaction to the activities of Europeans. It is also part of the history of the internal development of African communities and of inter-group relations in African history. This is why the colonial impact cannot be fully understood or assessed except in the context of African history. Thus it is difficult to agree with Professor Stengers that there could be 'a political entity brought into being on African soil completely by the will of a European'.[2] For even in the Congo, the colonial period represents only one episode in a long and eventful history.

[1] See, for example, Kathleen Mary Stahl, *History of the Chagga people of Kilimanjaro* (London, 1964).
[2] Jean Stengers, 'The Congo Free State and the Belgian Congo...', p. 261 in this volume: 'One would seek in vain for any African substructure, any autochthonous base for this state as it appeared towards the end of the nineteenth century...Its origins are to be found entirely in the will of one man.'

BIBLIOGRAPHY

Ajayi, J. F. A. *Christian missions in Nigeria, 1841–1891: the making of a new élite*. London, 1965.

'The continuity of African institutions under colonialism', in *Emerging themes in African history: proceedings of the International Historical Conference held at Dar es Salaam, 1965*, ed. T. O. Ranger. Nairobi, 1968.

Ajayi, J. F. A., and Robert S. Smith. *Yoruba warfare in the nineteenth century*. Cambridge University Press, 1964.

Johnston, Sir Harry H. *History of the colonization of Africa by alien races*. Cambridge University Press, 1899 (2nd ed., 1913; reprinted, 1930).

Jones, G. I. *The trading states of the Oil Rivers: a study of political development in Eastern Nigeria*. London, Oxford University Press, 1963.

Stahl, Kathleen Mary. *History of the Chagga people of Kilimanjaro*. London, 1964.

INDEX

Senegal (*cont.*)
194; trade of, 3, 13, 77, 177–83, 354 *passim*; *see also* Dakar
Senegal river, 13, 70, 81, 84, 86
Senegambia, 93, 358
Senoudébou, 150
Serae, 429, 433
Serer, 81
Serpa Pinto, Alexandre Alberto de la Rocha, 364
Serval, 133
Sétif, 137
Shaka (Zulu chief), 326, 500
Shembe (Zulu prophet), 317
Shepstone, Sir Theophilus, 329–30
Sherbo, 83, 90
Shire highlands, 466f.
Shire river, 363
Shoa, 14, 420ff., 426–36 *passim*, 444, 448–53 *passim*; Shoa treaty (1887), 426
Shona (Mashona), 309, 313f., 315, 319
Sierra Leone, 16, 94, 145, 151, 160, 207, 208; education in, 483; indigenous institutions in, 200; missions in, 483, 489; origins of, 464f.; Poro Society in, 50; revenue of, 89, 92; Sierra Leone People's Party, 200; trade of, 70, 75–7 *passim*, 82–3, 85, 92, 123, 135, 153, 208, 228, 245; *see also* Freetown
Sík, Endre, 109n.
Sikasso, 209
Siki (Nyamwezi chief), 409f.
Sinafe, 139
Skinner, Robert, 454
Slave Coast, 178, 394
Slave-trade, 2–5 *passim*, 12, 18, 46, 132–3, 221, 225, 249, 356, 361, 366, 453, 463–71 *passim*, 479ff., 485, 500–1, 504
Smuts, Jan Christiaan, 343, 348, 415
Social Democratic Party (Germany), 20
Socialism, 102–14 *passim*; African, 178
Société Commerciale, Industrielle et Agricole du Haut-Ogooué, 187–93 *passim*
Société Commerciale de L'Ouest
Société Flers Exportation, 153–4
Société Maurel and Prom, 167
Sociétés de Prévoyance, 194
Society, African, 8, 10, 123, 194, 248, 296, 480f., 484–5, 486, 488, 504
Society of Colonial and Maritime Studies, 142

Soddo, 451
Soden, Baron Julius von, 295–6
Soil, African, 100–2
Soji of Porto Novo, 214
Sokodé, 392ff.
Sokoto, 35, 72, 158, 199, 211, 227 and n., 244n., 251
Soleillet, Paul, 74, 137, 140, 142, 147
Somali, 5, 123, 321, 488
Somaliland, 424–46 *passim*; British, 442, 448; French, 439, 444f.; Italian, 424, 428f., 439
Songea of Ngoni, 315, 408, 411ff.
Souriau, 133
South Africa, 5–7 *passim*, 27, 123, 294, 325–60; African nationalism in, 320; Afrikaner nationalism in, 335–6, 348–9; antecedents of Boer war in, 339–45 *passim*; Boer war in (1899–1902), 16, 103, 382, 345–8, 371; British seize Cape in (1795 and 1806), 325; British retrocede Transvaal (1881), 331–2; Eastern Cape, 5, 325, 330; failure of confederal policy in, 328–9, 331; Jameson Raid (1895), 341–2; Majuba Hill, battle of (1881), 331; mineral discoveries in, 7, 100, 108–9, 327–8, 334f.; mining profits in, 108–9; missions in, 463, 466, 467, 469–70, 489, 492; National Convention in (1908), 349; racial discrimination in, 310, 349, 492; railways in, 334–5, 336, 338–40, 367; Union of, formed (1910), 348–50; *see also* names of individual territories
South African Republic, *see* Transvaal
South African Territories Limited, 387
South East Africa, 9f.
South West Africa, German, 17, 30, 333, 369, 467, 484
South West Africa Company, 387
Southern Rhodesia, *see* Rhodesia, Southern
Spain, 286, 465
Spanish Guinea, 157
Spiss, Cassian, 413
St Louis, 81–9 *passim*, 93, 133–4, 135, 147, 158, 180
Stanley, Sir Henry Morton, 141, 143, 154f., 157, 158, 267, 274f., 410, 470, 480
Stanley Falls, 143, 275
Stanley Pool, 143, 154f., 187, 402
State-building, 13, 500f., 504